Youth Mental Health

This book highlights the field of youth mental health and why it is a specialty distinct from both child and adolescent and adult mental health.

Youth Mental Health: Approaches to Emerging Mental Ill-Health in Young People examines issues such as mental health literacy, e-Health, family, psychological, vocational and pharmacological interventions. The authors also discuss issues that are particularly pertinent to young people, such as suicidality, substance abuse, gender identity and sexuality, attention deficit disorder and eating disorders. Taking a preventative focus, this book presents evidence for youth mental health as an important and growing field, makes the case for the reform of existing service structures to better serve this group and outlines the latest specialised approaches to treatment.

Drawing on the knowledge and expertise of leading thinkers in youth mental health, this book is instrumental for mental health professionals who wish to design new specialised mental health systems for young people.

Alison R. Yung is a professor of psychiatry at the Centre for Youth Mental Health, University of Melbourne, Australia.

Jack Cotter is an industry-based senior research scientist with expertise in mental health, neuropsychology and digital health.

Patrick D. McGorry is the executive director of Orygen and a professor of youth mental health at the University of Melbourne, Australia.

Youth Mental Health

Approaches to Emerging Mental Ill-Health in Young People

Edited by Alison R. Yung, Jack Cotter and Patrick D. McGorry

Routledge
Taylor & Francis Group
LONDON AND NEW YORK

First published 2021
by Routledge
2 Park Square, Milton Park, Abingdon, Oxon, OX14 4RN

and by Routledge
52 Vanderbilt Avenue, New York, NY 10017

Routledge is an imprint of the Taylor & Francis Group, an informa business

British Library Cataloguing-in-Publication Data
A catalogue record for this book is available from the British Library

Library of Congress Cataloging-in-Publication Data
A catalog record for this book has been requested

ISBN: 978-0-367-25061-4 (hbk)
ISBN: 978-0-367-25064-5 (pbk)
ISBN: 978-0-429-28580-6 (ebk)

Typeset in Baskerville
by Apex CoVantage, LLC

Contents

Contributors

Editors

Alison R. Yung; Affiliated with Orygen, The National Centre of Excellence in Youth Mental Health, Parkville, Australia; Centre for Youth Mental Health, University of Melbourne, Parkville, Australia; Division of Psychology and Mental Health, School of Health Sciences, University of Manchester, Manchester, UK

Jack Cotter; Affiliated with Orygen, The National Centre of Excellence in Youth Mental Health, Parkville, Australia; Centre for Youth Mental Health, University of Melbourne, Parkville, Australia

Patrick D. McGorry; Affiliated with Orygen, The National Centre of Excellence in Youth Mental Health, Parkville, Australia; Centre for Youth Mental Health, University of Melbourne, Parkville, Australia

Chapter authors

Jean Addington; Hotchkiss Brain Institute, Department of Psychiatry, University of Calgary, Calgary, Canada

Amanda L. Baker; School of Medicine and Public Health, University of Newcastle, Callaghan, Australia

Warrick Brewer; Orygen, The National Centre of Excellence in Youth Mental Health, Parkville, Australia; Centre for Youth Mental Health, University of Melbourne, Parkville, Australia

Sandra Bucci; Division of Psychology and Mental Health, School of Health Sciences, University of Manchester, Manchester, UK; Greater Manchester Mental Health NHS Foundation Trust, Manchester, UK

Lisa Butterly; Orygen, The National Centre of Excellence in Youth Mental Health, Parkville, Australia

Sadhbh Byrne; Orygen, The National Centre of Excellence in Youth Mental Health, Parkville, Australia

Grant I.G. Christie; Department of Psychological Medicine, Faculty of Medical and Health Sciences, University of Auckland, Auckland, New Zealand; CADS Youth Service Altered High, Waitemata District Health Board, Auckland, New Zealand

David Coghill; Departments of Paediatrics and Psychiatry, University of Melbourne, Melbourne, Australia; Murdoch Children's Research Institute, Melbourne, Australia

Georgina Cox; Department of Paediatrics, Monash University, Clayton, Victoria, Australia

Carmela Diaz-Arteche; Melbourne Neuropsychiatry Centre, Department of Psychiatry, University of Melbourne and Melbourne Health, Melbourne, Australia

David Fowler; School of Psychology, University of Sussex, Brighton, UK; Sussex Partnership NHS Foundation Trust, Swandean, West Sussex, UK

Paul French; Research and Innovation Department, Pennine Care NHS Foundation Trust, Manchester, UK; Faculty of Health, Psychology and Social Care, Manchester Metropolitan University, Manchester, UK

Dylan Gilbey; Telethon Kids Institute, University of Western Australia, Perth, Australia

Sarah Hetrick; Department of Psychological Medicine, University of Auckland, Auckland, New Zealand; Centre for Youth Mental Health, University of Melbourne, Parkville, Australia; Orygen, The National Centre of Excellence in Youth Mental Health, Parkville, Australia

Jo Hodgekins; Department of Clinical Psychology and Psychological Therapies, Norwich Medical School, University of East Anglia, Norwich, UK

Anthony F. Jorm; Centre for Mental Health, Melbourne School of Population and Global Health, University of Melbourne, Melbourne, Australia

Claire M. Kelly; Mental Health First Aid Australia, Parkville, Australia

Eóin Killackey; Orygen, The National Centre of Excellence in Youth Mental Health, Parkville, Australia; Centre for Youth Mental Health, University of Melbourne, Parkville, Australia

Betty A. Kitchener; Mental Health First Aid Australia, Parkville, Australia; Department of Psychology, Faculty of Health, Deakin University, Burwood, Australia

Ashleigh Lin; Telethon Kids Institute, University of Western Australia, Perth, Australia

Dan I. Lubman; Turning Point, Eastern Health, Richmond, Victoria, Australia; Eastern Health Clinical School, Monash University, Box Hill, Victoria,

Australia; Monash Addiction Research Centre, Monash University, Frankston, Victoria, Australia

David Marulanda; University of Calgary, Calgary, Canada

Catharine McNab; Orygen, The National Centre of Excellence in Youth Mental Health, Parkville, Australia

Cristina Mei; Orygen, The National Centre of Excellence in Youth Mental Health, Parkville, Australia; Centre for Youth Mental Health, University of Melbourne, Parkville, Australia

Brendan Murphy; Department of Psychiatry, Monash University, Melbourne, Victoria, Australia

Christos Pantelis; Melbourne Neuropsychiatry Centre, Department of Psychiatry, University of Melbourne and Melbourne Health, Melbourne, Australia; Florey Institute for Neuroscience and Mental Health, Melbourne, Australia

Alexandra G. Parker; Institute for Health and Sport, Victoria University, Melbourne, Australia; Centre for Youth Mental Health, University of Melbourne, Parkville, Australia; Orygen, The National Centre of Excellence in Youth Mental Health, Parkville, Australia

Paul Patterson; Forward Thinking Birmingham, Birmingham, UK

Yael Perry; Telethon Kids Institute, University of Western Australia, Perth, Australia

Rosemary Purcell; Orygen, The National Centre of Excellence in Youth Mental Health, Parkville, Australia; Centre for Youth Mental Health, University of Melbourne, Parkville, Australia

Renate L.E.P. Reniers; Institute of Clinical Sciences, College of Medical and Dental Sciences, University of Birmingham, Edgbaston, Birmingham, UK; Institute of Mental Health, School of Psychology, University of Birmingham, Edgbaston, Birmingham, UK

Debra Rickwood; headspace, The National Youth Mental Health Foundation, Melbourne, Australia; Faculty of Health, University of Canberra, Canberra, Australian Capital Territory, Australia

Jo Robinson; Orygen, The National Centre of Excellence in Youth Mental Health, Parkville, Australia

Penelope Strauss; Telethon Kids Institute, University of Western Australia, Perth, Australia

Andrew Thompson; Orygen, The National Centre of Excellence in Youth Mental Health, Parkville, Australia; Warwick Medical School, University of Warwick, Coventry, UK

Tracey Wade; College of Education, Psychology and Social Work, Flinders University, Adelaide, South Australia, Australia

Jon Wilson; Norfolk and Suffolk NHS Foundation Trust, Norwich, UK; Norwich Medical School, University of East Anglia, Norfolk, UK

Stephen J. Wood; Orygen, The National Centre of Excellence in Youth Mental Health, Parkville, Australia; Centre for Youth Mental Health, University of Melbourne, Parkville, Australia; School of Psychology, University of Birmingham, Birmingham, UK

Part I

Why focus on youth mental health?

1 Transition to adulthood

The changing landscape

Patrick D. McGorry and Alison R. Yung

Introduction

Mental health difficulties are the key health issue faced by adolescents and young adults in the developed world today, with the incidence and prevalence of mental disorders being highest in the 15–24 year age group.[1,2] Epidemiological studies have shown that 75% of all cases of mental illness begin before the age of 25, with most new onsets occurring in late adolescence and early adulthood.[1] Young people between the ages of 15 and 25 years also bear the brunt of the morbidity associated with the onset of mental ill-health, with 55% of the burden of disease in this age group being due to mental disorders. Furthermore, cohort studies indicate that 50% of young people will experience a diagnosable mental disorder at some stage during the transition from childhood to adulthood.[3] In line with international data, in Australia the prevalence of diagnosable mental disorders (including substance use) rises sharply from 9% before puberty to 19% afterwards,[4] and peaks in the early twenties at over 26% in any given 12-month period.[5]

Despite these disturbing statistics that emphasise their obvious need, young people are often reluctant to seek help from mainstream health services. The Australian National Survey of Mental Health and Wellbeing indicated that 75% of young people aged 16–24 years with a 12-month diagnosis of a common mental disorder did not seek professional help for their symptoms, with this figure rising to 87% in young men.[5] This is partly because our current health services are geared towards physical ill-health and are designed for children or independent adults, and they rarely cater for the specific needs of transition-age youth. Since young people are usually in good physical health, they often do not have a regular doctor, and when they do visit a general practitioner, they find it difficult to mention emotional concerns. Many factors contribute to this disengagement with our current health care system. These include poor mental health literacy, unhelpful beliefs involving personal strength and autonomy, and the level of their psychological symptoms. At a service level, issues of accessibility, confidentiality and cost, as well as the organisation of the services available, are critical barriers to accessing care for many young people.[6]

The impact of mental illness on young people

Mental ill-health in young people is all too often associated with ongoing disability, including impaired social functioning, poor educational achievement, unemployment, substance abuse, violence and victimisation, leading to a cycle of dysfunction and disadvantage that can be difficult to break.[2,3] In Australia, the annual financial cost of mental illness in young people has been estimated to be $10.6 billion, with the bulk of this cost attributed to lost productivity due to lower employment, as well as absenteeism and premature death. This equates to $10,544 per annum per young person with a mental health disorder.[7] These figures are likely to underestimate the true cost of emerging mental ill-health in young people as they do not account for school absenteeism and compromised educational achievement, which can have ramifications for future tertiary education and vocational pursuits.

An influential World Health Organization report on the global burden of disease estimated the peak age for the maximum negative social and economic impact of a disabling illness to be 22 years.[8] This is because our society invests heavily in its young people to enable them to reach adulthood and become socially and economically productive in their turn, and therefore any disabling illness that prevents a young person from fulfilling their potential is a social and economic calamity.[9] Mental disorder, precisely because its onset peaks in emerging adulthood and impacts on the most productive years of life, has recently been calculated to pose the greatest threat to the GDP of the developed and developing nations over the next 20 years, equal only to cardiovascular disease among the non-communicable diseases.[10,11] Given the personal, social and economic costs of mental ill-health in young people, a strong focus on prevention and early intervention in this age group has the potential to generate greater benefits than intervention at any other time during the lifespan.

Why are young people so vulnerable?

There are complex biological, psychological and sociological reasons why young people are uniquely vulnerable to, and often heavily impacted by, the onset of mental illness. During early adolescence, the physical and hormonal changes of puberty, together with the brain maturational processes that take place at this time of life, create a biological 'window of vulnerability' to the onset of mental illness. This vulnerability is further accentuated by the increasingly complex demands from the young person's social environment as they enter adolescence and begin the process of the transition to independent adulthood.

The activation of the hormonal systems that occurs during puberty has a significant influence on behaviour and emotional functioning. A sharp increase in the onset of depression, anxiety and substance abuse has been shown to occur around mid-puberty. In girls, pubertal stage predicts new cases of depression, as well as the persistence of depression. In boys, the rates of substance abuse, anxiety and conduct disorder all increase from early adolescence. Furthermore, children who enter puberty early have significantly higher rates of social and emotional difficulties. While much of this adolescent mental ill-health is relatively self-limiting, depression and anxiety tends to persist, with worry, obsessionality and anxiety being predictive of subsequent mental ill-health.[12]

Adolescence and early adulthood is a time of dynamic structural and functional change in the brain, driven by a series of maturational processes that result in the refinement of the neuronal circuitry, particularly in the frontal cortex.[13] The increased capacity for abstract rather than concrete thinking that occurs during early adolescence, along with young people's increased sensitivity to peer influence, creates a disjunction between their physical and intellectual maturity and their psychosocial maturity, which is exacerbated by the relatively slow maturation of the frontal cortex (see Chapter 2). This can be a source of considerable stress for young people and their families, as family and social roles must be renegotiated to accommodate the young person's developing sense of autonomy.

The process of the transition from childhood to independent adulthood has changed qualitatively and quantitatively in recent decades, particularly in Western societies. During this phase of life, young people must complete the tasks of defining their individuality and autonomy, which includes establishing their own social networks, beginning sexual relationships, completing their education and moving into employment. Each of these processes can be challenging.

As our lifespan has increased, this developmental phase has been stretched and made less secure in many ways, largely due to the rapid pace of change in our social, economic and technological environments. Financial independence in the current economic climate is particularly challenging, as during economic crises, youth unemployment rises faster and recovers more slowly than general unemployment. In 2012, there were 7.5 million 15–24-year-old and 6.5 million 25–29-year-old economically inactive young people in the European Union. Youth unemployment is estimated as 10–20% globally.[14] Thus this transitional phase of 'emerging adulthood' now often extends from prior to puberty into the late twenties before independent adulthood is securely achieved.[15,16]

Given the biological changes and sociological demands that young people must negotiate during the transition to adulthood, it is hardly surprising that mental illness, even when brief and relatively mild, can seriously disrupt this developmental trajectory and limit a young person's potential.

Prevention, early intervention and youth mental health

Early intervention is particularly relevant in the context of youth mental health, precisely because young people are so vulnerable to mental health problems. Early intervention aims to prevent, or at the least delay, the onset of a serious mental illness and therefore avoid or minimise the associated damage to a young person's social, educational and vocational functioning. Broadly speaking, preventive medicine relies on the concept of risk, and the availability of interventions to modify or counter the risk factors in question. In physical medicine, this concept has been widely adopted, and public health has benefited greatly from the proposal that preventive interventions – universal measures, selective measures or indicated prevention – could be targeted to particular population groups depending on an assessment of the risks, costs and benefits involved in each case.[17] Since many of the causal and/or modifiable risk factors for the onset of mental disorders are not well known, psychiatry has been slower to adopt a preventive approach. However, researchers have proposed that subthreshold syndromes be regarded as risk factors for full-threshold disorders and that these subthreshold syndromes could be targeted by preventive interventions as a step towards indicated prevention for serious mental illness.[18,19]

Because it is so prevalent in young people, preventive interventions that target mental ill-health in young people have an excellent chance of reducing the incidence of subsequent mental disorders and their associated morbidity and costs to the individual and society. Evidence supporting this argument has largely come from research into the treatment of early psychosis over the last two decades; early identification and intensive treatment of a first episode of psychosis was first proposed in the 1990s as a preventive strategy for the psychotic illnesses. Since then, a number of trials have shown that early intervention produces significantly better clinical and functional outcomes for individuals with first-episode psychosis,[20–23] as discussed in detail in Chapter 4. The success of this model of reform and its 'proof of concept' in a severe mental illness has encouraged the wider application of early diagnosis and specialised treatment for the full range of emerging disorders in young people, including the mood and anxiety disorders, substance use disorders, eating disorders and personality disorders.[24]

A clinical staging model for psychiatry

To maximise their chances of success, preventive interventions must be offered as early as possible. In physical medicine, where diagnostic criteria are often clearer, this can be a simpler process than it is in psychiatry, where the early stages of onset of mental illness have largely been ignored. This is at least in part because it is difficult to distinguish between normal, transitory changes in emotions and behaviour and the onset of what may develop into a persistent and disabling mental disorder, particularly in young people where emotional turmoil is so common. Our current diagnostic systems were largely derived from studies of chronic patients with well-established illness and do not consider the ebb and flow of symptoms and how they intensify during the early stages of illness; hence they lack criteria that clearly define the boundary between what should be considered normal and where some form of care should be offered. It is these early stages of illness that need to be targeted for preventive interventions to be most effective, and a clearer definition of these early stages is essential to guide clinicians in their selection of the most appropriate treatment. It is here that a clinical staging model has much to offer.

Put simply, clinical staging is a more refined form of diagnosis. Its value is widely recognised in physical medicine, where limiting the progression and impact of disease and improving quality of life all rely on the earliest possible delivery of effective treatments. The differentiation of early and milder clinical phenomena from those that accompany illness progression and chronicity lies at the heart of the staging model. This allows clinicians to select treatments most relevant to the stage of the illness, with the assumption that interventions delivered during the early stages of an illness will be both more effective and less harmful than treatments delivered later in the course of the illness. This model is particularly attractive in the context of youth mental health, since young people are most likely to experience the onset of mental illness, with new and evolving mixes of symptoms, distress and disability being the norm, which require different treatment considerations than the more established full-threshold syndromes.

How can we define the stages of a mental disorder?

In other medical conditions, clinical stages are defined by the extent and progression of the illness and its biological impact on the patient, which in turn must correlate with prognosis. This approach usually depends on a capacity to define pathologically, as well as clinically, the limits or extent of the disease process. We have proposed an initial clinical staging model for psychiatry that considers not only the symptoms that an individual experiences, as well as their severity, persistence and recurrence, but also the impact these symptoms have on the person's social relationships and daily functioning.

So what do the early stages of mental illness look like? Careful retrospective studies have shown that the major mental illnesses are preceded by a period of non-specific but increasingly severe symptoms, accompanied by a growing degree of distress and disability.[25,26] There are two common scenarios in young people; the first is where an adolescent has had problems earlier in childhood, and after entering adolescence these become more pronounced or evolve into different syndromes as the challenges of life increase and the social environment, especially high school, becomes more demanding. The second, and more common, scenario is that the young person has had an uneventful pre-pubertal period, yet begins to struggle later. Depression, irritability, anxiety, withdrawal and apathy are common features of this pre-onset phase, along with changes in cognitive functioning such as poor concentration, constant worrying or preoccupation with certain thoughts, and other non-specific symptoms, including sleep and appetite disturbance. Over time these symptoms may either intensify, eventually cohering into diagnosable syndromes, or remit and resolve.[9,24] While many of these symptoms are common in young people, fortunately they are often short-lived, and much of the distress associated with them resolves quickly. However, they should not be dismissed as trivial purely because they are so common; subthreshold symptoms strongly predict future illness.[18,26,27] For example, subsyndromal depression is a significant issue in young people, not only since it is a well-established risk factor for major depressive disorder, but also because of its prevalence and the impact of depressive symptoms on functioning.[27]

In the clinical staging model (Figure 1.1), Stage 0 represents an asymptomatic stage for those at increased risk of mental illness. For example, this population could include the first-degree adolescent relatives of those with a severe mental illness, who may themselves be at increased genetic risk. Potential interventions

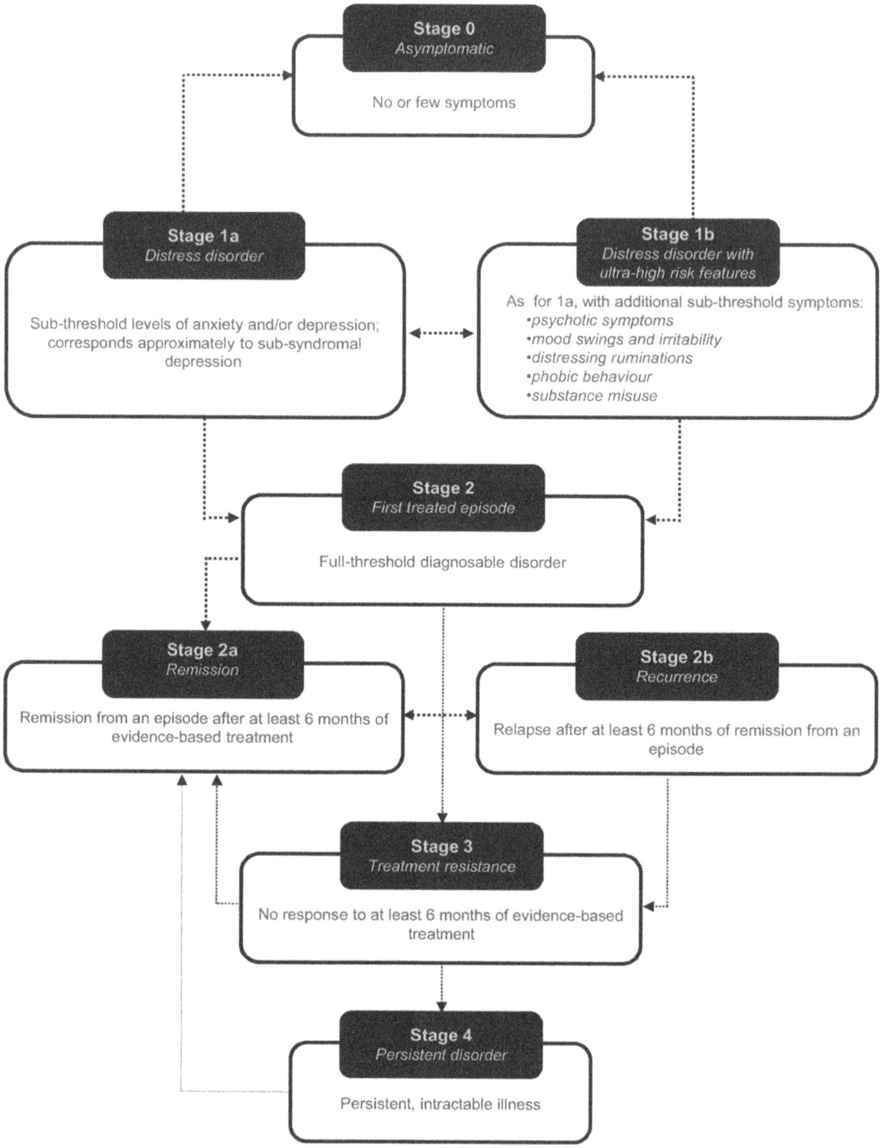

Figure 1.1 The clinical staging model

for this group might include improved mental health literacy, family education and drug education. Stage 1 represents the earliest stage of what could potentially develop into a serious mental illness and is best considered as a 'distress disorder' characterised by subthreshold levels of anxiety and/or depression, with associated distress and disruption to functioning. As this stage evolves, these symptoms intensify and may be accompanied by mood swings, irritability, sub-threshold psychotic symptoms and substance abuse. Potential interventions for this group include improving mental health literacy, formal cognitive therapy, psychoeducation, family therapy, active substance use reduction, benign treatments such as omega-3 fatty acids and, if symptoms or distress are severe, medication. Here, it should be stressed that remission (and relapse) is possible at any stage of illness, although this becomes less likely with progression through the stages of illness.

Stage 2 represents the first episode of a full-threshold diagnosable mental disorder, with moderate to severe symptoms and a serious decline in functioning. Interventions at this stage include all of those proposed for Stage 1 plus appropriate medication and vocational/educational rehabilitation. Stage 3 represents increasingly severe illness, where there has been no response to at least six months of best-practice, evidence-based treatment. Potential interventions here include an additional emphasis on medical and psychosocial strategies to manage symptoms and emphasise relapse prevention. Finally, Stage 4 represents severe, unremitting illness. Here, interventions should focus on medication, such as clozapine for psychosis, other tertiary treatments and encouraging social participation despite ongoing disability.

What are the potential benefits of staging?

Ultimately, as our knowledge of the biological factors underlying mental illness develops, this model could be expanded by mapping the relationships between the relevant biological markers and the stages of illness and allow a better definition of the interrelationships between symptoms and syndromes. On the clinical side, the staging model offers a new framework to guide clinicians in the selection of the most effective treatments that are relevant to the early stages of mental illness. This is particularly important for youth mental health, where the 'clinical landscape' is in a state of flux, with new and evolving syndromal patterns being the norm rather than the exception, and 'broad-spectrum' lower-risk treatments that focus on the young person's wider personal and psychosocial needs may often be the most appropriate form of intervention.

Most importantly, defining discrete stages according to the progression of disease creates a framework for the evaluation of interventions oriented towards prevention and cure. In order to achieve this, an accurate understanding of the social, biological and psychological risk and protective factors that influence progression from one stage to the next will be essential. Furthermore, we need to know the relative potency of these risk factors and which of them may be responsive to current interventions. Finally, by focusing on the early stages of mental illness, with their complex mix of symptoms that are yet to evolve into clearly defined syndromes, and testing broader psychosocial and more generic neuroprotective interventions, we may learn more about the subtle pathophysiology of the onset and persistence of disorder and distinguish this from vulnerability to illness on the one hand, and the consequences of illness on the other.

Future directions for the clinical staging model

The current clinical staging model is based on a young person's clinical picture, including symptoms and functioning. While this is a useful starting point, more research is needed to validate the 'cut points' between stages and assess the utility of the model for guiding treatment. The longitudinal courses of early symptoms and signs should be assessed and the effect of interventions at different stages examined.[28] One study has shown that while most young people presenting to mental health services will have transient syndromes, a subgroup characterised by more complex clinical presentations such as manic-like experiences and psychotic-like experiences are at increased risk of progression.[29]

Validation against neurobiological and other independent measures is needed too. This work is starting to get published, and recent evidence suggests that brain structure, neurocognition and circadian rhythm regulation are progressively more perturbed with increasing clinical stage.[28] For example, white matter integrity changes have been found in early stages of illness, and more significant disruptions were associated with illness progression.[30]

Preventive psychiatry and youth mental health

Over the last decade, the movement towards preventive psychiatry has been growing, and the clinical staging model has much to offer here. The success of the last two decades of reform in the treatment of early psychosis has encouraged the wider application of this model to the full range of emerging disorders in young people and has sparked a worldwide movement for service reform in youth mental health. Youth-specific services are needed that employ developmentally and culturally appropriate approaches to the management of emerging mental and substance abuse disorders and acknowledge the complex and evolving pattern of morbidity seen in this age group. Young peoples' unique life-stage issues, their individual and group identity, and their help-seeking needs and behaviours all need to be central to any service model. Part II of this book examines service systems more closely and discusses important elements of new models targeting youth. Part III focuses on specific interventions and how they may be tailored to young people. The final chapter of this book will explore future directions for a new youth mental health approach.

Box 1.1 Key points

- Most mental disorders begin before the age of 25
- Most disability in those aged 10–24 is due to mental disorders
- Biological, psychological and sociological challenges that begin around puberty and extend to the mid-twenties create a 'window of vulnerability' to mental disorders
- Mental disorders can disrupt and limit a young person's potential

- Early intervention to prevent, or at the least delay, the onset of mental illness could minimise the associated damage to a young person's social, educational and vocational functioning
- Interventions should be tailored to stage of illness. Early stages may benefit from more benign treatments such as improving mental health literacy, family work or psychological therapies. Later stages may need more robust treatments such as medication
- Youth-specific services are needed that employ developmentally and culturally appropriate approaches

References

1 Kessler RC, Berglund P, Demler O, Jin R, Merikangas KR, Walters EE. Lifetime prevalence and age-of-onset distributions of DSM-IV disorders in the National Comorbidity Survey Replication. *Archives of General Psychiatry* 2005;62(6):593–602.
2 McGorry PD, Purcell R, Goldstone S, Amminger GP. Age of onset and timing of treatment for mental and substance use disorders: implications for preventive intervention strategies and models of care. *Current Opinion in Psychiatry* 2011;24(4):301–6.
3 Gibb SJ, Fergusson DM, Horwood LJ. Burden of psychiatric disorder in young adulthood and life outcomes at age 30. *British Journal of Psychiatry* 2010;197(2):122–7.
4 Sawyer MG, Arney FM, Baghurst PA, Clark JJ, Graetz BW, Kosky RJ, et al. *The mental health of young people in Australia.* Canberra: Commonwealth Department of Health and Aged Care; 2000.
5 Statistics ABS. *National survey of mental health and wellbeing: summary of results.* Canberra: Australian Bureau of Statistics; 2008.
6 Rickwood DJ, Deane FP, Wilson CJ. When and how do young people seek professional help for mental health problems? *Medical Journal of Australia* 2007;187:S35–9.
7 Access Economics. *The economic impact of youth mental illness and the cost effectiveness of early intervention.* Melbourne: Access Economics; 2009.
8 Murray CJ, Lopez AD. *The global burden of disease.* Geneva: World Health Organization; 1996.
9 McGorry PD, Nelson B, Amminger GP, Bechdolf A, Francey SM, Berger G, et al. Intervention in individuals at ultra-high risk for psychosis: a review and future directions. *Journal of Clinical Psychiatry* 2009;70(9):1206–12.
10 Bloom DE, Cafiero ET, Jane-Llopis E, Abrahams-Gessel S, Bloom LR, Fathima S, et al. *The global economic burden of non-communicable disease.* Geneva: World Economic Forum; 2011.
11 Gore FM, Bloem PJN, Patton GC, Ferguson J, Joseph V, Coffey C, et al. Global burden of disease in young people aged 10–24 years: a systematic analysis. *Lancet* 2011;377(9783):2093–102.
12 Costello EJ, Copeland W, Angold A. Trends in psychopathology across the adolescent years: what changes when children become adolescents, and when adolescents become adults? *Journal of Child Psychology and Psychiatry* 2011;52(10):1015–25.
13 Paus T, Keshavan M, Giedd JN. Why do many psychiatric disorders emerge during adolescence? *Nature Reviews Neuroscience* 2008;9(12):947–57.
14 Scott J, Fowler D, McGorry P, Birchwood M, Killackey E, Christensen H, et al. Adolescents and young adults who are not in employment, education, or training: their problems are more than economic. *BMJ* 2013;347(7925):f5270.

15 Arnett JJ. *Emerging adulthood: the winding road from the late teens through the early twenties*. New York: Oxford University Press; 2004.
16 Eckersley RM. *Never better – or getting worse? The health and wellbeing of young Australians*. Canberra: Australia21; 2008.
17 Gordon RS, Jr. An operational classification of disease prevention. *Public Health Reports* 1983;98(2):107–9.
18 Eaton WW, Badawi M, Melton B. Prodromes and precursors: epidemiologic data for primary prevention of disorders with slow onset. *American Journal of Psychiatry* 1995;152(7):967–72.
19 Haggerty RJ, Mrazek PJ. Can we prevent mental illness? *Bulletin of the New York Academy of Medicine* 1994;71(2):300–6.
20 Bertelsen M, Jeppesen P, Petersen L, Thorup A, Øhlenschlaeger J, le Quach P, et al. Five-year follow-up of a randomized multicenter trial of intensive early intervention vs standard treatment for patients with a first episode of psychotic illness: the OPUS trial. *Archives of General Psychiatry* 2008;65(7):762–71.
21 Garety PA, Craig TK, Dunn G, Fornells-Ambrojo M, Colbert S, Rahaman N, et al. Specialised care for early psychosis: symptoms, social functioning and patient satisfaction: randomised controlled trial. *British Journal of Psychiatry* 2006;188:37–45.
22 Hegelstad WT, Larsen TK, Auestad B, Evensen J, Haahr U, Joa I, et al. Long-term follow-up of the TIPS early detection in psychosis study: effects on 10-year outcome. *American Journal of Psychiatry* 2012;169(4):374–80.
23 Thorup A, Petersen L, Jeppesen P, Ohlenschlaeger J, Christensen T, Krarup G, et al. Integrated treatment ameliorates negative symptoms in first episode psychosis – results from the Danish OPUS trial. *Schizophrenia Research* 2005;79(1):95–105.
24 McGorry PD, Hickie IB, Yung AR, Pantelis C, Jackson HJ. Clinical staging of psychiatric disorders: a heuristic framework for choosing earlier, safer and more effective interventions. *Australian and New Zealand Journal of Psychiatry* 2006;40(8):616–22.
25 Häfner H, Maurer K, Trendler G, an der Heiden W, Schmidt M. The early course of schizophrenia and depression*. *European Archives of Psychiatry and Clinical Neuroscience* 2005;255(3):167–73.
26 Yung AR, McGorry PD. The initial prodrome in psychosis: descriptive and qualitative aspects. *Australian and New Zealand Journal of Psychiatry* 1996;30(5):587–99.
27 Hetrick SE, Parker AG, Hickie IB, Purcell R, Yung AR, McGorry PD. Early identification and intervention in depressive disorders: towards a clinical staging model. *Psychotherapy and Psychosomatics* 2008;77(5):263–70.
28 Hickie IB, Scott EM, Carpenter JS, Iorfino F. The utility of clinical staging in youth mental health settings. In Uhlhaas PJ, Wood SJ (Eds) *Youth mental health: a paradigm for prevention and early intervention (Strüngmann Forum Reports (28))*. Cambridge, MA: The MIT Press; 2020. p 13–30.
29 Iorfino F, Scott EM, Carpenter JS, Cross SP, Hermens DF, Killedar M, et al. Clinical stage transitions in persons aged 12 to 25 years presenting to early intervention mental health services with anxiety, mood, and psychotic disorders. *JAMA Psychiatry* 2019;76(11):1167–75.
30 Lagopoulos J, Hermens DF, Hatton SN, Battisti RA, Tobias-Webb J, White D, et al. Microstructural white matter changes are correlated with the stage of psychiatric illness. *Translational Psychiatry* 2013;3:e248.

2 Adolescent brain development and implications for mental health

Stephen J. Wood, Renate L. E. P. Reniers, Carmela Diaz-Arteche and Christos Pantelis

Introduction

Adolescence is a formative period of human development, characterised by increases in affective reactivity, greater interest in and sensitivity towards peer-relationships, and an enhanced capacity to engage in behaviour directed towards long-term goals.[1] Although it comprises the teenage years from ages 13 to 19 and is heralded by the onset of puberty, it is not defined by specific events. Indeed, while puberty and adolescence are often used synonymously,[2] the two do not necessarily co-occur.[3] The developmental changes through this period promote the skills necessary for greater independence and enhance new forms of peer attachment, but they also create greater vulnerability to emotional and behavioural dysregulation.[4,5] Indeed, the transition into early adolescence is marked by a dramatic increase in morbidity and mortality, largely related to the emergence of mental disorders.[6] Schizophrenia and depression typically appear post-pubertally, with an average age of onset for both of around 20 years.[7,8] The prevalence of substance use disorder also follows a similar course,[9–11] suggesting that adolescence is a key maturational period that sets the stage for potentially a lifetime free from or full of psychopathology.

These behavioural developments are accompanied by major changes in brain structure and function.[12,13] The adolescent period is accompanied by extensive, but localised, brain maturation which takes the form of myelination and cortical synapse elimination and continues progressively into the third decade of life.[14–18] It has been suggested that as many as 30,000 synapses per second are lost during primate adolescence, resulting in a reduction of up to 40% in synapse density by adulthood.[19] The vast majority of these synapses are excitatory in nature, so it is unsurprising that removal of these synapses is associated with a decline in brain rates of glucose metabolism from the hypermetabolic state of childhood.[20] Indeed, the density of inhibitory interneurons seems to remain fairly stable across this developmental period.[21] Importantly, these studies show that these developmental changes do not occur concurrently in all brain regions, but rather in a series of regionally hierarchical waves. Synaptic pruning begins earlier in primary sensory areas such as visual, auditory and somatosensory cortices than in higher-order association areas such as prefrontal cortex,[17,22,23] while there is a graded progression of myelination from inferior to superior and posterior to anterior, with the cerebellum developing first and the frontal and temporal lobes last.[14,16] These two activity-dependent processes result in a refinement of the neural circuitry that is thought to strengthen the remaining functional connections and reduce competition from suboptimal associations. This is considered to substantially improve communication between distributed information systems, resulting in the development of the finely tuned circuits that characterise a mature brain as well as the emergence of mature cognitive function.[24–26] However, the hardwiring of neural networks, while improving communication between distributed systems, also reduces the redundancy available in the brain, thereby lowering capacity for learning and recovery from injury.[21] Disruptions in this process may also result in suboptimally tuned neural circuits which may ultimately lead to an increased vulnerability to neuropsychiatric disorders. For instance, impairment in plasticity-dependent synaptic refinement has been proposed as a potential common aetiological mechanism for failures in self-monitoring responsible for positive psychotic symptoms[27] and for the sequential appearance of the sensory, motor and cognitive disturbances in pre-schizophrenia individuals, which parallel the timing of normal brain maturation across development.[28] Environmental factors such as stress, particularly when chronic, and substance use also impact on this maturational process, resulting in decreased cognitive functioning and increased susceptibility to mental health problems such as anxiety and depression.[29–31]

Structural imaging

Recent advances in brain imaging have allowed the *in vivo* study of these maturational changes in brain structure during adolescence, with the most consistent findings being a significant decline in global grey matter volume and a contrasting increase in global white matter volume.[32,33] As predicted by the post-mortem and non-human primate studies, refinement of grey matter structure follows a heterochronous development, occurring latest in the prefrontal and parietal lobes.[32,34,35] This development is associated with 'thinning' of the cortex, with the most prominent grey matter reductions apparent in the dorsal, medial and lateral regions of the frontal lobes during adolescence.[36,37] Recent longitudinal studies have reported that different measures of cortical structure, such as cortical volume, thickness and surface area, follow distinct age-related trajectories across adolescent development, emphasising the need to consider their concurrent age-related changes independently.[38–40] Indeed, a study in 1189 youth aged 8–23 years old revealed that while grey matter volume and thickness decrease from young childhood to adulthood, grey matter density actually increases, consistent with the enhancement of neurocognitive performance that occurs during the transition from childhood to adolescence.[41] Therefore, while cortical volume and thickness have received the most attention in the literature, other measures of cortical structure may be as important when examining brain development. Despite the commonly reported loss of grey matter tissue, net brain volume continues to increase over adolescence due to an increase in global white matter volume – indeed this increase may continue into the fifth decade.[42,43] In contrast to the mostly non-linear changes in the cortex, white matter volume generally increases in a linear manner.[32,44,45] At least one study has suggested that white matter change during adolescence is seen most prominently in frontotemporal (specifically dorsal prefrontal-lateral temporal) and corticospinal pathways,[46] consistent with reported findings of striatal grey matter volume loss over the same period. These contrasting maturational changes are thought to enhance neural transmission between the motor connections of the striatal pathway with the frontal cortex, allowing for greater top-down mediation of behavioural output.[47,48]

However, the specific cognitive correlates of these anatomical changes remain unclear. Although structural maturation has been observed to largely parallel cognitive milestones across development,[49] only a few longitudinal studies have linked cortical development with cognitive development. One study looked specifically for an association between cortical thinning and development of general intellectual ability.[50] Using a longitudinal design, more than 300 participants aged between 6 and 19 were stratified on the basis of IQ into 'superior', 'high' and 'average' groups. Specific areas where there were differences in cortical development between the intelligence groups were found in the superior frontal gyri extending into the medial prefrontal cortex bilaterally, with further involvement of the middle and orbitofrontal gyri. Intriguingly, the superior intelligence group started from a relatively thinner cortex, but showed a marked increase up to age 11. All groups showed an overall decline in cortical thickness, but the age at which this decline started varied, being present across the age period studied in the average intelligence group, but only starting in early adolescence in those with superior intelligence. Burgaleta et al. provided further evidence for the association between changes in IQ and the dynamics of cortical thickness development,[51] with individuals showing large increases in IQ displaying the steepest declines in cortical thickness. When considering specific cognitive domains, developmental changes in prefrontal and parietal grey matter, including key nodes within the cognitive control network, have been linked to improvements in information processing, emotion identification, executive function and working memory during adolescence.[52–54] Other studies have correlated the development of fine motor skills and phonological processing skills to thinning in cortical motor regions and thickening in left hemispheric language areas respectively.[55,56] Social cognitive development shows a more widespread pattern and has been associated with reductions in grey matter volume and cortical thickness in medial prefrontal cortex, temporal parietal junction and posterior superior temporal sulcus, and increases in grey matter volume and cortical thickness in the anterior temporal cortex.[57] Clearly, although it is generally *thinning* which is regarded as the most reliable marker of maturation, areas of *thickening* play a role as well.

Another approach to the study of white matter maturation is diffusion tensor imaging (DTI). One measure commonly derived from this technique is fractional anisotropy (FA), which is thought to reflect the diameter, density and orientation of axons and provides information about the integrity of white matter more generally. An early exploration of diffusion tensor imaging in children and adults found age-related increases in FA within the frontal lobes.[58] Recent work has extended this finding to several principal fibre pathways, including the corpus callosum and the inferior fronto-occipital, superior and inferior longitudinal and uncinate fasciculi,[44,59–62] and has demonstrated that maturation of frontal association tracts underlying complex multimodal cognitive abilities continues beyond adolescence.[63,64] This age-related increase in FA has been ascribed primarily to reductions in radial diffusivity (diffusion perpendicular to the main axis of the tract) in cross-sectional studies[44] and is thought to reflect myelination.[65] However, a more recent longitudinal study of changes over 2.5 years suggests instead that increases in axial diffusivity (diffusion along the main axis of the tract) were responsible for the increases in FA, which would tend to indicate increases in the diameter of axons.[66] Interestingly, while the relationship between white matter volume and age is linear, this is not the case for diffusion measures.[44] FA in particular shows a steep increase through childhood which lessens during late adolescence, implying that different stages of development are associated with qualitatively different changes.[44,67,68]

It has been suggested that cortical thinning might be due to alterations at the boundary between cortical grey and white matter, such as proliferation of myelin into the cortical neuropil.[16] Such infiltration would alter the intensity of the voxels making up the grey and white matter on the image, potentially resulting in boundary grey matter voxels being reclassified as white matter. One cross-sectional study of adolescents has shown that the lower the grey matter density in the right frontal lobe, the higher the FA within white matter tracts connected to this region, consistent with the idea that increased myelination at the grey-white matter boundary could drive apparent cortical thinning.[60] In line with this, a recent study in 27 children (5–12 years old) and 30 adults (22–28 years old) suggested that apparent cortical thinning in the lateral ventral temporal cortex is actually driven by increasing myelination across development.[69] However, larger studies have yielded mixed findings. While one study revealed parallel age-related slope trajectories of coordinated white matter expansion and grey matter reductions within structurally connected networks in a 4–18-year-old sample,[70] two other studies that covered participants aged from 8 to 30 and 10 to 18 years of age, respectively, showed that cortical thinning and FA increases each have unique associations with age, and therefore, although there is an association between these measures, cortical thinning cannot be explained by white matter maturation alone.[71,72] Similarly, Whitaker and colleagues showed that changes in adolescent cortical shrinkage (particularly in regions within the association cortex) were significantly but not entirely mediated by age-related increases in intracortical myelination,[73] indicating that myelination is necessary but not sufficient to account for cortical shrinkage.

Functional imaging

Along with structural changes, there are important changes in brain activity during adolescence which can be assessed by functional MRI. For example, there is now consistent evidence to show that when performing tasks that require attentional control (such as Go/NoGo or Flanker tasks), young children typically activate larger and more diffuse regions of prefrontal cortex than adults.[74–77] More recently, studies have reported reductions in prefrontal engagement, together with increased recruitment of more focal, task-relevant areas, from childhood to adolescence, which in turn parallel the gradual transition to adult-level inhibitory control over adolescence.[78,79] This is consistent with the idea that, as synaptic pruning progresses through adolescence, immature and inefficient functional networks are lost,[80] thereby reducing metabolic demands. Indeed, studies have shown that activity that correlates with task performance becomes more focal with age, whereas activity not correlated with performance decreases with age.[76,81] Furthermore, for these kinds of inhibitory control tasks there is a clear differentiation between transient trial-specific activation, which is mature by adolescence, and sustained brain activation, which underlies the rate of successful inhibitory responding and develops over a much longer timespan.[82]

Similarly, functional MRI studies have also shown developmental changes in brain systems associated with reward across the adolescent period.[83–86] These seem to be related to under-activity during anticipation but over-activity following reward.[87,88] However, these findings have been questioned because of the variability in reward magnitude, probability or both, as well as the broad age range assessed and the way in which rewards were obtained.[89] More recent studies have tended to show that adolescents are indeed hypersensitive to reward, which is apparent through increased striatal activation when receiving rewards.[89,90] Compared to adults, they are more responsive to the immediacy and anticipation of reward.[91,92] Combined with reduced coordination between emotion and cognition, this may lead them to take more risks to obtain reward.[93,94]

Importantly, these associations with reward and risk-taking appear to be related to the presence or absence of peers.[95] In the study by Chein and colleagues,[96] three groups of participants (14–18-year-olds, 19–22-year-olds and 24–29-year-olds) were scanned while taking part in a virtual reality driving task. At each of 20 intersections, the participant had to decide whether or not to brake. Not braking (i.e., risk-taking) was encouraged by offering a monetary reward for quick completion of the course. The social context of risk-taking was manipulated by the presence or absence of two same-age peers, who were present in the scanner room for one of the two runs. Increasing age was significantly associated with increasing activity in a number of left prefrontal cortical regions. However, there was a much more striking interaction between age and social context in the ventral striatum and orbitofrontal cortex, which showed a sharp increase in activity in the adolescents when peers were present, which was not seen in the two older groups. A similar effect (i.e., greater ventral striatal engagement) was found in adolescents, but not adults, when performing a reward-processing gambling task with no risk involved in the presence of peers.[97] This suggests that adolescents are sensitised to reward when peers are present and may therefore explain the increased risky behaviour they display.[98,99]

Recent studies have extended these findings by demonstrating the impact of peer identity. Being told that an anonymous peer is watching you increased risk-taking behaviour on a delay discounting task compared to task performance when alone,[100] while the presence of a slightly older adult within a peer group versus a group of adolescent peers resulted in decreased risk-taking behaviour in adolescents similar to that observed when tested alone.[101] Others have shown that observation by a friend compared to observation by an experimenter reduced accuracy on a relational reasoning task,[102] while peer encouragement had a stronger impact on risk-taking behaviour than peer presence.[103] The impact of the quality of the peer relationship has been demonstrated by reports that the presence of uncontrollable stressors was associated with greater levels of sexual risk-taking among adolescents who reported low levels of supportive friendships.[104] Similarly, peer conflict has been associated with increased risk-taking behaviour, especially for adolescents who reported low peer support. Peer conflict was also associated with increased activation in neural regions involved in affect and reward processing (striatum and insula), especially among adolescents reporting low peer support.[105] Adolescents who reported low resistance to peer influence have also shown increased risk-taking after an episode of social exclusion.[106] This relationship was to some degree mediated by increased activation in right temporoparietal junction, suggesting increased attention to the presence of peers and mentalising. These findings provide tentative evidence that high levels of peer support may buffer the association between stressors and increased risk-taking behaviour. Indeed, there is emerging evidence from both behavioural and functional imaging studies suggesting that peer influence may also lead to positive psychosocial outcomes, such as explorative or adaptive prosocial behaviours, during adolescence.[107] In addition, having secured a personal identity may function as a buffer for risky behaviour, particularly in more controlling peer groups, while the degree to which adolescents have explored a variety of self-relevant values, beliefs and goals may operate as a buffer of general deviancy in more pressuring peer groups.[108]

Functional MRI of social cognition is also sensitive to developmental change through adolescence.[109] Adolescents demonstrate greater activity than adults in dorsal medial prefrontal cortex when engaged in mentalising tasks such as irony comprehension or intention understanding.[110] Similar differences are seen in the amygdala during face emotion processing.[111,112] Interestingly, compared to adults, adolescents show stronger connectivity within the social cognitive network to social emotions than to basic emotions, perhaps reflecting the relative importance of social engagement.[113] Reorganisation in the relationship between perceptual, motivational, affective and cognitive systems under the influence of pubertal hormones has been associated with this difference in connectivity and may improve performance on social information processing tasks such as face processing.[114] More specifically, the amygdala may mediate the shift in attribution of relevance of existing stimuli and contexts which causes the reweighting of functional interactions among regions within these social networks. This in turn may stimulate social and behavioural development.[115]

Connectivity

Functional connectivity can be studied by analysing correlations of spontaneous signal fluctuations between brain regions obtained from functional MRI, most frequently while the participant is lying still with eyes closed.[116] Interestingly, these functional connectivity patterns are not always directly related to anatomical connectivity.[117]

While many functional networks are already established by the start of puberty, there are important developmental changes through adolescence.[118,119] Long-distance connections become stronger with increasing age[118] and also display increasing amplitude.[120] Relationships within and between networks also develop with age, such that communication *within* networks becomes stronger, and that *between* networks more efficient.[121,122] However, not all networks show the same pattern of development. For example, frontoparietal networks appear not to change between childhood and adulthood, and while most networks show *increasing* connectivity with age (particularly those involved with higher cognitive functions related to language, attention and executive control), the visual and sensorimotor networks show *decreased* connectivity with development.[123]

It remains somewhat unclear how these changes in functional connectivity are related to structural changes in adolescence. Similar patterns of development can be seen by examining grey matter structural relationships across large-scale functional networks. This structural covariance technique has been applied in 300 children across four age categories (5–8 years, 8.5–11 years, 12–14 years and 16–18 years), examining eight distinct networks from sensory to executive control.[124] Consistent with expectations, primary visual, auditory and motor networks were already largely mature in the youngest age group, while language-related, salience and executive control networks showed marked developmental expansion up to late adolescence. Further evidence for a structure-function connectivity relationship comes from studies that have consistently reported age-related changes in both structural and functional connectivity of the amygdala-prefrontal cortex circuitry.[125–129] This circuitry continues to develop well into adolescence, indicative of a shift in affective control and regulation that is consistent with the emotional turmoil characteristic of the adolescent period.[130] Furthermore, synaptic pruning of inefficient or unused connections is thought to result in the shrinkage of grey matter,[21] while progressive myelination of these same areas leads to enhanced communication between functionally distributed systems.[131] Evidence for this latter point comes from a study that assessed a cohort of 30 subjects between the ages of 18 months and 18 years, using both DTI and resting functional MRI.[132] The authors examined a range of measures designed to characterise the capacity of the structural network to carry out functional segregation and functional integration. Segregation showed a significant age-related decline, implying an increase through development in global integration. Furthermore, the structure-function relationship in connectivity showed an age-related increase. In a recent paper by Baum et al. the development of structure-function coupling in 727 individuals aged 8–23 years was aligned with cortical hierarchies of functional specialisation,[133] suggesting that coupling between structural and functional connectivity remodels to support functional specialisation and higher-order cognition.

Implications for mental illness

The ultimate explanation for the adolescent onset of mental disorders is still unknown, but several lines of enquiry seem promising. Given the changes in brain structure and function through this developmental period, it is highly likely that maturational anomalies play a part.[134] Early onset schizophrenia, for example, has been associated with an exaggeration of the normal maturation process as demonstrated by a pattern of accelerated grey matter loss that correlates with psychotic symptom severity and mirrors the cognitive deficits associated with the illness,[135] as well as accelerated grey and white matter deterioration with age,[136] an age-related shift in the relationship between grey and white matter,[137] and network-based cortical thickness reductions throughout the course of the illness.[138] Excessive synaptic pruning has been hypothesised to underlie this process of abnormal maturation, although an alternative hypothesis suggests that schizophrenia may have a much earlier origin that is revealed as the brain prunes. Either way, the pruning process may assist in explaining the finding that the major psychiatric disorders of thought, mood and anxiety have their peak onset during this vulnerable period of development.

The role of maturational processes in the onset of adolescent mental disorders is likely being modified by psychosocial and environmental factors. One of the latter such factors that is still understudied is the relationship between the onset of puberty, sex hormones and brain development. This is a key issue, since there are notable sex differences in the incidence of specific pathological behaviours, with accidental deaths, suicide, substance abuse and violence being more likely amongst males,[139] while there is a similar female bias in the rates of mood, anxiety and eating disorders.[140] This female bias in particular seems related to puberty, since the sex differences only emerge after Tanner Stage III of pubertal development,[141] and pubertal status predicts the sex difference in prevalence better than age.[142]

There have been some preliminary efforts to relate changes in brain structure and function to pubertal measures and to demonstrate sexual dimorphism.[143–146] For example, one study has shown that boys display a positive association between testosterone and global grey matter, while females show a negative association with oestradiol,[147] although other findings show the opposite relationships.[148] Furthermore, the trajectory of development might be affected by sex steroids, as exemplified by the finding that expression levels of a gene encoding for the testosterone receptor were related to white matter maturation in males.[149]

Our own work has examined the relationship between pubertal timing, brain structure and depressive symptoms during early adolescence.[150] We found that a larger volume of the pituitary gland, a key component of the hypothalamic-pituitary-gonadal (HPG) and hypothalamic-pituitary-adrenal (HPA) axes, mediated the relationship between self- and parent-report measures of early pubertal timing and depressive symptoms in 155 adolescents (72 females). Similarly, larger pituitary gland volume has been shown to mediate the relationship between early adrenarche, as indexed by high levels of DHEA adrenarcheal hormone, and social anxiety symptoms in 95 children (50 females).[151] Furthermore, a recent study by Whittle et al. suggested a key role of adrenarcheal hormones (DHEA, DHEA-S and testosterone) on pituitary gland volume growth from late childhood into early adolescence particularly in females,[152] and alterations in pituitary gland volume have consistently been implicated in the development of a range of mental health problems including internalising symptoms, depression and psychosis.[153–157] These findings are consistent with neurobiological mechanisms being responsible for the link between early pubertal timing and psychopathology symptoms in adolescents. However, the focus on one brain region (the pituitary gland), although important, did not allow investigation of the role of brain anatomical development more broadly in these processes. When considering brain function, Whittle et al. found that blunted affect-related activation to happy faces in the posterior insula mediated the association between increased levels of DHEA and externalising symptoms in girls, but not in boys.[158]

Another area of great recent interest is in the developmental trajectories of functional and structural brain networks and how their compromise can lead to mental disorder. The idea of schizophrenia as a disease resulting from disconnectivity is not especially new, having first been suggested by Friston.[159] Indeed, there have been many recent reports of altered connectivity in the disorder,[160] both structural and functional.[138,161–165] In line with these findings, Whitaker et al. reported that the trajectory of coupled grey and white matter changes within topologically efficient networks during adolescence was strongly associated with a gene expression profile enriched for schizophrenia-related genes,[73] suggesting that the process of cortical hub consolidation may be relevant to the increased incidence of schizophrenia in young people. However, recent work has begun to suggest that altered patterns of connectivity might be features of other psychiatric disorders,[166] including depression, anxiety and attention-deficit/hyperactivity disorder.[167–169] Given the way in which structural and functional networks develop through adolescence, it is tempting to hypothesise that the cause of increased psychopathology in this period is a failure of networks subserving executive control, emotional processing or social cognition to mature normally. The exact nature of these altered trajectories would determine the particular symptoms – for example, a failure to develop executive control and emotional processing networks might result in the onset of mood symptoms. Determining this will require longitudinal imaging studies in childhood and adolescent samples to assess brain structural and functional trajectories as mental disorders develop.[170–171] Such studies should ideally assess individuals enriched to increase the rate of transition to serious mental illness.

References

1 Steinberg L. Cognitive and affective development in adolescence. *Trends in Cognitive Sciences* 2005;9(2):69–74.
2 Petersen AC. Adolescence. In Blechman EA, Brownell KD (Eds) *Behavioral medicine and women: a comprehensive handbook.* New York: Guilford Press; 1998. p 45–50.
3 Dubas JS. Cognitive abilities and physical maturation. In Lerner RM, Petersen AC, Brooks-Gunn J (Eds) *Encyclopedia of adolescence.* New York: Garland Publishing; 1991. p 133–8.
4 Andersen SL, Teicher MH. Stress, sensitive periods and maturational events in adolescent depression. *Trends in Neurosciences* 2008;31(4):183–91.
5 Dahl RE, Allen NB, Wilbrecht L, Suleiman AB. Importance of investing in adolescence from a developmental science perspective. *Nature* 2018;554(7693):441–50.

6 Dahl RE. Adolescent brain development: a period of vulnerabilities and opportunities. Keynote address. *Annals of the New York Academy of Sciences* 2004;1021:1–22.
7 Sham PC, MacLean CJ, Kendler KS. A typological model of schizophrenia based on age at onset, sex and familial morbidity. *Acta Psychiatrica Scandanavica* 1994;89(2):135–41.
8 Penninx BW, Nolen WA, Lamers F, Zitman FG, Smit JH, Spinhoven P, et al. Two-year course of depressive and anxiety disorders: results from the Netherlands Study of Depression and Anxiety (NESDA). *Journal of Affective Disorders* 2011;133(1–2):76–85.
9 Kessler RC, Berglund P, Demler O, Jin R, Merikangas KR, Walters EE. Lifetime prevalence and age-of-onset distributions of DSM-IV disorders in the National Comorbidity Survey Replication. *Archives of General Psychiatry* 2005;62(6):593–602.
10 McGorry PD, Purcell R, Goldstone S, Amminger GP. Age of onset and timing of treatment for mental and substance use disorders: implications for preventive intervention strategies and models of care. *Current Opinion in Psychiatry* 2011;24(4):301–6.
11 Kessler RC, Amminger GP, Aguilar-Gaxiola S, Alonso J, Lee S, Ustün TB. Age of onset of mental disorders: a review of recent literature. *Current Opinion in Psychiatry* 2007;20(4):359–64.
12 Paus T. Mapping brain maturation and cognitive development during adolescence. *Trends in Cognitive Sciences* 2005;9(2):60–8.
13 Dumontheil I. Adolescent brain development. *Current Opinion in Behavioral Sciences* 2016;10:39–44.
14 Benes FM, Turtle M, Khan Y, Farol P. Myelination of a key relay zone in the hippocampal formation occurs in the human brain during childhood, adolescence and adulthood. *Archives of General Psychiatry* 1994;51(6):477–84.
15 Huttenlocher PR. Synapse elimination and plasticity in developing human cerebral cortex. *American Journal of Mental Deficiency* 1984;88(5):488–96.
16 Yakovlev PI, Lecours AR. The myelogenetic cycles of regional maturation of the brain. In Minkowski A (Ed) *Regional development of the brain in early life*. Oxford: Blackwell; 1967. p 3–70.
17 Petanjek Z, Judaš M, Šimić G, Rašin MR, Uylings HBM, Rakic P, et al. Extraordinary neoteny of synaptic spines in the human prefrontal cortex. *Proceedings of the National Academy of Sciences* 2011;108(32):13281–6.
18 Grydeland H, Walhovd KB, Tamnes CK, Westlye LT, Fjell AM. Intracortical myelin links with performance variability across the human lifespan: results from T1-and T2-weighted MRI myelin mapping and diffusion tensor imaging. *Journal of Neuroscience* 2013;33(47):18618–30.
19 Rakic P, Bourgeois JP, Goldman-Rakic PS. Synaptic development of the cerebral cortex: implications for learning, memory and mental illness. In van Pelt J, Corner MA, Uylings HBM, Lopes da Silva FH (Eds) *Progress in brain research: The self-organizing brain: from growth cones to functional networks*. Amsterdam: Elsevier; 1994. p 227–43.
20 Chugani HT, Phelps ME, Mazziotta JC. Positron emission tomography study of human brain functional development. *Annals of Neurology* 1987;22(4):487–97.
21 Changeux JP, Danchin A. Selective stabilisation of developing synapses as a mechanism for the specification of neuronal networks. *Nature* 1976;264(5588):705–12.
22 Huttenlocher PR, Dabholkar AS. Regional differences in synaptogenesis in human cerebral cortex. *Journal of Comparative Neurology* 1997;387(2):167–78.
23 Huttenlocher PR. Morphometric study of human cerebral cortex development. *Neuropsychologia* 1990;28(6):517–27.
24 Menon V. Developmental pathways to functional brain networks: emerging principles. *Trends in Cognitive Sciences* 2013;17(12):627–40.

25 Selemon LD. A role for synaptic plasticity in the adolescent development of executive function. *Translational Psychiatry* 2013;3:e238.
26 Larsen B, Luna B. Adolescence as a neurobiological critical period for the development of higher-order cognition. *Neuroscience and Biobehavioral Reviews* 2018;94:179–95.
27 Stephan KE, Friston KJ, Frith CD. Dysconnection in schizophrenia: from abnormal synaptic plasticity to failures of self-monitoring. *Schizophrenia Bulletin* 2009;35(3): 509–27.
28 Forsyth JK, Lewis DA. Mapping the consequences of impaired synaptic plasticity in schizophrenia through development: an integrative model for diverse clinical features. *Trends in Cognitive Sciences* 2017;21(10):760–78.
29 Arain M, Haque M, Johal L, Mathur P, Nel W, Rais A, et al. Maturation of the adolescent brain. *Neuropsychiatric Disease and Treatment* 2013;9:449–61.
30 Holder MK, Blaustein JD. Puberty and adolescence as a time of vulnerability to stressors that alter neurobehavioral processes. *Frontiers in Neuroendocrinology* 2014;35(1): 89–110.
31 Romeo RD. The impact of stress on the structure of the adolescent brain: implications for adolescent mental health. *Brain Research* 2017;1654(B):185–91.
32 Giedd JN, Blumenthal J, Jeffries NO, Castellanos FX, Liu H, Zijdenbos A, et al. Brain development during childhood and adolescence: a longitudinal MRI study. *Nature Neuroscience* 1999;2(10):861–3.
33 Reiss AL, Abrams MT, Singer HS, Ross JL, Denckla MB. Brain development, gender and IQ in children: a volumetric imaging study. *Brain* 1996;119(5):1763–74.
34 Gogtay N, Giedd JN, Lusk L, Hayashi KM, Greenstein D, Vaituzis AC, et al. Dynamic mapping of human cortical development during childhood through early adulthood. *Proceedings of the National Academy of Sciences* 2004;101(21):8174–9.
35 Shaw P, Kabani NJ, Lerch JP, Eckstrand K, Lenroot R, Gogtay N, et al. Neurodevelopmental trajectories of the human cerebral cortex. *Journal of Neuroscience* 2008;28(14):3586–94.
36 Sowell ER, Thompson PM, Tessner KD, Toga AW. Mapping continued brain growth and gray matter density reduction in dorsal frontal cortex: inverse relationships during postadolescent brain maturation. *Journal of Neuroscience* 2001;21(22):8819–29.
37 Sowell ER, Peterson BS, Thompson PM, Welcome SE, Henkenius AL, Toga AW. Mapping cortical change across the human life span. *Nature Neuroscience* 2003;6(3):309–15.
38 Vijayakumar N, Allen NB, Youssef G, Dennison M, Yücel M, Simmons JG, et al. Brain development during adolescence: a mixed-longitudinal investigation of cortical thickness, surface area, and volume. *Human Brain Mapping* 2016;37(6):2027–38.
39 Tamnes CK, Herting MM, Goddings AL, Meuwese R, Blakemore SJ, Dahl RE, et al. Development of the cerebral cortex across adolescence: a multisample study of interrelated longitudinal changes in cortical volume, surface area, and thickness. *Journal of Neuroscience* 2017;37(12):3402–12.
40 Krongold M, Cooper C, Bray S. Modular development of cortical gray matter across childhood and adolescence. *Cerebral Cortex* 2017;27(2):1125–36.
41 Gennatas ED, Avants BB, Wolf DH, Satterthwaite TD, Ruparel K, Ciric R, et al. Age-related effects and sex differences in gray matter density, volume, mass, and cortical thickness from childhood to young adulthood. *Journal of Neuroscience* 2017; 37(20):5065–73.
42 Mills KL, Goddings AL, Herting MM, Meuwese R, Blakemore SJ, Crone EA, et al. Structural brain development between childhood and adulthood: convergence across four longitudinal samples. *NeuroImage* 2016;141:273–81.

43 Bartzokis G, Beckson M, Lu PH, Nuechterlein KH, Edwards N, Mintz J. Age-related changes in frontal and temporal lobe volumes in men: a magnetic resonance imaging study. *Archives of General Psychiatry* 2001;58(5):461–5.

44 Lebel C, Walker L, Leemans A, Phillips L, Beaulieu C. Microstructural maturation of the human brain from childhood to adulthood. *NeuroImage* 2008;40(3):1044–55.

45 Sowell ER, Trauner DA, Gamst A, Jernigan TL. Development of cortical and subcortical brain structures in childhood and adolescence: a structural MRI study. *Developmental Medicine and Child Neurology* 2002;44(1):4–16.

46 Paus T, Zijdenbos A, Worsley K, Collins DL, Blumenthal J, Giedd JN, et al. Structural maturation of neural pathways in children and adolescents: in vivo study. *Science* 1999;283(5409):1908–11.

47 Asato MR, Terwilliger R, Woo J, Luna B. White matter development in adolescence: a DTI study. *Cerebral Cortex* 2010;20(9):2122–31.

48 Sowell ER, Thompson PM, Holmes CJ, Jernigan TL, Toga AW. In vivo evidence for post-adolescent brain maturation in frontal and striatal regions. *Nature Neuroscience* 1999;2(10):859–61.

49 Casey BJ, Tottenham N, Liston C, Durston S. Imaging the developing brain: what have we learned about cognitive development? *Trends in Cognitive Sciences* 2005;9(3):104–10.

50 Shaw P, Greenstein D, Lerch J, Clasen L, Lenroot R, Gogtay N, et al. Intellectual ability and cortical development in children and adolescents. *Nature* 2006;440(7084):676–9.

51 Burgaleta M, Johnson W, Waber DP, Colom R, Karama S. Cognitive ability changes and dynamics of cortical thickness development in healthy children and adolescents. *NeuroImage* 2014;84:810–9.

52 Vijayakumar N, Whittle S, Yücel M, Dennison M, Simmons J, Allen NB. Prefrontal structural correlates of cognitive control during adolescent development: a 4-year longitudinal study. *Journal of Cognitive Neuroscience* 2014;26(5):1118–30.

53 Breukelaar IA, Antees C, Grieve SM, Foster SL, Gomes L, Williams LM, et al. Cognitive control network anatomy correlates with neurocognitive behavior: a longitudinal study. *Human Brain Mapping* 2017;38(2):631–43.

54 Tamnes CK, Walhovd KB, Grydeland H, Holland D, Østby Y, Dale AM, et al. Longitudinal working memory development is related to structural maturation of frontal and parietal cortices. *Journal of Cognitive Neuroscience* 2013;25(10):1611–23.

55 Lu L, Leonard C, Thompson P, Kan E, Jolley J, Welcome S, et al. Normal developmental changes in inferior frontal gray matter are associated with improvement in phonological processing: a longitudinal MRI analysis. *Cerebral Cortex* 2007;17(5):1092–9.

56 Sowell ER, Thompson PM, Leonard CM, Welcome SE, Kan E, Toga AW. Longitudinal mapping of cortical thickness and brain growth in normal children. *Journal of Neuroscience* 2004;24(38):8223–31.

57 Mills KL, Lalonde F, Clasen LS, Giedd JN, Blakemore SJ. Developmental changes in the structure of the social brain in late childhood and adolescence. *Social Cognitive and Affective Neuroscience* 2014;9(1):123–31.

58 Klingberg T, Vaidya CJ, Gabrieli JD, Moseley ME, Hedehus M. Myelination and organization of the frontal white matter in children: a diffusion tensor MRI study. *NeuroReport* 1999;10(13):2817–21.

59 Barnea-Goraly N, Menon V, Eckert M, Tamm L, Bammer R, Karchemskiy A, et al. White matter development during childhood and adolescence: a cross-sectional diffusion tensor imaging study. *Cerebral Cortex* 2005;15(12):1848–54.

60 Giorgio A, Watkins KE, Douaud G, James AC, James S, De Stefano N, et al. Changes in white matter microstructure during adolescence. *NeuroImage* 2008;39(1):52–61.

61 Schneiderman JS, Buchsbaum MS, Haznedar MM, Hazlett EA, Brickman AM, Shihabuddin L, et al. Age and diffusion tensor anisotropy in adolescent and adult patients with schizophrenia. *NeuroImage* 2009;45(3):662–71.

62 Uda S, Matsui M, Tanaka C, Uematsu A, Miura K, Kawana I, et al. Normal development of human brain white matter from infancy to early adulthood: a diffusion tensor imaging study. *Developmental Neuroscience* 2015;37(2):182–94.

63 Lebel C, Beaulieu C. Longitudinal development of human brain wiring continues from childhood into adulthood. *Journal of Neuroscience* 2011;31(30):10937–47.

64 Kochunov P, Williamson DE, Lancaster J, Fox P, Cornell J, Blangero J, et al. Fractional anisotropy of water diffusion in cerebral white matter across the lifespan. *Neurobiology of Aging* 2012;33(1):9–20.

65 Voss HU, Schiff ND. MRI of neuronal network structure, function and plasticity. *Progress in Brain Research* 2009;175:483–96.

66 Giorgio A, Watkins KE, Chadwick M, James S, Winmill L, Douaud G, et al. Longitudinal changes in grey and white matter during adolescence. *NeuroImage* 2010; 49(1):94–103.

67 Westlye LT, Walhovd KB, Dale AM, Bjørnerud A, Due-Tønnessen P, Engvig A, et al. Life-span changes of the human brain white matter: diffusion tensor imaging (DTI) and volumetry. *Cerebral Cortex* 2009;20(9):2055–68.

68 Lebel C, Gee M, Camicioli R, Wieler M, Martin W, Beaulieu C. Diffusion tensor imaging of white matter tract evolution over the lifespan. *NeuroImage* 2012;60(1):340–52.

69 Natu VS, Gomez J, Barnett M, Jeska B, Kirilina E, Jaeger C, et al. Apparent thinning of human visual cortex during childhood is associated with myelination. *Proceedings of the National Academy of Sciences* 2019;116(41):20750–9.

70 Bray S, Krongold M, Cooper C, Lebel C. Synergistic effects of age on patterns of white and gray matter volume across childhood and adolescence. *eNeuro* 2015;2(4):1–13.

71 Tamnes CK, Østby Y, Fjell AM, Westlye LT, Due-Tønnessen P, Walhovd KB. Brain maturation in adolescence and young adulthood: regional age-related changes in cortical thickness and white matter volume and microstructure. *Cerebral Cortex* 2010;20(3):534–48.

72 Wu M, Lu LH, Lowes A, Yang S, Passarotti AM, Zhou XJ, et al. Development of superficial white matter and its structural interplay with cortical gray matter in children and adolescents. *Human Brain Mapping* 2014;35(6):2806–16.

73 Whitaker KJ, Vértes PE, Romero-Garcia R, Váša F, Moutoussis M, Prabhu G, et al. Adolescence is associated with genomically patterned consolidation of the hubs of the human brain connectome. *Proceedings of the National Academy of Sciences* 2016;113(32):9105–10.

74 Bunge SA, Dudukovic NM, Thomason ME, Vaidya CJ, Gabrieli JDE. Immature frontal lobe contributions to cognitive control in children: evidence from fMRI. *Neuron* 2002;33(2):301–11.

75 Casey BJ, Trainor RJ, Orendi JL, Schubert AB, Nystrom LE, Cohen JD, et al. A developmental functional MRI study of prefrontal activation during performance of a go-no-go task. *Journal of Cognitive Neuroscience* 1997;9(6):835–47.

76 Durston S, Davidson MC, Tottenham N, Galvan A, Spicer J, Fossella JA, et al. A shift from diffuse to focal cortical activity with development. *Developmental Science* 2006;9(1):1–8.

77 Tamm L, Menon V, Reiss AL. Maturation of brain function associated with response inhibition. *Journal of the American Academy of Child and Adolescent Psychiatry* 2002;41(10):1231–8.

78 Rubia K, Lim L, Ecker C, Halari R, Giampietro V, Simmons A, et al. Effects of age and gender on neural networks of motor response inhibition: from adolescence to mid-adulthood. *NeuroImage* 2013;83:690–703.
79 Ordaz SJ, Foran W, Velanova K, Luna B. Longitudinal growth curves of brain function underlying inhibitory control through adolescence. *Journal of Neuroscience* 2013;33(46):18109–24.
80 Casey BJ, Galvan A, Hare TA. Changes in cerebral functional organization during cognitive development. *Current Opinion in Neurobiology* 2005;15(2):239–44.
81 Brown TT, Lugar HM, Coalson RS, Miezin FM, Petersen SE, Schlagger BL. Developmental changes in human cerebral functional organization for word generation. *Cerebral Cortex* 2005;15(3):275–90.
82 Velanova K, Wheeler ME, Luna B. The maturation of task set-related activation supports late developmental improvements in inhibitory control. *Journal of Neuroscience* 2009;29(40):12558–67.
83 Bjork JM, Knutson B, Fong GW, Caggiano DM, Bennett SM, Hommer DW. Incentive-elicited brain activation in adolescents: similarities and differences from young adults. *Journal of Neuroscience* 2004;24(8):1793–802.
84 May JC, Delgado MR, Dahl RE, Stenger A, Ryan ND, Fiez JA, et al. Event-related functional magnetic resonance imaging of reward-related brain circuitry in children and adolescents. *Biological Psychiatry* 2004;55(4):359–66.
85 Silverman MH, Jedd K, Luciana M. Neural networks involved in adolescent reward processing: an activation likelihood estimation meta-analysis of functional neuroimaging studies. *NeuroImage* 2015;122:427–39.
86 Richards JM, Plate RC, Ernst M. A systematic review of fMRI reward paradigms used in studies of adolescents vs. adults: the impact of task design and implications for understanding neurodevelopment. *Neuroscience and Biobehavioral Reviews* 2013;37(5):976–91.
87 Galvan A, Hare TA, Parra CE, Penn J, Voss HU, Glover GH, et al. Earlier development of the accumbens relative to orbitofrontal cortex might underlie risk-taking behavior in adolescents. *Journal of Neuroscience* 2006;26(25):6885–92.
88 Hoogendam JM, Kahn RS, Hillegers MH, van Buuren M, Vink M. Different developmental trajectories for anticipation and receipt of reward during adolescence. *Developmental Cognitive Neuroscience* 2013;6:113–24.
89 Van Leijenhorst L, Zanolie K, Van Meel CS, Westenberg PM, Rombouts SA, Crone EA. What motivates the adolescent? Brain regions mediating reward sensitivity across adolescence. *Cerebral Cortex* 2010;20(1):61–9.
90 Braams BR, van Duijvenvoorde AC, Peper JS, Crone EA. Longitudinal changes in adolescent risk-taking: a comprehensive study of neural responses to rewards, pubertal development, and risk-taking behavior. *Journal of Neuroscience* 2015;35(18):7226–38.
91 Mitchell SH, Schoel C, Stevens AA. Mechanisms underlying heightened risk taking in adolescents as compared with adults. *Psychonomic Bulletin & Review* 2008;15(2):272–7.
92 Galvan A, Hare T, Voss H, Glover G, Casey BJ. Risk-taking and the adolescent brain: who is at risk? *Developmental Science* 2007;10(2):F8–14.
93 Steinberg L. A social neuroscience perspective on adolescent risk-taking. *Developmental Review* 2008;28(1):78–106.
94 Shulman EP, Smith AR, Silva K, Icenogle G, Duell N, Chein J, et al. The dual systems model: review, reappraisal, and reaffirmation. *Developmental Cognitive Neuroscience* 2016;17:103–17.
95 Albert D, Chein J, Steinberg L. The teenage brain: peer influences on adolescent decision making. *Current Directions in Psychological Science* 2013;22(2):114–20.

96 Chein J, Albert D, O'Brien L, Uckert K, Steinberg L. Peers increase adolescent risk taking by enhancing activity in the brain's reward circuitry. *Developmental Science* 2011;14(2):F1–10.
97 Smith AR, Steinberg L, Strang N, Chein J. Age differences in the impact of peers on adolescents' and adults' neural response to reward. *Developmental Cognitive Neuroscience* 2015;11:75–82.
98 Steinberg L, Albert D, Cauffman E, Banich MT, Graham S, Woolard J. Age differences in sensation seeking and impulsivity as indexed by behavior and self-report: evidence for a dual systems model. *Developmental Psychology* 2008;44(6):1764–78.
99 van Duijvenvoorde AC, Peters S, Braams BR, Crone EA. What motivates adolescents? Neural responses to rewards and their influence on adolescents' risk taking, learning, and cognitive control. *Neuroscience and Biobehavioral Reviews* 2016;70:135–47.
100 Weigard A, Chein J, Albert D, Smith A, Steinberg L. Effects of anonymous peer observation on adolescents' preference for immediate rewards. *Developmental Science* 2014;17(1):71–8.
101 Silva K, Chein J, Steinberg L. Adolescents in peer groups make more prudent decisions when a slightly older adult is present. *Psychological Science* 2016;27(3):322–30.
102 Wolf LK, Bazargani N, Kilford EJ, Dumontheil I, Blakemore SJ. The audience effect in adolescence depends on who's looking over your shoulder. *Journal of Adolescence* 2015;43:5–14.
103 Reynolds EK, MacPherson L, Schwartz S, Fox NA, Lejuez CW. Analogue study of peer influence on risk-taking behavior in older adolescents. *Prevention Science* 2014;15(6):842–9.
104 Brady SS, Dolcini MM, Harper GW, Pollack LM. Supportive friendships moderate the association between stressful life events and sexual risk taking among African American adolescents. *Health Psychology* 2009;28(2):238–48.
105 Telzer EH, Fuligni AJ, Lieberman MD, Miernicki ME, Galván A. The quality of adolescents' peer relationships modulates neural sensitivity to risk taking. *Social Cognitive and Affective Neuroscience* 2014;10(3):389–98.
106 Peake SJ, Dishion TJ, Stormshak EA, Moore WE, Pfeifer JH. Risk-taking and social exclusion in adolescence: neural mechanisms underlying peer influences on decision-making. *NeuroImage* 2013;82:23–34.
107 van H, van Hoorn J, Fuligni A, Crone E, Galván A. Peer influence effects on risk-taking and prosocial decision-making in adolescence: insights from neuroimaging studies. *Current Opinion in Behavioral Sciences* 2016;10:59–64.
108 Dumas TM, Ellis WE, Wolfe DA. Identity development as a buffer of adolescent risk behaviors in the context of peer group pressure and control. *Journal of Adolescence* 2012;35(4):917–27.
109 Kilford EJ, Garrett E, Blakemore SJ. The development of social cognition in adolescence: an integrated perspective. *Neuroscience and Biobehavioral Reviews* 2016;70:106–20.
110 Blakemore SJ. The social brain in adolescence. *Nature Reviews Neuroscience* 2008; 9(4):267–77.
111 Burnett S, Sebastian C, Cohen Kadosh K, Blakemore SJ. The social brain in adolescence: evidence from functional magnetic resonance imaging and behavioural studies. *Neuroscience and Biobehavioural Reviews* 2011;35(8):1654–64.
112 Hare TA, Tottenham N, Galvan A, Voss HU, Glover GH, Casey BJ. Biological substrates of emotional reactivity and regulation in adolescence during an emotional go-nogo task. *Biological Psychiatry* 2008;63(10):927–34.
113 Burnett S, Blakemore SJ. Functional connectivity during a social emotion task in adolescents and in adults. *European Journal of Neuroscience* 2009;29(6):1294–301.

114 Scherf KS, Behrmann M, Dahl RE. Facing changes and changing faces in adolescence: a new model for investigating adolescent-specific interactions between pubertal, brain and behavioral development. *Developmental Cognitive Neuroscience* 2012;2(2):199–219.
115 Scherf KS, Smyth JM, Delgado MR. The amygdala: an agent of change in adolescent neural networks. *Hormones and Behavior* 2013;64(2):298–313.
116 Fox MD, Raichle ME. Spontaneous fluctuations in brain activity observed with functional magnetic resonance imaging. *Nature Reviews Neuroscience* 2007;8(9):700–11.
117 Honey CJ, Sporns O, Cammoun L, Gigandet X, Thiran JP, Meuli R, et al. Predicting human resting-state functional connectivity from structural connectivity. *Proceedings of the National Academy of Science* 2009;106(6):2035–40.
118 Fair DA, Cohen AL, Dosenbach NUF, Church JA, Miezin FM, Barch DM, et al. The maturing architecture of the brain's default network. *Proceedings of the National Academy of Science* 2008;105(10):4028–32.
119 Di Martino A, Fair DA, Kelly C, Satterthwaite TD, Castellanos FX, Thomason ME, et al. Unraveling the miswired connectome: a developmental perspective. *Neuron* 2014;83(6):1335–53.
120 Stevens MC, Kiehl KA, Pearlson GD, Calhoun VD. Functional neural networks underlying response inhibition in adolescents and adults. *Behavioral Brain Research* 2007;181(1):12–22.
121 Stevens MC, Pearlson GD, Calhoun VD. Changes in the interaction of resting-state neural networks from adolescence to adulthood. *Human Brain Mapping* 2009;30(8): 2356–66.
122 Baum GL, Ciric R, Roalf DR, Betzel RF, Moore TM, Shinohara RT, et al. Modular segregation of structural brain networks supports the development of executive function in youth. *Current Biology* 2017;27(11):1561–72.
123 Jolles DD, van Buchem MA, Crone EA, Rombouts SA. A comprehensive study of whole-brain functional connectivity in children and young adults. *Cerebral Cortex* 2011;21(2):385–91.
124 Zielinski BA, Gennatas ED, Zhou J, Seeley WW. Network-level structural covariance in the developing brain. *Proceedings of the National Academy of Science* 2010;107(42): 18191–6.
125 Swartz JR, Carrasco M, Wiggins JL, Thomason ME, Monk CS. Age-related changes in the structure and function of prefrontal cortex – amygdala circuitry in children and adolescents: a multi-modal imaging approach. *NeuroImage* 2014;86:212–20.
126 Jalbrzikowski M, Larsen B, Hallquist MN, Foran W, Calabro F, Luna B. Development of white matter microstructure and intrinsic functional connectivity between the amygdala and ventromedial prefrontal cortex: associations with anxiety and depression. *Biological Psychiatry* 2017;82(7):511–21.
127 Gee DG, Humphreys KL, Flannery J, Goff B, Telzer EH, Shapiro M, et al. A developmental shift from positive to negative connectivity in human amygdala – prefrontal circuitry. *Journal of Neuroscience* 2013;33(10):4584–93.
128 Gabard-Durnam LJ, Flannery J, Goff B, Gee DG, Humphreys KL, Telzer E, et al. The development of human amygdala functional connectivity at rest from 4 to 23 years: a cross-sectional study. *NeuroImage* 2014;95:193–207.
129 Wu M, Kujawa A, Lu LH, Fitzgerald DA, Klumpp H, Fitzgerald KD, et al. Age-related changes in amygdala – frontal connectivity during emotional face processing from childhood into young adulthood. *Human Brain Mapping* 2016;37(5):1684–95.
130 Tottenham N, Galván A. Stress and the adolescent brain: amygdala-prefrontal cortex circuitry and ventral striatum as developmental targets. *Neuroscience and Biobehavioral Reviews* 2016;70:217–27.

131 Paus T. Growth of white matter in the adolescent brain: myelin or axon? *Brain and Cognition* 2010;72(1):26–35.
132 Hagmann P, Sporns O, Madan N, Cammoun L, Pienaar R, Wedeen VJ, et al. White matter maturation reshapes structural connectivity in the late developing human brain. *Proceedings of the National Academy of Science* 2010;107(44):19067–72.
133 Baum GL, Cui Z, Roalf DR, Ciric R, Betzel RF, Larsen B, et al. Development of structure-function coupling in human brain networks during youth. *bioRxiv* 2019:729004.
134 Paus T, Keshavan M, Giedd JN. Why do many psychiatric disorders emerge during adolescence? *Nature Reviews Neuroscience* 2008;9(12):947–57.
135 Thompson PM, Vidal C, Giedd JN, Gochman P, Blumenthal J, Nicolson R, et al. Mapping adolescent brain change reveals dynamic wave of accelerated gray matter loss in very early-onset schizophrenia. *Proceedings of the National Academy of Sciences* 2001;98(20):11650–5.
136 Cropley VL, Klauser P, Lenroot RK, Bruggemann J, Sundram S, Bousman C, et al. Accelerated gray and white matter deterioration with age in schizophrenia. *American Journal of Psychiatry* 2016;174(3):286–95.
137 Di Biase MA, Cropley VL, Cocchi L, Fornito A, Calamante F, Ganella EP, et al. Linking cortical and connectional pathology in schizophrenia. *Schizophrenia Bulletin* 2018;45(4):911–23.
138 Wannan CMJ, Cropley VL, Chakravarty MM, Bousman C, Ganella EP, Bruggemann JM, et al. Evidence for network-based cortical thickness reductions in schizophrenia. *American Journal of Psychiatry* 2019;176(7):552–63.
139 Forum on Child and Family Statistics. *America's children: key national indicators of well-being.* Washington, DC: US Government Printing Office; 2009.
140 Green H, McGinnity A, Meltzer H, Ford T, Goodman R. *Mental health of children and young people in Great Britain, 2004.* Basingstoke, UK: Palgrave Macmillan; 2004.
141 Angold A, Costello EJ. Puberty and depression. *Child and Adolescent Psychiatric Clinics of North America* 2006;15(4):919–37.
142 Patton GC, Hibbert ME, Carlin J, Shao Q, Rosier M, Caust J, et al. Menarche and the onset of depression and anxiety in Victoria, Australia. *Journal of Epidemiology and Community Health* 1996;50(6):661–6.
143 Goddings AL, Beltz A, Peper JS, Crone EA, Braams BR. Understanding the role of puberty in structural and functional development of the adolescent brain. *Journal of Research on Adolescence* 2019;29(1):32–53.
144 Vijayakumar N, Op de Macks Z, Shirtcliff EA, Pfeifer JH. Puberty and the human brain: insights into adolescent development. *Neuroscience and Biobehavioral Reviews* 2018;92:417–36.
145 Herting MM, Sowell ER. Puberty and structural brain development in humans. *Frontiers in Neuroendocrinology* 2017;44:122–37.
146 Blakemore SJ, Burnett S, Dahl RE. The role of puberty in the developing adolescent brain. *Human Brain Mapping* 2010;31(6):926–33.
147 Peper JS, Brouwer RM, Schnack HG, van Baal GC, van Leeuwen M, van den Berg SM, et al. Sex steroids and brain structure in pubertal boys and girls. *Psychoneuroendocrinology* 2009;34(3):332–42.
148 Neufang S, Specht K, Hausmann M, Güntürkün O, Herpertz-Dahlmann B, Fink GR, et al. Sex differences and the impact of steroid hormones on the developing human brain. *Cerebral Cortex* 2009;19(2):464–73.
149 Perrin JS, Hervé PY, Leonard G, Perron M, Pike GB, Pitiot A, et al. Growth of white matter in the adolescent brain: role of testosterone and androgen receptor. *Journal of Neuroscience* 2008;28(38):9519–24.

150 Whittle S, Yücel M, Lorenzetti V, Byrne ML, Simmons JG, Wood SJ, et al. Pituitary volume mediates the relationship between pubertal timing and depressive symptoms during adolescence. *Psychoneuroendocrinology* 2012;37(7):881–91.
151 Murray CR, Simmons JG, Allen NB, Byrne ML, Mundy LK, Seal ML, et al. Associations between dehydroepiandrosterone (DHEA) levels, pituitary volume, and social anxiety in children. *Psychoneuroendocrinology* 2016;64:31–9.
152 Whittle S, Barendse M, Pozzi E, Vijayakumar N, Simmons J. Pubertal hormones predict sex-specific trajectories of pituitary gland volume during the transition from childhood to adolescence. *NeuroImage* 2019;204:116256.
153 Zipursky AR, Whittle S, Yücel M, Lorenzetti V, Wood SJ, Lubman DI, et al. Pituitary volume prospectively predicts internalizing symptoms in adolescence. *Journal of Child Psychology and Psychiatry* 2011;52(3):315–23.
154 MacMaster FP, Kusumakar V. MRI study of the pituitary gland in adolescent depression. *Journal of Psychiatric Research* 2004;38(3):231–6.
155 MacMaster FP, Russell A, Mirza Y, Keshavan MS, Taormina SP, Bhandari R, et al. Pituitary volume in treatment-naive pediatric major depressive disorder. *Biological Psychiatry* 2006;60(8):862–6.
156 MacMaster FP, Leslie R, Rosenberg DR, Kusumakar V. Pituitary gland volume in adolescent and young adult bipolar and unipolar depression. *Bipolar Disorders* 2008;10(1):101–4.
157 Garner B, Pariante CM, Wood SJ, Velakoulis D, Phillips L, Soulsby B, et al. Pituitary volume predicts future transition to psychosis in individuals at ultra-high risk of developing psychosis. *Biological Psychiatry* 2005;58(5):417–23.
158 Whittle S, Simmons JG, Byrne ML, Strikwerda-Brown C, Kerestes R, Seal ML, et al. Associations between early adrenarche, affective brain function and mental health in children. *Social Cognitive and Affective Neuroscience* 2015;10(9):1282–90.
159 Friston KJ. The disconnection hypothesis. *Schizophrenia Research* 1998;30(2):115–25.
160 Keshavan MS, Paus T. Neurodevelopmental trajectories, disconnection, and schizophrenia risk. *JAMA Psychiatry* 2015;72(9):943–5.
161 Zalesky A, Fornito A, Seal ML, Cocchi L, Westin CF, Bullmore ET, et al. Disrupted axonal fiber connectivity in schizophrenia. *Biological Psychiatry* 2011;69(1):80–9.
162 Roalf DR, de la Garza AG, Rosen A, Calkins ME, Moore TM, Quarmley M, et al. Alterations in white matter microstructure in individuals at persistent risk for psychosis. *Molecular Psychiatry* 2019; in press.
163 Zalesky A, Pantelis C, Cropley V, Fornito A, Cocchi L, McAdams H, et al. Delayed development of brain connectivity in adolescents with schizophrenia and their unaffected siblings. *JAMA Psychiatry* 2015;72(9):900–8.
164 Fornito A, Yoon J, Zalesky A, Bullmore ET, Carter CS. General and specific functional connectivity disturbances in first-episode schizophrenia during cognitive control performance. *Biological Psychiatry* 2011;70(1):64–72.
165 Tian Y, Zalesky A, Bousman C, Everall I, Pantelis C. Insula functional connectivity in schizophrenia: subregions, gradients, and symptoms. *Biological Psychiatry: Cognitive Neuroscience and Neuroimaging* 2019;4(4):399–408.
166 Broyd SJ, Demanuele C, Debener S, Helps SK, James CJ, Sonuga-Barke EJ. Default-mode brain dysfunction in mental disorders: a systematic review. *Neuroscience and Biobehavioural Reviews* 2009;33(3):279–96.
167 Greicius MD, Flores BH, Menon V, Glover GH, Solvason HB, Kenna H, et al. Resting-state functional connectivity in major depression: abnormally increased contributions from subgenual cingulate cortex and thalamus. *Biological Psychiatry* 2007;62(5):429–37.

168 Zhao XH, Wang PJ, Li CB, Hu ZH, Xi Q, Wu WY, et al. Altered default mode network activity in patients with anxiety disorders: an fMRI study. *European Journal of Radiology* 2007;63(3):373–8.
169 Castellanos FX, Magulies DS, Kelly C, Uddin LQ, Ghaffari M, Kirsch A, et al. Cingulate-precuneus interactions: a new locus of dysfunction in adult attention-deficit/hyperactivity disorder. *Biological Psychiatry* 2008;63(3):332–7.
170 Gogtay N, Vyas NS, Testa R, Wood SJ, Pantelis C. Age of onset of schizophrenia: perspectives from structural neuroimaging studies. *Schizophrenia Bulletin* 2011;37(3):504–13.
171 Testa R, Pantelis C. The role of executive functions in psychiatric disorders. In Wood SJ, Allen NB, Pantelis C (Eds) *The neuropsychology of mental illness*. Cambridge, UK: Cambridge University Press; 2009. p 117–37.

Part II

Mental health systems: do we need specialised services for youth?

3 Help-seeking in young people

Debra Rickwood

Introduction

One of the greatest challenges to intervening early and taking a preventive approach to mental disorders is the reluctance of young people to seek professional mental health care. Paradoxically, the life-stage between 12 and 25 years of age is characterised by both the highest level of need for effective mental health care and the lowest level of service use. Unique developmental factors impact on the help-seeking beliefs and behaviours of adolescents and young adults, and these must be understood so that associated barriers to seeking professional help can be overcome and young people can access early the mental health care they need. The high level of need for appropriate care in terms of the prevalence and major impact of mental disorder, reluctance to seek professional help and social and psychological factors unique to adolescent and early adult development mean that special emphasis is needed on help-seeking at this particular stage of life.

The high need for mental health care among young people is well established, with emerging consensus that about one-quarter will experience a clinically relevant mental disorder each year. In Australia, as elsewhere, large-scale surveys reveal that the adolescent and early adult years are periods of peak prevalence and incidence of most mental disorders. The Australian National Survey of Mental Health and Wellbeing revealed that 26% of 16–24-year-olds had experienced an anxiety, affective or substance use disorder in the past 12 months.[1] A large national US survey showed that the prevalence of mental disorder with severe impairment was 22% among 13–18-year-olds,[2] and the US national comorbidity study showed that 75% of all mental disorders emerge by 24 years of age.[3]

The high prevalence of mental disorder in this age group should be matched by a commensurate level of help-seeking behaviour. Instead, there is a marked mismatch between the prevalence of disorder and professional help-seeking. Figure 3.1 plots the percentage of Australians, from the National Survey of Mental Health and Wellbeing, experiencing mental disorder within a 12-month period and the relative proportion of those with disorder who sought professional help.[1] This clearly reveals that the mismatch between prevalence and service use is greatest for the 16–24-year-olds and decreases with age. For males aged 16–24 years, there were 23% who reported mental disorder, but only 13% of these young men

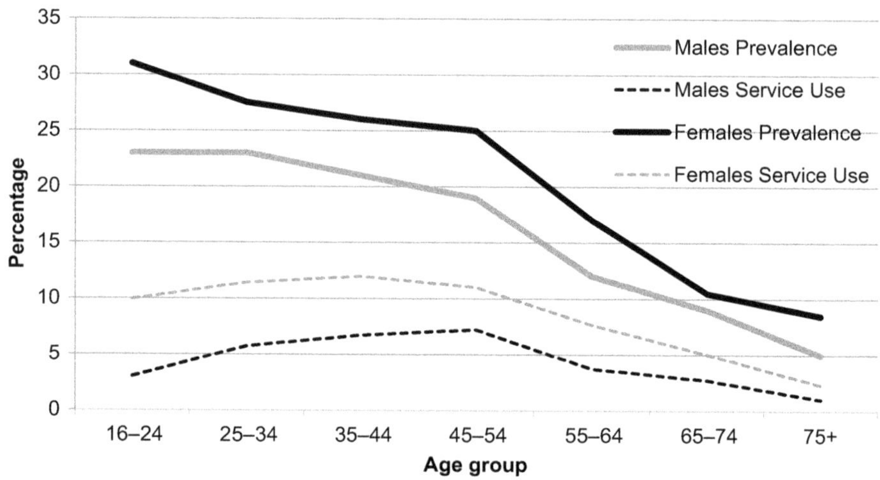

Figure 3.1 Prevalence of 12-month mental disorder and relative proportion who had sought professional help, by gender and age group

had sought professional help (about 3% overall); for the females in this age group, 31% experienced mental disorder and 30% of these young women had sought professional help (about 10% overall).

The reluctance of young people to seek professional mental health care is evident internationally. For example, in Norway, a large study of 15–16-year-olds showed that only 34% of those with high levels of depression and anxiety had sought professional help.[4] In Switzerland, a large, nationally representative sample of young adults aged 16–20 years revealed that only 13% who needed psychological help had consulted general health care.[5] Even in countries with good access to health care, the marked disinclination of young people to access professional care for mental health problems is clearly evident.

The help-seeking process

The term 'help-seeking' is used to refer to actively seeking assistance through problem-focused coping attempts. Help-seeking entails approaching other people and resources to obtain information, understanding, advice, treatment and general support in response to a problem.[6,7] Help can be sought from a wide range of sources that vary in their level of formality and expertise. *Informal help-seeking* is through informal social networks, such as friends and family. *Formal help-seeking* is from professionals who have a legitimate role in providing relevant advice, support and/or treatment. Formal help-seeking is itself diverse and can include teachers, youth workers and clergy, as well as generalist health and specialist mental health care providers. There is a growing focus on self-managed *self-help*, especially by incorporating the use of technology at early help-seeking stages.[7]

Help-seeking is not simply the act of responding to symptoms by accessing a source of health care, but rather is a complex and temporal process. It includes symptom recognition, the decision to seek help, the choice of a source of help and accessing and engaging with the chosen help-source until goals are attained. These multiple decision points are evident in most help-seeking models,[8,9] comprising some form of the elements shown in Figure 3.2. The help-seeking process for mental disorders begins with the development of symptoms, which need to be recognised by the person experiencing the symptoms or significant others and appraised as something that requires help-seeking action. Decisions must then be made about the type of help that is available and appropriate. For service access to occur, the decision to seek help must be actualised. Increasingly, help-seeking is conceptualised beyond the first point of service access, as effective help-seeking requires engagement with services until the needs and goals of the client are met. The help-seeking process generally aligns with the Transtheoretical Stages of Change Model, corresponding to the precontemplation, contemplation, preparation, action and maintenance stages.[10]

While Figure 3.2 implies a linear progression through the help-seeking process, this is not necessarily the case, and people progress in different ways and at different rates. Notably, however, no research has applied a prospective longitudinal design to validate all the stages of the proposed process. Most research has been cross-sectional, investigating either future intentions to seek help or past help-seeking behaviour, and, consequently, empirical knowledge of the process is limited and there is no accepted model or theory of help-seeking.

At each point in the process a range of factors can help or hinder effective help-seeking, and circumstances may accelerate or regress progress. A systematic review of barriers and facilitators to help-seeking in young people, derived from both qualitative and quantitative studies of young people's perspectives, identified the major barriers as problems recognising symptoms, a preference for self-reliance and perceived stigma and embarrassment.[11] Facilitators were shown to be mostly unresearched, but those for which there was some evidence were positive

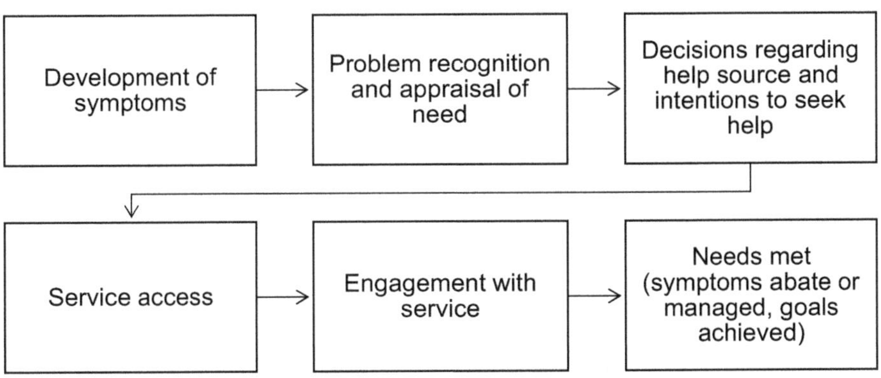

Figure 3.2 Help-seeking process

past experiences and encouragement from others as aids to seeking help. While these barriers and facilitators are relevant across the lifespan, they have particular salience for young people.

Problem recognition

The initiator of help-seeking is the development of symptoms, although the presence of symptoms alone does not automatically start the process. This is clearly demonstrated by the many studies showing that the majority of young people with significant psychological disorder do not access professional help. In a large study of Norwegian adolescents (n = 11,154), even at the highest percentile of anxiety and depression, only one-third had sought help; and within the highest tenth percentile only one-quarter reported seeking professional help.[4] The study revealed a very weak association, or dose response, between level of symptoms and professional help-seeking. Although awareness of symptoms has long been acknowledged as the first filter in the help-seeking process,[12] many factors affect whether symptoms are perceived as a problem that requires professional help and whether actual help is subsequently sought.

One of the factors that works against symptoms initiating help-seeking for young people is difficulty distinguishing 'normal' from 'abnormal' thoughts, feelings and behaviour. Because the teenage years are seen as a period of emotional lability and often challenging behaviours,[13] distinguishing between normal teenage issues and a mental health problem is difficult for young people themselves, their families and others in close contact with them. Importantly, compared distress has been shown to be a strong correlate of help-seeking; a large-scale study in the US revealed that even among people who were highly distressed by symptoms, it was those who perceived themselves to be *more* distressed than others who were likely to seek help. It is social comparison and recognition that distress and symptoms are outside the norm that facilitate seeking help.[14] Consequently, the acceptance of some of the symptoms of mental ill-health as common adolescent issues works against seeking help in a unique way for young people: if symptoms are attributed to normal teenage behaviour or other causal factors, such as peer pressure or substance use, rather than as an indication of a mental health problem, then the help-seeking process is not likely to commence.

Good mental health literacy,[15] particularly the 'ability to recognise specific disorders', enables help-seeking for young people and their families. In a large sample of Australian young people, better accuracy in labelling vignettes showing depression or psychosis was associated with choosing appropriate professional health care as the preferred response.[16] Better problem recognition is argued to account for the gender difference that is often observed in help-seeking intentions and behaviour.[17] Studies that have investigated early stages of the help-seeking process show that it is greater symptom recognition and perception of need for help that account for the increased propensity of young women to seek help compared with young men.[18] Many studies show that females have better mental health literacy than males at all ages, but particularly during adolescence and young adulthood.[19–21] Part of this comprises greater emotional competence, meaning that young women are better able to acknowledge and express their feelings and emotional world than young men.

Help-negation

Help-seeking is inhibited further by the very nature of the mental health problems that are most commonly experienced by young people. Help-negation is the opposite of help-seeking and was first noted in relation to the effect of suicidal ideation, whereby strong suicidal thoughts were shown to be associated with actively avoiding seeking help.[22] Help-negation has been defined as 'the refusal to accept or access available helping resources' and is argued to be a function of 'hopelessness, pessimism and cynicism regarding the efficacy of treatment'[23] (p. 499). The effect has been well established for suicidal thoughts, even at lower levels of ideation,[24,25] and young people are especially vulnerable due to the high prevalence of suicidal ideation at this stage of life.

The help-negation effect operates for other mental health problems commonly experienced by youth and adolescents, namely depression, anxiety, substance misuse and self-harm.[26] The social withdrawal and hopelessness that often accompany depression can impede seeking help, and studies show that young people are more likely to seek help from no one as depressive symptoms increase.[27] The help-negation effect of anxiety disorders has not been well studied, but the likely impact of symptoms of social anxiety and agoraphobia on accessing traditional in-person mental health services is clear.

The effect on help-seeking of the generally illicit nature of substance use and the highly stigmatised nature of substance use disorders was evident in the Australian National Survey of Mental Health and Wellbeing. This showed that for respondents of all ages, consulting a health professional for a mental health problem was lowest for those with a substance use problem at 24%, compared with 38% of those with an anxiety disorder and 59% of those with an affective disorder.[1] For respondents aged 16–24 years, these disparities were even more striking, with only 11% of those with a substance use problem seeking help, compared with 32% of those with anxiety disorders and 49% of those with an affective disorder.[28] Since substance use disorders were the most prevalent disorder for those aged 16–24 years, the reluctance to seek help for these disorders substantially accounts for the lower level of mental health care use in this age group.

Although less common, mental disorders with psychotic features have their peak period of incidence in late adolescence and early adulthood, and these disorders are often accompanied by social withdrawal, lack of insight, loss of touch with reality and paranoia, all of which can actively work against seeking professional help.[29] Only a minority of people experiencing psychosis initiate help-seeking themselves, and there are both help-seeking and health system delays to accessing treatment.[30] A small qualitative study revealed that young people with psychosis repeatedly attempted to ignore or hide their symptoms, generally thinking they were normal and would go away.[31] In areas without specific youth early intervention psychosis services, long durations of untreated first episode psychosis are well documented, and entry to health care is often triggered by the emergence of positive symptoms and crisis, when family members and others intervene to access health care.[32] More insidious onset is associated with longer delay and acute onset with a shorter treatment delay.[33]

Consequently, the very nature of mental disorder in the 12–25 year age range works against help-seeking; it is difficult for young people and their families to differentiate symptoms from 'normal' feelings, and the most common symptoms work against a young person wanting to seek out other people, and professionals in particular, for mental health care. To facilitate appropriate professional help-seeking for young people, good mental health literacy is paramount so that young people and their families are able to determine what signs indicate a mental health problem and what the appropriate responses might be. In concert, active outreach and opportunistic screening are required to help identify young people who may be unaware that they could benefit from mental health interventions.

Self-reliance

Another major barrier to young people accessing professional health care is their preference to deal with problems themselves.[34] Even at high levels of distress, young people usually define their symptoms as something that should be managed on their own. For example, in a large, nationally representative sample of Australian adolescents aged 13–17 years, the most common reason, reported by 38%, for not seeking professional help was preference to manage the problem alone.[35] Similarly, a large US study reported that a third of adolescents with serious suicidal ideation, depression or substance use problems felt that they should deal with problems themselves without outside help.[36] Studies of more marginalised young people show that the importance of self-reliance can be even stronger. A small qualitative study of homeless adolescents revealed that they placed a very high priority on self-sufficiency and were particularly distrustful of professional services.[37]

That self-reliance repeatedly emerges as a key barrier to seeking professional help is not surprising as the development of independence and self-reliance is one of the main goals of adolescence and a valued attainment in early adulthood. Becoming an independently functioning adult entails increasingly making one's own decisions, including health decisions. While developing independence is equally important for both boys and girls, it has been suggested that the focus on self-reliance is a stronger barrier to boys seeking help than for girls and is another factor that accounts for gender differences in help-seeking.[19,38]

Interestingly, young people are more predisposed to seek help for others than for themselves. This has been termed the 'personal service gap' and was demonstrated in a large Israeli study which showed that adolescents will refer peers to a psychologist more readily than themselves.[39] Peer support is an important avenue in promoting professional help-seeking and using the focus on aiding a friend has been suggested as an effective pathway for conveying help-seeking information to young people.

Informal social support

Encouragement from others is one of the most well-established facilitators of professional health care.[11] The informal support network of parents, friends and family is a critical part of the help-seeking process, as most people turn first to their informal social networks before accessing professional help. Furthermore, it is those people closest to a young person who are most likely to notice unusual changes in behaviour that may indicate a need for mental health care, and those with a close and trusted relationship are able to encourage seeking professional help.[40] When professional care is sought, three-quarters of people have had someone in their social network recommend it.[41]

Developmental patterns in help-seeking show that early in adolescence both boys and girls are most likely to seek help for their mental health problems from their parents, usually their mother.[6] Over the high school years, seeking help from parents decreases, which is developmentally appropriate as young people become increasingly independent from family.[41] For girls, this reduction is compensated for by increased reliance on friends, whereas boys increasingly rely on no one but themselves.[6] Internationally, the preference for young people to turn to informal social support for mental health problems is well established, as is the increasing reluctance of boys to disclose to anyone at all.[42]

Not surprisingly, the younger the adolescent the more influential parents are in the help-seeking process.[43] In childhood, parental perception of problems is usually the starting point for referral to professional services.[44] The capacity for self-referral develops during adolescence along with increasing autonomy from parents, but parents continue to play a vital role in accessing professional treatment for most adolescents and many young adults.

The preference for informal support stems from two main reasons. Firstly, most young people believe that informal support is sufficient and the most appropriate source of help for personal and emotional problems.[45] Such beliefs are particularly strong among young people who are not part of mainstream Western cultures. Many of those from culturally and linguistically diverse backgrounds have strong norms regarding keeping personal information within family. For example, a study of teenage refugees from seven different countries found that most were very reluctant to go beyond their close social relationships to seek help for psychosocial problems.[46]

The second reason is that young people prefer to disclose problems to those they know well and trust.[6] Young people are especially reluctant to talk to strangers about very personal issues; they find it embarrassing, intrusive and anxiety-provoking. They also believe that people they do not know, particularly health professionals who tend to be much older, will not understand them and their issues, and that it is only within their informal networks of friends and family that their problems will be understood.[6]

Family and friends are not the only sources of support available to young people that they know and trust. Young people are in regular contact with a range of other adults, including teachers, coaches and youth workers. Such people have been called gatekeepers, or gateway providers, being the adults within young people's formal networks who, although not mental health professionals, can be the first to identify a problem and guide young people to appropriate treatment.[47] This can be especially important for young people who are marginalised, or who cannot confide in their family. For example, young homeless people reported that they would rely exclusively on their youth worker for support with mental health problems.[48] Trusted adults in formal roles in the broader context of young people's lives, like teachers, youth workers and coaches, can play a vital role in encouraging young people to access appropriate mental health care. However, the mental health literacy, role perceptions and help-seeking intentions of these gateway providers themselves need to be supportive of seeking help before they are able to facilitate young people's service access.[49]

Stigma and confidentiality

One of the most commonly reported reasons why young people prefer to keep their mental health problems to themselves, or within their closest personal networks, is the stigma of mental illness. Stigma has long been recognised as a key barrier to mental health care for people of all ages.[50] Stigma is a broad concept, however, with several distinct forms. Public stigma is the negative stereotypes and prejudice commonly held within the community about people with mental illness, perceived public stigma is an individual's perception of public stigma and self-stigma is when a person identifies with the stigmatised group and internalises the stigmatising characteristics.[51]

A large-scale survey of young people from 13 different universities in the US revealed that it was only personally held stigmatising attitudes that were related to reluctance to seek help, rather than perceptions of what others believe in the form of public stigma.[52,53] Similarly, a systematic review concluded that it was mostly concerns about what others, including the help providers, would think of them personally that were the basis of fears of stigma related to seeking help,[11] rather than concerns about public stigma toward people with mental illness in general. Personal and self-stigma seem to be the greatest barriers to help-seeking,[54] although these are influenced by the generally perceived public attitudes toward people with mental illness and mental health service use within the community.

Fears of personally being identified as having a mental illness and being a service user are more salient during youth and adolescence than at other stages of life. Fundamentally, the primacy of peers means that confidentiality from the general peer group regarding mental health problems is essential to maintain peer group status. Peers become increasingly important as a social reference point during adolescence and have maximal effect in middle adolescence,[55] at the same time that mental health problems are rapidly rising. Secondly, identity development is a central issue during adolescence, and the strong self-stigma associated with mental illness means that young people are very unwilling to adopt a mental illness identity.

Deriving from fears of personal stigma and the need to protect identity, confidentiality is a major concern of young people seeking mental health care.[6] Not surprisingly, this is especially true in settings where exposure to others of one's seeking help is more likely, such as in rural and school communities.[56,57] Greater fear of stigma is another reason why young men are more reluctant to seek help than young women, as they have been shown to have substantially higher scores on measures of stigma than girls.[19] Consequently, anonymity can be an important facilitator of seeking help, particularly in the initial stages and especially for boys and young men.[8]

The online and technology-enabled environment is a setting that has substantial capacity to reduce stigma, enable confidentiality and increase help-seeking for young people.[58] Computer-assisted help-seeking does not need to involve the direct person-to-person contact inherent in most other forms of support and can be engaged with incognito. This highly valued anonymity is achievable via online communication formats and is suitable for seeking information, many prevention interventions and online and crisis counselling. Interestingly, young people using online counselling say they find it easier to write than talk about deeply personal issues and sensitive topics and prefer online to telephone counselling.[59,60] An entire spectrum of interventions to support youth mental health is emerging via computer-mediated technologies, and the anonymity, ease of access and wide reach of these rapidly expanding initiatives make them vital links in the help-seeking process.[61]

Perceptions of professional help

Closely aligned with stigma are negative perceptions of mental health care and professional services. Foremost, there is a pervasive belief that professional help does not work; the view that traditional forms of mental health care are not effective is held by most young people, along with their parents.[62] Thinking that 'nothing could help' was the second most endorsed barrier to accessing mental health care in the Australian National Survey of Mental Health and Wellbeing.[1] In parallel, a large Dutch study showed that beliefs that treatment *can* help were associated with an *increased* likelihood of mental health service use.[63] Similarly, experimental research with a large sample of youth aged 14–22 years showed that a counter-stereotypical message showing a person with depression who had been successfully treated had a robust effect on reducing stigma to encourage help-seeking.[64]

Issues related to problem recognition extend to recognition of the need for professional health care. Even when symptoms are acknowledged, this is often not translated into a need for professional intervention, and the decision of no need for care is frequently made.[65] Many young people believe that symptoms are self-limiting and that self-care or informal support are all that is required. A common belief is that professional mental health care will do more harm than good,[66] and there are particularly negative views regarding the use of psychotropic medication.[67] Young people are more likely to endorse social support (including helping each other), generic counselling and general stress reduction as effective interventions than specialist mental health care.[62] Furthermore, young people are selective regarding to whom they will talk about what type of problem and match the source of help to the type of problem when they have the opportunity to do so. Frequently, traditional health and mental health services are not deemed appropriate to their issues.[68]

Negative impressions of past experiences of professional mental health care contribute to such views. Not surprisingly, young people who have had a poor past experience are much less likely to intend to access professional health care again.[57] The main factors accounting for negative experiences include not being helped, not feeling listened to and not being taken seriously. Notably, the initial experience of mental health care is critical; if the first impression is not positive, then the young person is unlikely to return.[6] Young people express the desire for 'an attentive, trusting and non-judgemental professional who showed respect towards young people'[69] (p. 18). With young people increasingly sharing their experiences through social media, negative service experiences and perceptions can rapidly be widely shared.

In Australia, as in many other countries, specialist mental health care is rarely accessed directly, but rather through primary health or counselling services. Generalist services, themselves, provide a substantial proportion of mental health care. General practitioners (GPs) and school counsellors are the services attended by most young people with mental health problems; in the child and adolescent component of the Australian National Survey of Mental Health and Wellbeing, over half the sample with mental health problems had attended such generalist services, while only 17% had attended a psychiatrist, mental health clinic or hospital-based department of psychiatry.[35]

General practice and school health, counselling and guidance services have a critical role in youth mental health; they are major providers of mental health care, and GPs are the formal gatekeepers to most specialist care. However, despite their prominent role, young people are often reluctant to seek such help. In a large study of where young Australians would seek help, few young people saw the GP as a preferred source of help; GPs were mentioned by only 4–13% of adolescents and 19–34% of young adults.[70] Similar findings have come from the UK.[71] In contrast, parents much more frequently mention the GP as a preferred source, comprising 40–72% of the parents of adolescents and 61–76% of the parents of young adults.[70]

Although young people tend not to see general practice as a preferred source of mental health care, primary care nevertheless has an essential role in promoting effective help-seeking. Importantly, most young people access primary care at least once a year, providing an opportunity for screening for mental health problems, which is warranted given the high prevalence of mental disorder and low level of recognition at this stage of life.[72] This need is especially relevant for young people without a strong informal network.[40] Furthermore, the high accessibility of primary care for parents is important to support because it is parents who are often the first to recognise the need for professional help. Enhanced general practice–based service models are an essential component of a mental health service system that provides effective primary care and enables timely access to appropriate specialist mental health care.[72]

School-based pastoral care and counselling services are a critical component of mental health care for young people still at school,[57] and the high school years are a period of peak vulnerability. Unique barriers to accessing school services have been identified, including concerns regarding confidentiality, specialisation of support staff and integration with teaching roles, and negative experiences of young people seeking school-based support. Schools need to be well informed regarding youth mental health, provide appropriate responses within the school setting and be well linked with local primary care and specialist services. Notably, schools need to prioritise the mental health literacy of all staff and students and have access to the most recent evidence-based online approaches to be able to fulfil their critical role in the mental health help-seeking process.

Interventions to increase help-seeking

In response to widespread recognition of the high level of need for professional mental health care for young people but their reluctance to seek it, interventions to increase help-seeking behaviour have proliferated. These generally focus on improving mental health literacy and reducing stigma. Growing activity in this field became evident about a decade ago,[21] and the trend has accelerated. We now have evidence that interventions that improve mental health literacy include whole-of-community campaigns, interventions in educational settings, Mental Health First Aid training and information websites.[73] Importantly, effective interventions need to adhere closely to established models of health promotion that identify appropriate elements for attitude and behaviour change, as change in knowledge alone without other supports does not translate into changes in actual help-seeking behaviour.

Significant focus has been placed on improving mental health literacy for young people in schools, as these are ideal settings through which to efficiently reach large numbers of young people. A systematic review of school-based interventions revealed that they need to be embedded within a whole-school approach, build teacher capacity, include links to parents and the wider community and be sustainable.[74] More recently, the mental health of tertiary students and the role of higher education settings have been recognised as a priority.[75] For older adolescents and young adults in these settings, peer-based and peer-led programs, like batyr@uni (Australia), jack.org (Canada) and Student Minds (UK) show promise as effective approaches.[75,76]

Another main avenue targeted for increasing help-seeking is the online environment, as young people are constantly connected to their digital worlds. However, a systematic review of the effectiveness of online services in facilitating mental health help-seeking in young people concluded that there are few studies that examine effects on actual help-seeking and further research is needed, and most of the current studies did not reveal significant effects on service use.[77] For example, a randomised controlled trial among community-based young adults yielded no evidence that providing depression information through health e-cards had an effect on help-seeking.[78]

Interestingly, the factors influencing online help-seeking itself have been shown to be quite distinct from those affecting help-seeking from traditional in-person services. In the online environment young people navigate independently from an early age without the influence of significant others, like parents, who have a strong influence on traditional service use.[43] Further, to date, the online environment has been shown to be much more attractive to young women than young men.[79] Consequently, online interventions need to be able to appropriately guide and facilitate self-navigation, including for the youngest adolescents and with targeted approaches for young men. This means that safe, evidence-based and moderated online pathways are required.

Essential elements promoting help-seeking

Current understanding of young people's help-seeking identifies key factors that promote appropriate service use, with the essential elements summarised in Figure 3.3.

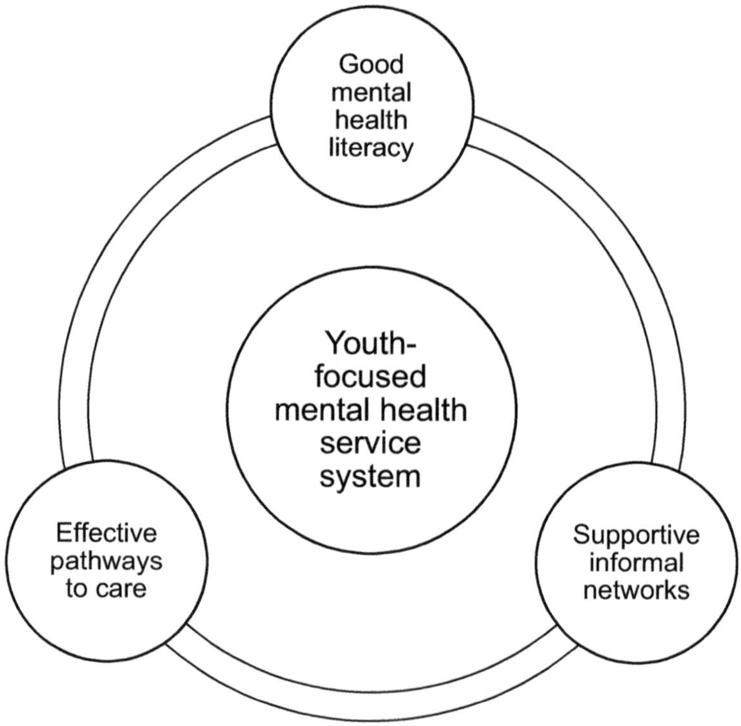

Figure 3.3 Essential elements for promoting young people's help-seeking

This shows four main areas of intervention, in which a range of approaches in different settings are needed to facilitate young people's help-seeking behaviour.

Firstly, young people need help to recognise and acknowledge their need for mental health care in response to symptoms of mental health disorders. This requires good mental health literacy overall, but specifically in relation to beliefs in the need for professional care and that such care is effective. Multiple communication avenues need to be used to convince young people of two main messages – that mental health problems are real and not an inevitable part of adolescence and emerging adulthood that has to be endured, and that they can be effectively treated. This requires reaching out with appropriate messages and information to engage young people in the settings they are most likely to be found: online, at home and through schools, workplaces and community services.

Secondly, young people's informal networks need to be engaged in encouraging symptom recognition and appropriate service use. The effect of friends and families on professional help-seeking is somewhat contradictory: they can both help and hinder the process. It needs to be acknowledged that while the support of friends and family is very valuable, it is generally not sufficient to deal effectively with the symptoms and functional impacts of a mental health disorder. Concerns regarding personal and self-stigma must be reduced so that young people are prepared to disclose potential symptoms to others in their social network, and friends and family need to be skilled in useful ways to respond. This requires improved mental health literacy for friends, families and significant others and also clearly signposted and easy access to appropriate evidence-based services.

Thirdly, effective pathways to the services young people require must be in place. This entails reliable and high-quality evidence-based information and advice, screening, outreach and non-specialist care be available. Effective pathways need to be facilitated through general practice and other primary health care settings, but also through the education, work and community-based settings in which young people spend their time. Alongside the health system, the broader network of formal supports needs to be engaged so that the trusted adults that young people are in regular contact with, who may become aware when a young person is in need of mental health care, have the skills and knowledge to encourage and support access to appropriate interventions. Increasingly, online settings provide some of the most efficient and potentially effective opportunities to inform and engage young people in the pathways to seeking help.

Finally and fundamentally, however, the main challenge to improving young people's professional help-seeking for mental health problems is providing the type of mental health and wellbeing services that adolescents and young adults are prepared to access and engage with. There is no point encouraging help-seeking if appropriate, youth-focused, easily accessible service options are not in place. If the professional services that meet young people's specific needs are available, then they will use them. This has been clearly demonstrated in Australia with the extraordinary uptake of *headspace* services, the national initiative in youth mental health care built on sound understanding of young people's mental health needs and help-seeking preferences, barriers and facilitators.[80,81] *headspace* is part of a strong and growing international movement that has emerged advocating for the provision of youth mental health service systems, which is based on understanding of the principles that underpin what works specifically for adolescents and young adults.[82] Services that young people will use are those that: are youth-friendly by truly listening to and responding to young people's views and presenting issues; intervene early in the developmental course of mental health problems so as to be maximally effective; and provide confidential, non-stigmatising, easily-accessible, holistic and effective treatments that respect and support young people's emerging adult status.

References

1 Slade T, Johnston A, Teesson M, Whiteford H, Burgess P, Pirkis J, et al. *The mental health of Australians 2: report on the 2007 National Survey of Mental Health and Wellbeing*. Canberra: Department of Health and Ageing; 2009.

2 Merikangas KR, He J, Burstein M, Swanson SA, Avenevoli S, Cui L, et al. Lifetime prevalence of mental disorders in U.S. adolescents: results from the National Comorbidity Survey Replication – Adolescent Supplement (NCS-A). *Journal of the American Academy of Child and Adolescent Psychiatry* 2010;49(10):980–9.

3 Kessler RC, Amminger AG, Aguilar-Gaxiola S, Alonso J, Lee S, Utsun TB. Age of onset of mental disorders: a review of recent literature. *Current Opinion in Psychiatry* 2007;20(4):359–64.

4 Zachrisson HD, Rödje K, Mykletun A. Utilization of health services in relation to mental health problems in adolescents: a population based survey. *BMC Public Health* 2006;6:34.

5 Mauerhofer Al, Berchtold A, Michaud PA, Suris JC. GPs' role in the detection of psychological problems of young people: a population-based study. *British Journal of General Practice* 2009;59(566):e308–14.

6 Rickwood D, Deane FP, Wilson CJ, Ciarrochi J. Young people's help-seeking for mental health problems. *Advances in Mental Health* 2005;4(3):1–34.

7 Rickwood D, Thomas K. Conceptual measurement framework for help-seeking for mental health problems. *Psychology Research and Behavior Management* 2012;5:173–83.

8 Rickwood D. Responding effectively to support the mental health and well-being of young people. In Wyn J, Cahill H (Eds) *Handbook of children and youth studies*. Singapore: Springer; 2015. p 139–54.

9 Scott SE, Walter FM, Webster A, Sutton S, Emery J. The model of pathways to treatment: conceptualization and integration with existing theory. *British Journal of Health Psychology* 2012;18(1):45–64.

10 Tanielian T, Jaycox LH, Paddock SM, Chandra A, Meredith LS, Burnam MA. Improving treatment seeking among adolescents with depression: understanding readiness for treatment. *Journal of Adolescent Health* 2009;45(5):490–8.

11 Gulliver A, Griffiths KM, Christensen H. Perceived barriers and facilitators to mental health help-seeking in young people: a systematic review. *BMC Psychiatry* 2010;10:113.

12 Goldberg D, Huxley P. *Mental illness in the community: the pathway to psychiatric care*. London: Tavistock; 1980.

13 Offer D, Schonert-Reichl KA. Debunking the myths of adolescence: findings from recent research. *Journal of the American Academy of Child and Adolescent Psychiatry* 1992;31(6):1003–14.

14 Biddle L, Donovan J, Sharp D, Gunnell D. Explaining non-help-seeking amongst young adults with mental distress: a dynamic interpretive model of illness behaviour. *Sociology of Health & Illness* 2007;29(7):983–1002.
15 Jorm AF, Korten AE, Jacomb PA, Christensen H, Rodgers B, Pollitt P. "Mental health literacy": a survey of the public's ability to recognise mental disorders and their beliefs about the effectiveness of treatment. *Medical Journal of Australia* 1997;166(4):182–6.
16 Wright A, Jorm AF, Harris MG, McGorry PD. What's in a name? Is accurate recognition and labelling of mental disorders by young people associated with better help-seeking and treatment preferences? *Social Psychiatry and Psychiatric Epidemiology* 2007;42(3):244–50.
17 Zwaanswijk M, Van der Ende J, Verhaak PF, Bensing JM, Verhulst FC. Factors associated with adolescent mental health service need and utilization. *Journal of the American Academy of Child and Adolescent Psychiatry* 2003;42(6):692–700.
18 Zwaanswijk M, Van der Ende J, Verhaak PF, Bensing JM, Verhulst FC. The different stages and actors involved in the process leading to the use of adolescent mental health services. *Clinical Child Psychology and Psychiatry* 2007;12(4):567–82.
19 Rice SM, Purcell R, McGorry PD. Adolescent and young adult male mental health: transforming system failures into proactive models of engagement. *Journal of Adolescent Health* 2018;62(3):S9–17.
20 Cotton SM, Wright A, Harris MG, Jorm AF, McGorry PD. Influence of gender on mental health literacy in young Australians. *Australian and New Zealand Journal of Psychiatry* 2006;40(9):790–6.
21 Kelly CM, Jorm AF, Wright A. Improving mental health literacy as a strategy to facilitate early intervention for mental disorders. *Medical Journal of Australia* 2007;187(7):S26–30.
22 Clark D, Fawcett B. Review of empirical risk factors for evaluation of the suicidal patient. In Bongar B (Ed) *Suicide: guidelines for assessment, management, and treatment.* New York: Oxford University Press; 1992.
23 Rudd MD, Joiner TE, Rajab MH. Help negation after acute suicidal crisis. *Journal of Consulting and Clinical Psychology* 1995;63(3):499–503.
24 Wilson CJ, Deane FP. Help-negation and suicidal ideation: the role of depression, anxiety and hopelessness. *Journal of Youth and Adolescence* 2010;39(3):291–305.
25 Wilson CJ, Deane FP, Marshall KL, Dalley A. Adolescents' suicidal thinking and reluctance to consult general medical practitioners. *Journal of Youth and Adolescence* 2010;39(4):343–56.
26 Rickwood D, White A, Eckersley R. Overview of current trends in mental health problems for Australia's youth and adolescents. *Clinical Psychologist* 2007;11(3):72–8.
27 Wilson CJ, Rickwood D, Deane FP. Depressive symptoms and help-seeking intentions in young people. *Clinical Psychologist* 2007;11(3):98–107.
28 Australian Bureau of Statistics. *Customised report.* Canberra: Australian Bureau of Statistics; 2010.
29 Larsen TK, Joa I, Langeveld J, Johannessen JO. Optimizing health-care systems to promote early detection of psychosis. *Early Intervention in Psychiatry* 2009;3(1):S13–6.
30 O'Callaghan E, Turner N, Renwick L, Jackson D, Sutton M, Foley SD, et al. First episode psychosis and the trail to secondary care: help-seeking and health-system delays. *Social Psychiatry and Psychiatric Epidemiology* 2010;45(3):381–91.
31 Boydell KM, Gladstone BM, Volpe T. Understanding help seeking delay in the prodrome to first episode psychosis: a secondary analysis of the perspectives of young people. *Psychiatric Rehabilitation Journal* 2006;30(1):54–60.

32 Corcoran C, Gerson R, Sills-Shahar R, Nickou C, McGlashan T, Malaspina D, et al. Trajectory to a first episode of psychosis: a qualitative research study with families. *Early Intervention in Psychiatry* 2007;1(4):308–15.
33 Compton MT, Chien VH, Leiner AS, Goulding SM, Weiss PS. Mode of onset of psychosis and family involvement in help-seeking as determinants of duration of untreated psychosis. *Social Psychiatry and Psychiatric Epidemiology* 2008;43(12):975–82.
34 Farrand P, Perry J, Lee C, Parker M. Adolescents' preference towards self-help: implications for service development. *Primary Care and Community Psychiatry* 2006;11(2):73–9.
35 Sawyer MG, Arney FM, Baghurst PA, Clark JJ, Graetz BW, Kosky RJ, et al. *Child and adolescent component of the National Survey of Mental Health and Wellbeing: the mental health of young people in Australia.* Canberra: Commonwealth Department of Health and Aged Care; 2000.
36 Gould MS, Velting D, Kleinman M, Lucas C, Thomas JG, Chung M. Teenagers' attitudes about coping strategies and help-seeking behaviour for suicidality. *Journal of the American Academy of Child and Adolescent Psychiatry* 2004;43(9):1124–33.
37 Collins P, Barker C. Psychological help-seeking in homeless adolescents. *International Journal of Social Psychiatry* 2009;55(4):372–84.
38 Jorm AF, Kelly CM, Wright A, Parslow RA, Harris MG, McGorry PD. Belief in dealing with depression alone: results from community surveys of adolescents and adults. *Journal of Affective Disorders* 2006;96(1–2):59–65.
39 Raviv A, Raviv A, Vago-Gefen I, Fink AS. The personal service gap: factors affecting adolescents' willingness to seek help. *Journal of Adolescence* 2009;32(3):483–99.
40 Frojd S, Marttunen M, Pelkonen M, von der Pahlen B, Kaltiala-Heino R. Adult and peer involvement in help-seeking for depression in adolescent population. *Social Psychiatry and Psychiatric Epidemiology* 2007;42(12):945–52.
41 Gray S, Daraganova G. Adolescent help-seeking. In *LSAC Annual Statistical Report 2017 chapter.* Melbourne: Australian Institute of Family Studies; 2018.
42 Barker G. *Adolescents, social support and help-seeking behaviour: an international literature review and programme consultation with recommendations for action.* Geneva: World Health Organization; 2007.
43 Rickwood DJ, Mazzer KR, Telford NR. Social influences on seeking help from mental health services, in-person and online, during adolescence and young adulthood. *BMC Psychiatry* 2015;15:40.
44 Sayal K. Annotation: pathways to care for children with mental health problems. *Journal of Child Psychology and Psychiatry* 2006;47(7):649–59.
45 Kuhl J, Jarkon-Horlick L, Morrisey RF. Measuring barriers to help-seeking behaviour in adolescents. *Journal of Youth and Adolescence* 1997;26(6):637–50.
46 De Anstiss H, Ziaian T. Mental health help-seeking and refugee adolescents: qualitative findings from a mixed-methods investigation. *Australian Psychologist* 2010;45(1):29–37.
47 Stiffman AR, Pescosolido B, Cabassa LJ. Building a model to understand youth service access: the gateway provider model. *Mental Health Services Research* 2004;6(4):189–98.
48 Keys Young. *Research and consultation among young people on mental health issues: final report.* Canberra: Commonwealth Department of Health and Family Services; 1997.
49 Mazzer KR, Rickwood DJ. Teachers' and coaches' role perceptions for supporting young people's mental health: multiple group path analyses. *Australian Journal of Psychology* 2014;67(1);10–19.
50 Clement S, Schauman O, Graham T, Maggioni F, Evans-Lacko S, Bezborodovs N, et al. What is the impact of mental health-related stigma on help-seeking? A systematic review of quantitative and qualitative studies. *Psychological Medicine* 2014;45(1):11–27.

51 Corrigan PW, Watson AC, Barr L. The self-stigma of mental illness: implications for self-esteem and self-efficacy. *Journal of Consulting and Clinical Psychology* 2006;25(8): 875–84.
52 Eisenberg D, Downs MF, Golberstein E, Zivin K. Stigma and help seeking for mental health among college students. *Medical Care Research and Review* 2009;66(5):522–41.
53 Golberstein E, Eisenberg D, Gollust SE. Perceived stigma and help-seeking behavior: longitudinal evidence from the healthy minds study. *Psychiatric Services* 2009;60(9):1254–6.
54 Corrigan PW, Druss BG, Perlick DA. The impact of mental illness stigma on seeking and participating in mental health care. *Psychological Science in the Public Interest* 2014;15(2):37–70.
55 Monahan KC, Steinberg L, Cauffman E. Affiliation with antisocial peers, susceptibility to peer influence, and antisocial behavior during the transition to adulthood. *Developmental Psychology* 2009;45(6):1520–30.
56 Boyd C, Francis K, Aisbett D, Newnham K, Sewell J, Dawes G, et al. Australian rural adolescents' experiences of accessing psychological help for a mental health problem. *Australian Journal of Rural Health* 2007;15(3):196–200.
57 Rickwood DJ. Supporting young people at school with high mental health needs. *Australian Journal of Guidance and Counselling* 2005;15(2):137–55.
58 Burns JM, Durkin LA, Nicholas J. Mental health of young people in the United States: what role can the internet play in reducing stigma and promoting help seeking? *Journal of Adolescent Health* 2009;45(1):95–7.
59 Bradford SA, Rickwood DJ. Acceptability and utility of an electronic psychosocial assessment (myAssessment) to increase self-disclosure in youth mental healthcare: a quasi-experimental study. *BMC Psychiatry* 2015;15:305.
60 Gould MS, Greenberg T, Munfakh JL, Kleinman M, Lubell K. Teenagers' attitudes about seeking help from telephone crisis services (hotlines). *Suicide and Life-Threatening Behavior* 2006;36(6):601–13.
61 Rickwood D. Entering the e-spectrum. *Youth Studies Australia* 2012;31(4):17–26.
62 Jorm AF, Morgan AJ, Wright A. A comparison of clinician, youth, and parent beliefs about helpfulness of interventions for early psychosis. *Psychiatric Services* 2008;59(10):1115–20.
63 Vanheusden K, van der Ende J, Mulder CL, van Lenthe FJ, Verhulst FC, Mackenbach JP. Beliefs about mental health problems and help-seeking behavior in Dutch young adults. *Social Psychiatry and Psychiatric Epidemiology* 2009;44(3):239–46.
64 Romer D, Bock M. Reducing the stigma of mental illness among adolescents and young adults: the effects of treatment information. *Journal of Health Communication* 2008;13(8):742–58.
65 Vanheusden K, Mulder CL, van der Ende J, van Lenthe FJ, Mackenbach JP, Verhulst FC. Young adults face major barriers to seeking help from mental health services. *Patient Education and Counseling* 2008;73(1):97–104.
66 ten Have M, de Graaf R, Ormel J, Vilagut G, Kovess V, Alonso J, et al. Are attitudes towards mental health help-seeking associated with service use? Results from the European Study of Epidemiology of Mental Disorders. *Social Psychiatry and Psychiatric Epidemiology* 2010;45(2):153–63.
67 Wright A, Harris MG, Wiggers JH, Jorm AF, Cotton SM, Harrigan SM, et al. Recognition of depression and psychosis by young Australians and their beliefs about treatment. *Medical Journal of Australia* 2005;183(1):18–23.
68 Marcell AV, Halpern-Felsher BL. Adolescents' beliefs about preferred resources for help vary depending on the health issue. *Journal of Adolescent Health* 2007;41(1):61–8.

69 Cohen A, Medlow S, Kelk N, Hickie I. Young people's experiences of mental health care: implications for the Headspace National Youth Mental Health Foundation. *Youth Studies Australia* 2009;28(1):13–20.
70 Jorm AF, Wright A, Morgan AJ. Where to seek help for a mental disorder? National survey of the beliefs of Australian youth and their parents. *Medical Journal of Australia* 2007;187(10):556–60.
71 Biddle L, Donovan JL, Gunnell D, Sharp D. Young adults' perceptions of GPs as a help source for mental distress: a qualitative study. *British Journal of General Practice* 2006;56(533):924–31.
72 Hickie IB, Fogarty AS, Davenport TA, Luscombe GM, Burns J. Responding to experiences of young people with common mental health problems attending Australian general practice. *Medical Journal of Australia* 2007;187(7):S47–52.
73 Jorm A. Mental health literacy: empowering the community to take action for better mental health. *American Psychologist* 2012;67(3):231–43.
74 Weare K, Nind M. Mental health promotion and problem prevention in schools: what does the evidence say? *Health Promotion International* 2011;26(1):i29–69.
75 Orygen. *Under the radar: the mental health of Australian university students.* Melbourne: Orygen, The National Centre of Excellence in Youth Mental Health; 2018.
76 Gilham C, Austen EL, Wei Y, Kutcher S. Improving mental health literacy in post-secondary students: field testing the feasibility and potential outcomes of a peer-led approach. *Canadian Journal of Community Mental Health* 2018;37(1):1–12.
77 Kauer SD, Mangan C, Sanci L. Do online mental health service improve help-seeking for young people: a systematic review. *Journal of Medical Internet Research* 2014;16(3):e66.
78 Costin DL, Mackinnon AJ, Griffiths KM, Batterham PJ, Bennett AJ, Bennett K, et al. Health e-cards as a means of encouraging help seeking for depression among young adults: randomized controlled trial. *Journal of Medical Internet Research* 2009;11(4):e42.
79 Rickwood D, Webb M, Kennedy V, Telford N. Who are the young people choosing online mental health support? Findings from the implementation of Australia's national online youth mental health service, eheadspace. *JMIR Mental Health* 2016;3(3):e40.
80 Rickwood D, Paraskakis M, Quin D, Hobbs N, Ryall V, Trethowan J, et al. Australia's innovation in youth mental health care – the headspace centre model. *Early Intervention in Psychiatry* 2019;13(1):159–66.
81 Perera S, Hetrick S, Cotton S, Parker A, Rickwood D, Davenport T, et al. Awareness of headspace youth mental health centres across Australian communities between 2008 and 2015. *Journal of Mental Health* 2019; in press.
82 Hetrick SE, Bailey AP, Smith KE, Malla A, Mathias S, Singh SP, et al. Integrated (one-stop shop) youth health care: best available evidence and future directions. *Medical Journal of Australia* 2017;207(10):S5–18.

4 Early psychosis services

Jean Addington, Eóin Killackey and David Marulanda

Introduction

Over the last 15–20 years there has been a worldwide movement to detect and intervene as early as possible for those with psychotic illness. Unparalleled progress has been made in program and service development with a wide range of research results, outcome studies, treatment approaches and new initiatives for those individuals experiencing a first episode of psychosis.[1] More recently, similar efforts have focused on the pre-psychotic or "prodromal" stage of illness which has been defined as the period marked by changes from a person's premorbid mental state and level of functioning up to the appearance of psychotic features.[2]

Since psychosis typically begins in late adolescence or early adulthood, its onset may complicate or interfere with many of the developmental tasks that the young adult is attempting to accomplish at this time. Typical developmental tasks of early adulthood include individuating from the family; developing interests, hobbies and skills; discovering and experimenting with sexuality; forming and maintaining relationships; and engaging in further and/or higher education and vocational activities. It is not difficult to envisage the often devastating effects that psychosis and even the early pre-psychotic phase can have on what is a normal struggle with adult developmental tasks. When these young individuals develop a psychosis they often fall out of step with their peers, become socially isolated, have an altered self-perception and are unable to complete their education. The potential for achievements is reduced and, as the gap between these individuals and their peers widens, catching up becomes more difficult. The potential for achievement is further reduced if these individuals delay completion of their education or vocational training because of difficulties resulting from their illness. Thus, failure or difficulty in accomplishing these developmental tasks, along with any experiences of stigma, has a major impact on the young person over and above the psychosis itself.

Typical ages for those at their first episode are 15–25 and for those in the pre-psychotic phase are 12–23. These ages typically cross the traditional split of child and adolescent services and adult services. This chapter will first give an overview of psychosis and the importance of and rationale for early intervention. It will then address key components of early intervention for those young people experiencing a first episode of psychosis including timing, setting and the wide range of both psychosocial and pharmacological treatments. The chapter will then address those young people who appear to be at risk for developing a psychotic illness. Although services do exist that are clearly youth-friendly, there needs to be a system change within the mental health field in order to best meet the needs of these young people.

First episode psychosis

As mentioned, the onset of psychosis tends to happen between the ages of 15 and 25 years, a feature in common with the onset of higher prevalence mental illnesses such as depression and anxiety. Psychosis is a non-diagnostic title used to describe a range of illness features such as hallucinations and delusions as well as negative symptoms which may be present. The purpose of using the word psychosis rather than a diagnostic label such as schizophrenia is firstly to avoid premature judgment about the course of illness as there is a very high rate of diagnostic instability after presentation for treatment. Secondly, there is a need to avoid the stigma attached to the illness label for young people with psychosis, carers and clinicians. This stigma around the label can have serious and deleterious influences on the interactions between the young person and clinician, clinician and carer, and carer and young person, as well as reducing the belief that the individual has the ability to recover, which can run the risk of becoming a self-fulfilling prophecy if not checked early.

Rationale for early intervention

In nearly all other areas of life and medicine, early intervention is seen as an intuitive and sensible way to limit damage and to prevent greater problems requiring greater solutions down the track. Until relatively recently, psychiatry, particularly in relation to psychotic illnesses, stood alone in being dominated by a culture that merely managed acute behavioural crises until the development of chronic illness. This approach was largely driven by a therapeutic nihilism with notions of schizophrenia as an illness of inevitable decline. Despite this, the idea that the early phase of psychotic illness is an opportune target of intervention has a long history in psychiatry. However, it was not until 1992 that the field of early psychosis research and practice really began to develop.[3]

Increasingly it became understood that an early and comprehensive intervention is very important. The work of Max Birchwood and others has illustrated this through the concept of the critical period.[4] The critical period is the first five years after the onset of the illness. It is during this time that the disability associated with psychotic illness develops. The phase of life in which the onset of illness tends to occur is also a key developmental period across a range of life domains which are all associated with the establishment of independence and identity. Severe interruption of, or failure in, these developmental tasks leads to psychosocial disabilities associated with psychotic illnesses such as unemployment, homelessness, singleness and social exclusion.[5] It is also the key risk time in the course of illness for suicide. Intensive and sustained intervention in this period has the potential to impede the progress of illness and, importantly, prevent the development of disability. The concept of early intervention in psychosis is no longer a fringe idea and has been adopted and recommended in several international treatment guidelines.[6,7]

Timing and duration of early intervention

A key concept in the first episode psychosis literature is the duration of untreated psychosis (DUP). While there are definitely a number of complexities around measuring DUP,[8] as a concept it refers to the period of time between the emergence of psychotic symptoms and the beginning of treatment for those symptoms. DUP was seen as a potentially important factor as it was one of the few malleable variables that could be identified. The theory was that reducing DUP would lead to better outcomes. For a number of years there were arguments for and against this proposition.[5] Several studies and meta-analyses have resolved this, finding that while controlling for other variables that may also have been implicated in outcome, DUP did have an independent contribution in explaining outcome, with shorter DUP leading to better outcomes.[9–11] These results accord with the intuitive idea that the best time to intervene is as soon as possible after the onset of the psychosis.

In the 1990s as clinical and research work in early intervention was developing, early research showed that there were long delays in accessing treatment for people with first episode psychosis. In many cases there was often over a year between the emergence of symptoms and the onset of treatment.[5] Studies have shown that with a concerted education and communication strategy and the availability of early intervention services the DUP can be reduced by two thirds.[12] The best way to reduce DUP is to have services for those who are potentially at risk for developing psychosis (addressed later) which links into, or is even a part of, a first episode service. Such an arrangement can see DUP reduced to nothing as treatment is seamless and continuous. In any case, the presence of psychotic symptoms with duration of more than one week requires treatment in an early intervention setting.

Since the first five years after onset is the period when maximal disability levels are reached, duration of treatment also requires consideration. In ideal situations, close monitoring and provision of a broad mixture of treatments would be provided in a continuous manner throughout the entire critical period in a specialized early intervention service. This would limit the development of disability and promote maximal symptomatic and functional recovery. However, in many situations, this is currently more of a goal than a reality. Typically, most current programs have between 18 months and three years of tenure with patients. Research has shown that while the outcomes are better at the end of the specialized intervention for first episode psychosis, most of this gain is lost after a few years in generic adult mental health services.[13] This suggests that greater duration of specialized treatment is required to see people through the critical period.

Setting for early intervention

One of the key recommendations in guidelines published by the National Institute for Health and Care Excellence in the UK is to approach the treatment of schizophrenia with optimism about potential outcome.[6] In relation to first episode psychosis, the importance of an optimistic approach cannot be overemphasized. This applies not only to the treatment team, but also to the treatment setting. As is the case for all people with psychotic illnesses, people with first episode psychosis should be treated in the least restrictive setting in which they are safe.[14] If possible, such treatment should occur in the community, at home or in youth friendly settings such as a youth health clinic. The greater the degree of specialization of the clinic (i.e., where for example the clinic sees only people with first episode psychosis), the better the outcome.[15] On the occasions when young people with first episode psychosis need to be hospitalized, optimal treatment is in a separate ward from people with chronic illness, or at least in a separated area of an adult ward if a separate ward is not available. In both inpatient and outpatient settings there needs to be a very low threshold to access services to encourage the earliest possible presentation.[16]

Treatments for first episode psychosis

Three areas of treatment for first episode psychosis will be briefly covered; medication, psychological interventions and psychosocial interventions. Because of the broad multi-domain nature of the disability brought about by psychosis, it is important that treatment is equally broad in its coverage. Treatment should target equally psychotic symptoms and psychological and functional domains.

Medication

Initiation of medication in first episode psychosis needs to be conducted in a safe and supportive environment. This may be in the community where adequate outreach is available, or it may be in hospital. The provision of benzodiazepines in this process may be a useful adjunct.[7] People who are experiencing first episode psychosis are more likely to be sensitive to the effects of medication as well as being more prone to experiencing side effects.[13] Therefore in relation to medication, guidelines suggest starting with a low dose and patiently titrating up to therapeutic levels.[6] Despite some research findings which cast doubt on the superior value of atypical antipsychotic medications in chronic schizophrenia,[17,18] and while there are no dramatic efficacy advantages,[19] most but not all clinical guidelines recommend that the atypical antipsychotics are used as a first line treatment owing to their better tolerability and lower side-effect profiles than older drugs.

Adequate trials of medication need to be given. This may mean up to six weeks in some cases. If a first atypical proves unsuccessful, it is recommended a second is tried for an adequate period. If unsuccessful, consideration should be given to a trial of injectable medication, especially if adherence is questionable despite psychosocial endeavours in this direction, and also an early trial of clozapine if treatment resistance is apparent. There may be a place for milder neuroprotective agents in the future to augment recovery at this stage of illness, but further research is required.[20]

There should be careful discussions with the young person and their carers, informing them of the side effects and benefits of medication and, where possible, including their opinion in decision-making.[6] Side effects of atypical antipsychotics can include impaired glucose tolerance, sexual side effects and weight gain. Serial monitoring of weight, BMI and metabolic parameters is an essential part of routine care given the medical comorbidity that steadily accrues, exacerbated in part by adverse effects of antipsychotic medications.[21] In addition to aiming for remission of positive symptoms, other key syndromes such as major depression and mania should be carefully diagnosed and treated with antidepressants or mood-stabilizers for several months at least.[22]

As in many illnesses, lack of adherence is common. There may be simply resolved reasons (such as morning dosing causing drowsiness), or a resolution may require more intense methods such as a psychological therapy. Where this does not help, a small number of people may need to be given a slow-release injectable form of their medication.

Psychological interventions in first episode psychosis

Cognitive behaviour therapy

Cognitive behaviour therapy (CBT) was originally developed for the treatment of depression. Studies more recently which have applied CBT to first episode psychosis have found encouraging results.[23,24] The basic principle of CBT for psychosis is that faulty thinking about a perception, either real in the case of a delusion, or perceived to be real in the case of a hallucination, causes distress. The distress in turn reinforces the faulty thinking. The reduction of this distress through the challenging of the faulty thinking then becomes the target of the therapy rather than the removal of the symptom. A good example of how this works is in the movie *A Beautiful Mind* in which the central character realizes that the people he sees in his hallucinations do not ever age. A CBT therapist would use this to challenge the belief that the hallucination is real. Obviously this requires good rapport and specialist skills in the provision of CBT. While a full discussion of CBT for psychosis is beyond the scope of this chapter, there are a number of good manuals and reviews of these manuals for the conduct of CBT with schizophrenia and first episode psychosis.[25,26]

Cognitive remediation

Another cognitive intervention which is being used more often in first episode psychosis is cognitive remediation (sometimes known as cognitive rehabilitation). The aim of cognitive remediation is to address the cognitive impairments of patients with schizophrenia, for example, distractibility, memory problems, lack of vigilance, attentional deficits and limitations in planning and decision-making.[27] Although there is some suggestion that there are better outcomes achieved through cognitive remediation in first episode psychosis than in more established illness, the research is still at a very preliminary stage.[28,29]

Psychosocial interventions in first episode psychosis

Psychoeducation

Psychoeducation is a means whereby the consumer of mental health services (and/or their family) is educated about their illness and its treatment. In order that the patient may participate in decisions on their treatment to the fullest degree possible, psychoeducation is a necessary process. In first episode psychosis psychoeducation has been shown to lead to a number of better outcomes including improving adherence to treatment, better management of subsequent relapse, lower readmission rates and having a positive effect on patient's wellbeing.[30]

Family interventions

Family, broadly defined, often play an important role in both caring for the patient with first episode psychosis and helping them care for themselves. However, this is a role that is often considerably stressful and has the potential to lead to strain in the relationship, if not alienation. Family interventions cover a wide variety of practices, which are conducted in a range of situations. They can be psychoeducational, therapeutic or skills based; can be conducted with or without the patient present, in multifamily groups or with one family alone; and can be brief in duration (e.g., single or few sessions) or conducted over an extended period. Family interventions have a range of positive effects including decreasing relapse, reducing hospital admission and encouraging medication compliance.[31] The effect on families was to reduce the burden of illness, increase knowledge and decrease expressed emotion. There is evidence that multifamily groups may be better than single family groups; however, families may have a preference for single family groups, and this should be respected where possible. Local and national support groups are also effective in supporting the family, and referrals to consumer and carer networks are recommended.

Vocational interventions

The onset of psychosis most often falls in a key period of vocational development. Often the practical results of this are that education is either not completed or completed at a standard lower than may have otherwise been achieved, or that employment is not gained or maintained. In the absence of a mental illness, not finishing high school and a lack of employment experience are two of the largest barriers to entering the competitive labour market. Despite wanting to work, over 40% of people with first episode psychosis are unemployed,[32] and even in the presence of a specialized mental health service this does not improve. Unemployment is associated with an increase in marginalization, poorer health outcomes, lower self-esteem and increased substance use.[33] Further, a study has found that functional recovery at 14 months post start of treatment predicts symptom and functional recovery at 7.5 years.[34]

Employment is an important path back to other areas of functioning such as social and economic participation.[33] Functional recovery is increasingly being recognized as being equally important to symptomatic recovery. The opportunity to reduce functional disability is one of the most important elements of the early intervention paradigm.[35] The method of vocational recovery that has the most evidence underpinning is called "supported employment", the most defined form of which is called "individual placement and support".[36] Randomized controlled trials and a number of less controlled studies have found very promising results with this approach.[32,37,38] Vocational recovery is covered in more detail in Chapter 13 in this book.

Summary of early intervention for first episode psychosis

Although it has its critics,[39] early intervention in psychosis is an evidence-based practice which shows great benefits for those who are treated according to this paradigm. Its focus on not only treating psychotic symptoms of psychosis, but the entire functional injury caused by psychosis means that people with psychosis have the best possible chance of recovery and participation in the community. For its optimal implementation it requires a specialized service which has the ability to provide interventions that cover a range of domains and which can be continued for a sustained period – ideally up to five years. Its emphasis on a low threshold for access and optimistic view about outcome are a major departure from "normal" psychiatric practice with its focus on management of acute phase illness.

High risk for psychosis

Recent research developments have allowed us to identify those who may be at risk for psychosis, that is, potentially be in the prodromal period of a psychotic illness.[40] The prodromal phase of a psychotic illness refers to the signs and symptoms that a person experiences prior to the onset of a full-blown illness. Reliable criteria have been developed to identify individuals who may be at risk of developing psychosis and thus experiencing a potential prodrome for psychosis.[2,41] These criteria include three possible syndromes. The first is based on the presence of at least one symptom at an attenuated level (i.e., of insufficient severity to meet diagnostic criteria for a psychotic disorder) such as unusual thought content, suspiciousness, grandiose ideas, perceptual abnormalities or disorganized communication. A second criterion includes having genetic risk and recent functional deterioration, and the third is the presence of very brief intermittent psychotic symptoms. Current evidence indicates that approximately 36% of individuals meeting those criteria will go on to develop a full-blown illness after three years.[42]

These young people often present with other concerns in addition to complaints of attenuated positive psychotic symptoms. Many have comorbid diagnoses, in particular anxiety, depression and substance use disorders.[43–45] High levels of negative symptoms, significant impairments in academic performance and occupational functioning and difficulties with interpersonal relationships are often observed.[45–48] Negative and/or non-specific symptoms may be present for years before attenuated positive psychotic symptoms emerge.

Treatment programs

Currently treatment is being offered to these young people in a range of different ways.[41] Some programs may only be research related, and to obtain treatment young people have to participate in the research. Other research programs investigating the pre-psychotic period have been implemented in mental health clinics, integrating research into the clinical service. Internationally, the first such research clinic was the Personal Assessment and Crisis Evaluation (PACE) clinic in Melbourne, Australia. Like PACE, there are already in the USA, Canada, Australia and several European countries specialized integrated research and service clinics. These "prodromal" or high-risk clinics may offer combinations of treatment packages including engagement, supportive therapy, case management, stress management, cognitive behavioural therapy, family-based treatment and pharmacotherapy. However, the possibly more common alternative may be that some of these young people may be being seen within services for adults, often with more chronic mental illness. The need for treatment for those with an "at-risk mental state" has high importance for youth mental health. The typical age of this high-risk period is 14 to 23 and sometimes even as young as 12.

Nevertheless, recruitment in this population is known to be an elusive and challenging process. A key challenge to obtain referrals for these clinics may be first to educate potential referrers about the aims of the clinics as well as the clinical services offered. Educational campaigns need to reach out to all possible gatekeepers, family physicians, psychiatrists and paediatricians, relevant community agencies, school and college counselling as well as the general public. But most importantly the service needs to have appeal for these young individuals that most need help.

These young people are help-seeking, but their concerns and difficulties are neither well understood nor addressed adequately in a regular mental health clinic. Understandably, it is difficult to seek help when the symptoms and concerns are so often ill-defined and non-specific. Many do seek help, often having been advised by a school counselor or family physician or initiated by family members. However, it may be difficult for individuals, families and professionals alike to really know the best place for these young people to get help.

Of course a common problem is that not everyone who is at risk is willing to engage with treatment. Reluctance to engage in therapy may be due to anxiety, unfamiliarity with mental health professionals, or it may stem from unsuccessfully seeking help in the past. Creating an atmosphere of safety and trust as well as offering a sense of hope will not only encourage engagement, but it will also form the basis for a strong therapeutic alliance. Poor social functioning is also common in the early course of psychoses and may represent a potential barrier to engagement as well. Pre-psychotic symptoms such as unusual thoughts or persecutory ideas have the potential to impact communication, trust or the client's cognitive processing, and thus interfere with engagement as well. The client may also be presenting already with mild cognitive impairments such as problems with understanding or producing speech, problems with abstract thinking or difficulty dividing attention. Thus, improving their awareness and understanding of the impact of their symptoms, thoughts and worries in a warm and empathic manner will help reduce the "fear of going crazy" and encourage engagement.

Despite their mental health concerns and problems, many of those who are at risk do not have diagnosable mental health problems, and so treatment for these individuals should be offered in a "neutral environment" that is not associated with a medical or psychiatric setting, especially one where chronically ill individuals are receiving treatment. Concerns regarding the stigma associated with mental illness may be counterproductive to engagement and treatment adherence. In addition, many young adults learn about mental health from the distorted accounts provided by the media. Flexible scheduling is also important since many of these individuals still attend school. Interpersonal difficulties are common in this population, and many struggle to place trust in others.

Interventions for the "at-risk" group

A range of treatment studies have suggested that intervention before a potential first episode of psychosis may possibly delay the onset of psychosis and may improve symptoms. The effectiveness of antipsychotics has been studied with results suggesting that they reduced both symptoms and conversion rates,[49,50] although issues have been raised with respect to the use of antipsychotics in this "at-risk" population.[51] Other RCTs[52,53] have studied the effectiveness of psychological interventions, in particular cognitive behaviour therapy. In general, results demonstrated reduction in attenuated positive symptoms, enhanced social adjustment, improvements in anxiety and depression and, in some cases, a significantly lower risk of progressing to psychosis.[53] Although longitudinal studies are rare, some of these benefits persisted at a 3-year follow-up.[54] However, the testing of effective treatments still needs much more work to determine what would be the best treatment for which person.[55] However, in terms of the outcome of existing trials, at the moment we can say that receiving any focused treatment is associated with a lower risk of developing psychosis if compared with no treatment.[56]

In response to concerns about what types of treatments should be offered, McGorry and colleagues suggest employing a clinical staging model in which the intensity of treatment is matched to the stage and severity of the psychiatric disorder.[57] This has been addressed in more detail earlier in this book. Although the issue of acceptability of certain treatments for those at risk of psychosis has been raised, to our knowledge no studies to date have actually addressed this issue with respect to "at-risk" individuals.

In terms of treatment, the emphasis has typically been on the risk of conversion and understanding the evolution of the psychotic illness. Likewise, treatment studies have focused on preventing or reducing conversion through the use of antipsychotic medications or with psychological interventions. There has been less emphasis on improving the outcome and/or presenting concerns of these help-seeking individuals.[47] In fact, recent studies have demonstrated that although only around a third of these at-risk patients go on to develop a psychotic illness, at least one third do not fully recover from their initial subthreshold symptoms and functional difficulties.[58] Although current trials are not equivocal in what treatments may or not be more effective, they have offered some valuable insights as to how we should best be helping these young people at the present time.

Monitoring

For some young people just having their symptoms monitored may be enough. Interestingly, monitoring was used as a control treatment in the Manchester Early Detection and Intervention Evaluation (EDIE) study[53] and, although CBT may have been the more effective treatment, many young people benefitted from simply being monitored. Retrospectively, those in the monitoring condition received warm, empathetic and non-judgemental face-to-face contact, as well as supportive listening and referrals to appropriate local services for unmet needs and crisis management when needed.

Similarly, the ADAPT (Access, Detection and Psychological Treatment) study demonstrated that the control treatment, which was supportive therapy, was also beneficial for these at-risk youth.[52] The supportive therapy focused on assisting individuals to cope with current problems. There was an emphasis on listening, reflecting and empathizing, and demonstrating uncritical acceptance and genuineness. Psychoeducational information about psychosis and managing stress was also offered. Participants in the supportive therapy group demonstrated significant improvements in attenuated symptoms, depression and anxiety.

Cognitive behaviour therapy

Several arguments have been put forward in support of CBT as a beneficial psychological intervention for young people at high risk.[59] It has been shown to be effective for helping those with schizophrenia to cope with psychotic symptoms and to reduce associated distress as well as the risk of relapse. There is extensive evidence for its effectiveness in the treatment of mood and anxiety disorders and even with substance use problems. Evidence also suggests it can target problems with metacognitions and self-schemas, psychological processes also affected in the UHR population.[60] Finally, CBT interventions fit well in a stress-vulnerability model and may be an invaluable therapy to teach the types of coping strategies that may offer protection against environmental stressors that could potentially precipitate conversion. The collaborative nature of CBT, in that it is problem-orientated and involves working towards shared goals, may make it more acceptable to young adults, particularly since they often express a preference for psychological interventions and to participate in trials of psychological interventions.[60,61] Thus, it appears that CBT could be the model of psychological intervention that holds the greatest promise for being effective during this high-risk period. Recent trials have demonstrated improvement in a range of functioning and symptom measures among those receiving this option.

Family work

Family work for the at-risk group is in its early stages. An association between symptomatic improvement and lower reduced expressed emotion has been observed.[62] Better problem-solving and communications skills between at-risk young patients and their family have also been associated with lower symptom ratings at follow-up.[63] Results such as these suggest that the family environment should be a specific target for treatment. Building on this work a framework for family work with young people at risk has been proposed.[64] This framework is based on a recovery model and it focuses on (i) managing the presenting symptoms (e.g., social isolation, attenuated positive symptoms), (ii) monitoring for the possible emergence of psychosis, (iii) development and maintenance of psychological wellbeing and adaptive functioning in family members. To date, the only RCT that used a family intervention was completed by Miklowitz and colleagues comparing three sessions of psychoeducation on stress management to family-focused therapy.[65] Family-focused therapy consisted of 18 sessions that focused on symptom management, communication and problem-solving. Findings demonstrated that over six months, in the family-focused therapy condition there was a decrease in attenuated psychotic symptoms, an improvement in constructive communication and a reduction of family conflict behaviours compared to enhanced care.

Peer support

The idea of peer support has not been formally addressed with this group. The effectiveness of group therapy across a wide variety of mental disorders (including schizophrenia) is well documented. The Early Recognition and Intervention Centre for Mental Crises (FETZ) is an outpatient program that offers short-term group therapy as part of their program. The intervention uses a wide range of didactic and cognitive-behavioural strategies and aims to address the young person's global functioning, social functioning and coping skills. It contains three modules: (i) positive mood and enjoyment, (ii) social perception and social skills training and (iii) mastering difficult situations. The effectiveness of this program is under current evaluation, but early preliminary findings reveal symptomatic and functional improvements.

The need for a youth-friendly approach for those at high risk of psychosis

In summary there are several key issues described previously that point to the need for this group to be treated as a separate group and not in part in child and adolescent services and in part in adult services;

- Early signs and symptoms are developmentally disruptive
- Outcome of the "at-risk state" is not clear
- Outcomes are not disorder specific
- Recruitment and engagement are difficult
- Referrers are more likely to refer to a youth program that is not disorder specific
- Young people themselves are more likely to be willing to seek help in a non-stigmatizing and nontraditional mental health setting
- Effective treatments may be as benign as observational, monitoring and supportive
- Since CBT may be effective for a range of more specific concerns, it can be delivered in a problem- and not disorder-specific way
- There are more opportunities for families to be involved and learn from one another
- Peer support could be readily available

Conclusion

In this chapter we have presented an overview of both research and clinical endeavours for the treatment of early psychosis. The leaders in this field from the outset advocated for early treatment that was synonymous with a comprehensive approach for youth. For those at high risk of developing psychosis there are internationally several specialized programs dedicated to treatment and research that clearly are designed with youth in mind. However, going forward with new initiatives it will be important that further development for early psychosis services, programs or even interventions ensure that such initiatives need to be youth-relevant and youth-friendly.

References

1 Addington J. The promise of early intervention. *Early Intervention in Psychiatry* 2007; 1(4):294–307.
2 Yung AR, McGorry PD. The initial prodrome in psychosis: descriptive and qualitative aspects. *Australian and New Zealand Journal of Psychiatry* 1996;30(5):587–99.
3 Killackey E, Yung AR. Effectiveness of early intervention in psychosis. *Current Opinion in Psychiatry* 2007;20(2):121–5.
4 Birchwood M, Fiorillo A. The critical period for early intervention. *Psychiatric Rehabilitation Skills* 2000;4(2):182–98.
5 Birchwood M, McGorry P, Jackson H. Early intervention in schizophrenia. *British Journal of Psychiatry* 1997;170:2–5.

6 National Institute for Health and Care Excellence (NICE). *Psychosis and schizophrenia in children and young people: recognition and management.* London: NICE; 2013.
7 Galletly C, Castle D, Dark F, Humberstone V, Jablensky A, Killackey E, et al. Royal Australian and New Zealand College of Psychiatrists clinical practice guidelines for the management of schizophrenia and related disorders. *Australian and New Zealand Journal of Psychiatry* 2016;50(5):410–72.
8 Norman RM, Malla AK. Duration of untreated psychosis: a critical examination of the concept and its importance. *Psychological Medicine* 2001;31(3):381–400.
9 Marshall M, Lewis S, Lockwood A, Drake R, Jones P, Croudace T. Association between duration of untreated psychosis and outcome in cohorts of first-episode patients: a systematic review. *Archives of General Psychiatry* 2005;62(9):975–83.
10 Penttilä M, Jääskeläinen E, Hirvonen N, Isohanni M, Miettunen J. Duration of untreated psychosis as predictor of long-term outcome in schizophrenia: systematic review and meta-analysis. *British Journal of Psychiatry* 2014;205(2):88–94.
11 Ran MS, Xiao Y, Chui CHK, Hu XZ, Yu YH, Peng MM, et al. Duration of untreated psychosis (DUP) and outcome of people with schizophrenia in rural China: 14-year follow-up study. *Psychiatry Research* 2018;267:340–5.
12 Larsen TK, Melle I, Auestad B, Friis S, Haahr U, Johannessen JO, et al. Early detection of first-episode psychosis: the effect on 1-year outcome. *Schizophrenia Bulletin* 2006;32(4):758–64.
13 Bertelsen M, Jeppesen P, Petersen L, Thorup A, Øhlenschlaeger J, le Quach P, et al. Five-year follow-up of a randomized multicenter trial of intensive early intervention vs standard treatment for patients with a first episode of psychotic illness: the OPUS trial. *Archives of General Psychiatry* 2008;65(7):762–71.
14 Lehman AF, Lieberman JA, Dixon LB, McGlashan TH, Miller AL, Perkins DO, et al. Practice guideline for the treatment of patients with schizophrenia, second edition. *American Journal of Psychiatry* 2004;161(2):1–56.
15 Fowler D, Hodgekins J, Howells L, Millward M, Ivins A, Taylor G, et al. Can targeted early intervention improve functional recovery in psychosis? A historical control evaluation of the effectiveness of different models of early intervention service provision in Norfolk 1998–2007. *Early Intervention in Psychiatry* 2009;3(4):282–8.
16 Early Psychosis Guidelines Writing Group and EPPIC National Support Program. *Australian clinical guidelines for early psychosis.* 2nd ed. Melbourne: Orygen, The National Centre of Excellence in Youth Mental Health; 2016.
17 Jones PB, Barnes TR, Davies L, Dunn G, Lloyd H, Hayhurst KP, et al. Randomized controlled trial of the effect on quality of life of second- vs first-generation antipsychotic drugs in schizophrenia: cost utility of the latest antipsychotic drugs in schizophrenia study (CUtLASS 1). *Archives of General Psychiatry* 2006;63(10):1079–87.
18 Lieberman JA, Stroup TS, McEvoy JP, Swartz MS, Rosenheck RA, Perkins DO, et al. Effectiveness of antipsychotic drugs in patients with chronic schizophrenia. *New England Journal of Medicine* 2005;353(12):1209–23.
19 Kahn RS, Fleischhacker WW, Boter H, Davidson M, Vergouwe Y, Keet IP, et al. Effectiveness of antipsychotic drugs in first-episode schizophrenia and schizophreniform disorder: an open randomised clinical trial. *Lancet* 2008;371(9618):1085–97.
20 Berger GE, Proffitt TM, McConchie M, Yuen H, Wood SJ, Amminger GP, et al. Ethyl-eicosapentaenoic acid in first-episode psychosis: a randomized, placebo-controlled trial. *Journal of Clinical Psychiatry* 2007;68(12):1867–75.
21 De Hert M, Detraux J, van Winkel R, Yu W, Correll CU. Metabolic and cardiovascular adverse effects associated with antipsychotic drugs. *Nature Reviews Endocrinology* 2011;8(2):114–26.

22 International Early Psychosis Association Writing Group. International clinical practice guidelines for early psychosis. *British Journal of Psychiatry Supplement* 2005;48:s120–4.
23 Jackson HJ, McGorry PD, Killackey E, Bendall S, Allott K, Dudgeon P, et al. Acute-phase and 1-year follow-up results of a randomized controlled trial of CBT versus befriending for first-episode psychosis: the ACE project. *Psychological Medicine* 2008;38(5):725–35.
24 Tarrier N, Lewis S, Haddock G, Bentall R, Drake R, Kinderman P, et al. Cognitive-behavioural therapy in first-episode and early schizophrenia. 18-month follow-up of a randomised controlled trial. *British Journal of Psychiatry* 2004;184:231–9.
25 Addington J, Gleeson J. Implementing cognitive-behavioural therapy for first-episode psychosis. *British Journal of Psychiatry Supplement* 2005;48:s72–6.
26 Addington J, Haarmans M. Cognitive behavioral therapy for individuals recovering from a first episode of psychosis. *Journal of Contemporary Psychotherapy* 2006;36(1): 43–9.
27 Wykes T, Huddy V, Cellard C, McGurk SR, Czobor P. A meta-analysis of cognitive remediation for schizophrenia: methodology and effect sizes. *American Journal of Psychiatry* 2011;168(5):472–85.
28 Eack SM, Hogarty GE, Cho RY, Prasad KM, Greenwald DP, Hogarty SS, et al. Neuroprotective effects of cognitive enhancement therapy against gray matter loss in early schizophrenia: results from a 2-year randomized controlled trial. *Archives of General Psychiatry* 2010;67(7):674–82.
29 Deste G, Barlati S, Galluzzo A, Corsini P, Valsecchi P, Turrina C, et al. Effectiveness of cognitive remediation in early versus chronic schizophrenia: a preliminary report. *Frontiers in Psychiatry* 2019;10:236.
30 Xia J, Merinder LB, Belgamwar MR. Psychoeducation for schizophrenia. *Cochrane Database of Systematic Reviews* 2011;6:CD002831.
31 Pharoah F, Mari J, Rathbone J, Wong W. Family intervention for schizophrenia. *Cochrane Database of Systematic Reviews* 2010;12:CD000088.
32 Killackey E, Jackson HJ, McGorry PD. Vocational intervention in first-episode psychosis: individual placement and support v. treatment as usual. *British Journal of Psychiatry* 2008;193(2):114–20.
33 Killackey E. Something for everyone: employment interventions in psychotic illness. *Acta Neuropsychiatrica* 2008;20(5):277–9.
34 Álvarez-Jiménez M, Gleeson JF, Henry LP, Harrigan SM, Harris MG, Killackey E, et al. Road to full recovery: longitudinal relationship between symptomatic remission and psychosocial recovery in first-episode psychosis over 7.5 years. *Psychological Medicine* 2011;42(3):595–606.
35 Killackey E, Yung AR, McGorry PD. Early psychosis: where we've been, where we still have to go. *Epidemiologia e psichiatria sociale* 2007;16(2):102–8.
36 Becker D, Drake R. *A working life for people with severe mental illness*. New York: Oxford University Press; 2003.
37 Nuechterlein KH, Subotnik KL, Turner LR, Ventura J, Becker DR, Drake RE. Individual placement and support for individuals with recent-onset schizophrenia: integrating supported education and supported employment. *Psychiatric Rehabilitation Journal* 2008;31(4):340–9.
38 Rinaldi M, Killackey E, Smith J, Shepherd G, Singh SP, Craig T. First episode psychosis and employment: a review. *International Review of Psychiatry* 2010;22(2):148–62.
39 Bosanac P, Patton GC, Castle DJ. Early intervention in psychotic disorders: faith before facts? *Psychological Medicine* 2010;40(3):353–8.

40 Fusar-Poli P, Borgwardt S, Bechdolf A, Addington J, Riecher-Rössler A, Schultze-Lutter F, et al. The psychosis high-risk state: a comprehensive state-of-the-art review. *JAMA Psychiatry* 2013;70(1):107–20.
41 McGlashan TH, Addington J, Cannon T, Heinimaa M, McGorry P, O'Brien M, et al. Recruitment and treatment practices for help-seeking "prodromal" patients. *Schizophrenia Bulletin* 2007;33(3):715–26.
42 Fusar-Poli P, Bonoldi I, Yung AR, Borgwardt S, Kempton MJ, Valmaggia L, et al. Predicting psychosis: meta-analysis of transition outcomes in individuals at high clinical risk. *Archives of General Psychiatry* 2012;69(3):220–9.
43 Woods SW, Addington J, Cadenhead KS, Cannon TD, Cornblatt BA, Heinssen R, et al. Validity of the prodromal risk syndrome for first psychosis: findings from the North American Prodrome Longitudinal Study. *Schizophrenia Bulletin* 2009;35(5): 894–908.
44 Fusar-Poli P, Nelson B, Valmaggia L, Yung AR, McGuire PK. Comorbid depressive and anxiety disorders in 509 individuals with an at-risk mental state: impact on psychopathology and transition to psychosis. *Schizophrenia Bulletin* 2014;40(1):120–31.
45 Yung AR, Nelson B, Stanford C, Simmons MB, Cosgrave EM, Killackey E, et al. Validation of "prodromal" criteria to detect individuals at ultra high risk of psychosis: 2 year follow-up. *Schizophrenia Research* 2008;105(1–3):10–7.
46 Addington J, Penn D, Woods SW, Addington D, Perkins DO. Social functioning in individuals at clinical high risk for psychosis. *Schizophrenia Research* 2008;99(1–3):119–24.
47 Cotter J, Drake RJ, Bucci S, Firth J, Edge D, Yung AR. What drives poor functioning in the at-risk mental state? A systematic review. *Schizophrenia Research* 2014;159(2–3):267–77.
48 Lencz T, Smith CW, Auther A, Correll CU, Cornblatt B. Nonspecific and attenuated negative symptoms in patients at clinical high-risk for schizophrenia. *Schizophrenia Research* 2004;68(1):37–48.
49 McGlashan TH, Zipursky RB, Perkins D, Addington J, Miller T, Woods SW, et al. Randomized, double-blind trial of olanzapine versus placebo in patients prodromally symptomatic for psychosis. *American Journal of Psychiatry* 2006;163(5):790–9.
50 McGorry PD, Yung AR, Phillips LJ, Yuen HP, Francey S, Cosgrave EM, et al. Randomized controlled trial of interventions designed to reduce risk of progression to first-episode psychosis in a clinical sample with subthreshold symptoms. *Archives of General Psychiatry* 2002;59(10):921–8.
51 Bentall RP, Morrison AP. More harm than good: the case against using anti-psychotic drugs to prevent severe mental illness. *Journal of Mental Health* 2002;11(4):351–6.
52 Addington J, Epstein I, Liu L, French P, Boydell KM, Zipursky RB. A randomized controlled trial of cognitive behavioral therapy for individuals at clinical high risk of psychosis. *Schizophrenia Research* 2011;125(1):54–61.
53 Morrison AP, French P, Walford L, Lewis SW, Kilcommons A, Green J, et al. Cognitive therapy for the prevention of psychosis in people at ultra-high risk: randomised controlled trial. *British Journal of Psychiatry* 2004;185:291–7.
54 Morrison AP, French P, Parker S, Roberts M, Stevens H, Bentall RP, et al. Three-year follow-up of a randomized controlled trial of cognitive therapy for the prevention of psychosis in people at ultrahigh risk. *Schizophrenia Bulletin* 2007;33(3):682–7.
55 Addington J, Devoe DJ, Santesteban-Echarri O. Multidisciplinary treatment for individuals at clinical high risk of developing psychosis. *Current Treatment Options in Psychiatry* 2019;6(1):1–16.
56 Preti A, Cella M. Randomized-controlled trials in people at ultra high risk of psychosis: a review of treatment effectiveness. *Schizophrenia Research* 2010;123(1):30–6.

57 McGorry PD, Hickie IB, Yung AR, Pantelis C, Jackson HJ. Clinical staging of psychiatric disorders: a heuristic framework for choosing earlier, safer and more effective interventions. *Australian and New Zealand Journal of Psychiatry* 2006;40(8):616–22.
58 Addington J, Stowkowy J, Liu L, Cadenhead KS, Cannon TD, Cornblatt BA, et al. Clinical and functional characteristics of youth at clinical high-risk for psychosis who do not transition to psychosis. *Psychological Medicine* 2019;49(10):1670–7.
59 French P, Morrison AP. *Early detection and cognitive therapy for people at high risk of developing psychosis*. Chichester: John Wiley & Sons Ltd; 2004.
60 Addington J, Addington D. Clinical trials during the prodromal stage of schizophrenia. *American Journal of Psychiatry* 2005;162(7):1387.
61 Morrison AP, Renton JC, Williams S, Dunn H, Knight A, Kreutz M, et al. Delivering cognitive therapy to people with psychosis in a community mental health setting: an effectiveness study. *Acta Psychiatrica Scandinavica* 2004;110(1):36–44.
62 O'Brien MP, Zinberg JL, Bearden CE, Daley M, Niendam TA, Kopelowicz A, et al. Psychoeducational multi-family group treatment with adolescents at high risk for developing psychosis. *Early Intervention in Psychiatry* 2007;1(4):325–32.
63 O'Brien MP, Zinberg JL, Ho L, Rudd A, Kopelowicz A, Daley M, et al. Family problem solving interactions and 6-month symptomatic and functional outcomes in youth at ultra-high risk for psychosis and with recent onset psychotic symptoms: a longitudinal study. *Schizophrenia Research* 2009;107(2–3):198–205.
64 Collins AA, Addington J. Working with families following the diagnosis of an at risk mental state. In Addington J, Francey SM, Morrison AP (Eds) *Working with people at risk of developing psychosis: a treatment handbook*. Chichester: John Wiley & Sons Ltd; 2006. p 153–68.
65 Miklowitz DJ, O'Brien MP, Schlosser DA, Addington J, Candan KA, Marshall C, et al. Family-focused treatment for adolescents and young adults at high risk for psychosis: results of a randomized trial. *Journal of the American Academy of Child and Adolescent Psychiatry* 2014;53(8):848–58.

5 Neuro-informed psychotherapy, a manualised intervention for accessing marginalised youth

Clinical rationale, theoretical underpinnings and practice

Warrick Brewer and Brendan Murphy

Overview

Personality disorders are longstanding maladaptive patterns of perceiving and relating to people and stressful situations. Antisocial personality disorder (ASPD), one of the commonest personality disorders, is characterised by a gross disparity between behaviour and the prevailing social norms and a pervasive pattern of disregard for, and violation of, the rights of others that begins in childhood or early adolescence and continues into adulthood.[1] It is strongly associated with interpersonal and social impairment, offending behaviours and increased risk of mental and physical health problems, particularly alcohol and other drug misuse. Many more individuals do not possess the full disorder and are said to have antisocial traits (such as irresponsibility, deceitfulness, recklessness, impulsivity, irritability and aggression), while an even greater proportion only exhibit such traits when exposed to stress.

Although the role of genetics and environment in causing the disorder is inconclusive, it is clear that both ASPD and borderline personality disorder (BPD) are common outcomes of childhood trauma[2,3] and that 'resilience' may explain inter-individual differences in those exposed to the same trauma.[4] People with both disorders often have a background of parental conflict. Harsh and inconsistent parenting can lead to acting out at school, truancy, other delinquent behaviour and early substance misuse and associated psychosis.

ASPD is usually associated with a previous diagnosis of oppositional defiant disorder, conduct disorder, attention-deficit/hyperactivity disorder, and low educational attainment. Conduct disorder itself is associated with childhood trauma.[5,6] While the rate of conversion from conduct disorder to ASPD varies from 40% to 70%,[7–10] the fact that the risk factor most predictive of adult antisocial personality is the severity and extent of prior conduct symptoms suggests that childhood and adolescence should be a focus for early intervention strategies to prevent ASPD. This is important as ASPD frequently results in adverse outcomes including unstable relationships, unemployment, unstable housing, imprisonment and premature death through reckless behaviour.[1] People with ASPD are also at greater risk of depression, self-harm and suicide, in part due to drug and alcohol misuse. The characteristic pattern of recidivistic behaviour not only impacts on self-concept and marginalises the person, further limiting life opportunities;[11] it also traumatises families and has wider societal costs. Violent and offending behaviour impacts victims, and there are the costs of policing and other initiatives to curb antisocial behaviour and general costs to the criminal justice system, including the costs of detention and other punitive measures.

Unlike those with borderline personality disorder, those with ASPD are 'treatment rejecting' rather than 'treatment seeking' and when they do present it is often under coercion and/or for treatment of a comorbid condition.[12] They are therefore difficult to retain in treatment. Engagement is paramount. Guidelines for the treatment of ASPD concluded that the experience of many people with ASPD was of being excluded from services and from decision-making concerning their care.[1] Furthermore, when those with ASPD present for treatment of comorbidities, they are less likely to be treated, even though standard evidence-based interventions are just as likely to be effective. If they are seen by mental health services, much of the focus remains around risk, when it is clear that many need treatment of comorbid mental disorders including depression, anxiety, psychosis and substance misuse in addition to wider issues including physical health, vocation, housing, welfare and relationship and parenting needs, requiring linkage to other services.

While a range of therapies have been developed for BPD[13–15] and early intervention services established,[16] pharmacological and psychological interventions for ASPD are limited.[17,18] Cognitive behavioural approaches have gained prominence,[1] principally to reduce offending though there is little supporting evidence.[19–23] The National Institute for Health and Clinical Excellence (NICE) reviewed the literature and found only one suitable trial of psychological treatment for ASPD in the community,[24] a CBT intervention on 39 participants. The study found no effect for CBT on anger or verbal aggression compared with treatment as usual but did find a small, non-significant effect for social functioning and physical aggression. Similarly, for the treatment of symptoms or behaviour associated with ASPD, NICE found one trial that investigated 'anger management' on 31 offenders[25] but was deemed too low quality to provide recommendations. There was consistent evidence that group-based cognitive and behavioural interventions were effective for the treatment of offending behaviour in people aged under 17 in community and institutional settings and adult males over 21 in criminal justice settings. However, there was no effect on those aged 18–20 years.

The lack of interventions aimed at the underlying precursors relative to 'management' of end-state symptoms highlights an imperative for trialling alternative approaches. We outline the rationale and key elements of a six-hour intervention targeted at young people with ASPD. While the original target group was a 15–25-year-old, predominately male cohort, suffering with a first episode psychosis and ASPD traits, the principles underlying the intervention are applicable to other externalising disorders, with or without psychosis.

Key elements of emotional processing

Understanding the normative function of anger is crucial to the intervention and distinguishes it from traditional anger 'management' techniques. As a fundamental emotion, anger is characterised as a bioregulatory device with which we are equipped to maximise survival.[26] Survival incorporates the abilities to adapt and control internal and external environments for the purpose of predictability. As such, anger can be framed as an instinctive immune system–like emotional arousal that effectively energises an organism to act via a 'flight or fight' response to neutralise the impact of a perceived threat. The degree of arousal (mediated by subconscious limbic processes) is hypothesised to be proportional to the degree of perceived threat (mediated by conscious prefrontal processes). The functional release of arousal returns the organism to a position of homeostasis or 'being at rest'. Should the functional release be thwarted (e.g., when a child is powerless to stop parental assault) or remain unconscious (e.g., immature language development preventing the mediation of focused action), the anger becomes compounded and experienced as anxiety. As the foreboding sense of loss of control increases, further emotional resources are generated to 'manage' the instinct for release rather than attend to the primary threat, thereby establishing a negative feedback loop. A key aim is to teach the client to regulate this process based on the principle that increased knowledge of their emotional self and how they came to be in crisis is the most efficient way of restoring a sense of control (Box 5.1; Figure 5.1). This involves working with clients to articulate an organised account of key aspects of identity, the role of developmental risks and the meaning of crisis. It seeks to move away from pathologising clients and dispelling their perceptions of challenges to their self-control by giving them the tools to help themselves. Thus, rather than it being something else 'done' to them, it becomes a client-driven process. By using information elicited via cognitive, personality, schema and symptom evaluation, it allows them to construct a personalised account of self-development and an organised sense of self. This is supplemented by psychoeducation focusing on emotional intelligence and the functional roles of anger, enabling the client to construct a realistic understanding of strengths and weaknesses across core aspects of self-identity, to identify early warning signs of crisis and to articulate healthier response options in the event that early warning signs are detected. The impact of the intervention draws on the powerful therapeutic benefit of the adolescent becoming more confident using the tools of language to regain internal control. The aim is to harness the diverted energy that has been driving behavioural disturbance for the purpose of constructing more functional scaffolding to the developing self.

Box 5.1 Key aims of intervention

- Provide clients with an understanding of their emotional processing
- Work with clients to construct an organised account of sense of self
- Reduce chaos/offending behaviour by attenuating secondary distress
- Model functional attachment with the therapist as an exemplar for future relationships
- Develop a crisis plan to facilitate pre-emptive treatment response
- Provide a behavioural management plan for ongoing therapeutic support

- Inform on the relative weighting of Axis I (clinical) and Axis II (personality) disorders
- Reduce the incidence of serious mental disorder and its secondary impact
- Provide a treatment package for individuals in the youth justice system

Frustrated and intense levels of emotion are also likely to overwhelm the delicate maturational processes of the prefrontal brain that begin around adolescence, contributing to any neurodevelopmental arrest. The stress of the growing mismatch between chronological age and delayed emotional maturity exacerbates the normal instability of adolescence, leaving the adolescent more vulnerable to decompensation. In this context, the client is assisted to reframe the otherwise negative impact of traumatic events in such a way as to validate the triggers for crisis as healthy and normal.

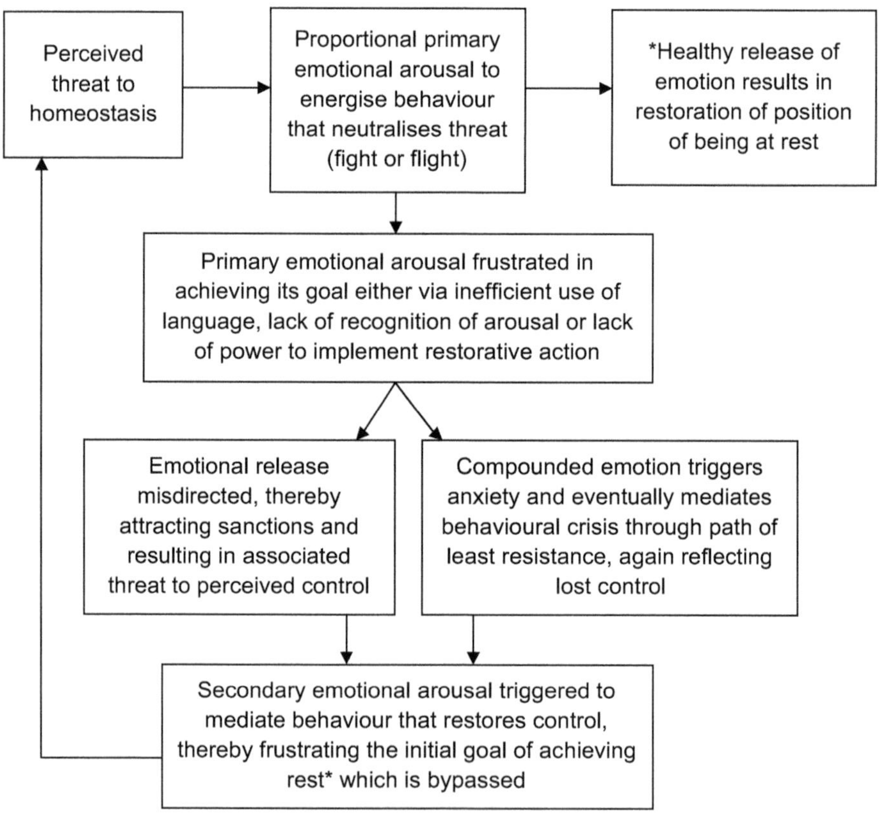

Figure 5.1 Primary emotional response and the negative feedback loop of compounded secondary emotion

Theoretical rationale

The predominant brain region maturing during adolescence is the frontal lobes, such that the development of the neuropsychological and social cognitive functions they mediate becomes relevant to disorders emerging during this stage,[27–29] including ASPD. These functions include higher-order executive processes such as strategic planning, problem-solving, inhibitory control, cognitive flexibility, abstract thinking, concept formation, working memory and self-monitoring,[30] and relationship skills associated with emerging self-consciousness such as awareness of the impact of self on others and the capacity to efficiently identify and articulate emotional processes in oneself and others. All of these functions are necessary for successful independent, goal-directed, volitional behaviour and the navigation of independent relationships.[31]

In engaging young people it is important to understand that normal adolescent behaviour is highly dynamic, apparently unstable and characterised by novelty-seeking, risk-taking and peer-directed social interactions that foster the development of adult independence.[32] These processes occur more rapidly than the development of executive skills, leading to a mismatch between drive and self-regulation.[33] In order to place any developmental insult (including childhood trauma) into perspective, the nature, extent, and timing of associated deficits need to be considered within a maturational context. In turn, the identification of developmental functional compromise provides clues as to the timing and nature of any insult; this is important as clients are often unable to recall trauma.[30]

It is important, then, to clearly identify the point at which thwarted emotion began to deviate toward a dysfunctional trajectory.

Brain structural abnormalities

There is emerging evidence that conduct disorder, ASPD and psychopathy are all associated with brain structural abnormalities with whole brain volumes, prefrontal including left orbitofrontal cortex (OFC), putamen and temporal lobes including the amygdala and hippocampus implicated.[34–38] These abnormalities fall within regions mediating emotional and learning processes. In addition, lesion studies suggest that early insult to the OFC often leads to the spontaneous development of antisocial behaviours such as pathological lying, irresponsibility, shallow or flattened affect and a lack of guilt and remorse.[39] Furthermore, the amygdala is primarily implicated in the emotional response to fear-inducing stimuli and is critical to the development of stimulus-response conditioning.[40] Such conditioning is crucial to the development of socialisation in children so that they learn to avoid engaging in behaviours that have the potential to harm either themselves or others.[40,41] Structural abnormalities of the amygdala are therefore implicated in the developmental arrest of fear conditioning, leading to the development of the callous, instrumental aggression that appears to be a hallmark of ASPD.[42]

Brain functional abnormalities

Investigation of neuropsychological functioning has suggested that frontal lobe dysfunction is common to all Cluster B personality disorders (including ASPD and BPD), with ASPD correlated with the greatest degree of hypofrontality,[43] which is bilateral.[44] Paradoxically, ASPD has been associated with increased activity in the dorsolateral prefrontal cortex during emotional processing tasks.[45–47] This region is implicated in executive cognition suggesting that people with ASPD use greater deliberative 'higher order' cognitive resources to process automatic 'lower order' affective information.[48] A number of neural imaging studies have also demonstrated reduced amygdaloid functioning in ASPD, especially during tasks involving emotional decision-making.[48,49]

Neuropsychological abnormalities

Cognitive abnormalities in verbal intellect and executive functions have been demonstrated in clients with ASPD.[50,51] These deficits implicate prefrontal neural compromise including reduced activity in the OFC and amygdala.[52] Since the OFC mediates emotional control, hypofrontality of these regions would be expected to be associated with poor emotional regulation, particularly during frustrating or stressful situations, a profile that has been observed in individuals with ASPD.

Pilot data

A core adolescent rite of passage is harnessed when sense of self-control is achieved. A key function of personality development is to acquire an ordered/ predictable sense of internal emotional awareness. This facilitates acquisition of the tools for effective decision-making (control), particularly those relating to typical challenges of adolescence / early adulthood, including navigating successful peer relationships. A second characteristic germane to the adolescent brain is alert reorientation to novel phenomena. To harness this, delivery of engagement style is designed to contradict the expectations of clients who have a history of eliciting anxiety-induced responses and associated inflexible boundaries from others. Finally, acting out behaviour and its impact of indiscriminate attachment and chaotic disorganisation is reframed such that the client is instinctively seeking an externalised boundary that would successfully contain otherwise intolerable anxiety levels.

This neuro-informed psychotherapeutic approach was piloted clinically at the Early Psychosis Prevention and Intervention Centre (EPPIC),[53] a clinic for clients with first episode psychosis (age 15–24 years) in Melbourne, Australia. An intensive case management subprogram was developed to provide assertive outreach to young people at high risk due to their level of risk to self or others, disengagement or suboptimal recovery. These clients typically presented with high levels of comorbidity, ambivalence about treatment and numerous social and functional handicaps. Intensive case management clients were characterised by a family history of mental illness, high levels of family break-up at a young age, high levels of physical and sexual abuse, and forensic history including violence to others. Forty-one percent of clients had comorbidity, a high proportion were on Community Treatment Orders and/or depot medication, their intelligence fell towards the low end of the average range and there were very high levels of illicit drug use. Risk ratings ranked most clients as being at significant or serious risk, particularly for suicide and violence. Engagement with the structured intervention outlined in this chapter, in addition to treatment as usual, resulted in attenuation of psychosis within 3–6 months, facilitating opportunities for early discharge from EPPIC for high risk clients with comorbid ASPD. Evaluation of treatment effectiveness of 120 consecutive referrals to intensive case management compared to 50 EPPIC treatment as usual clients revealed significant advantages for intensive case management clients in reducing admissions, bed days and crisis contacts. Clients demonstrated significant improvements in risk ratings, psychopathology and psychosocial outcomes over the course of treatment.[54]

Intensive case management – a brief overview

Pre-engagement

Prior to the first session, the therapist should begin to structure an understanding of the client using any available information. This includes medical records and reports from referring agencies or treating team and collateral history from family. The aim is to formulate the most probable weighting of Axis I (clinical) and Axis II (personality) disorders. Aim to understand the behaviour in the context of normal emotional reactions. Find out who the client is and how they came to be in crisis. This will show the client you care by investing time in trying to understand them before you have even met. It also allows the client to begin to establish an organised autobiography, a validating sense of self and an informed insight into intact and dysfunctional aspects of identity. It also validates the client's unique emotional experience and serves to reflect a consistent, containing approach in the therapist.

In a team situation, having a shared formulation alleviates individual therapist distress from 'sitting with' high-risk clients and structures distributed responsibility of coping with the distress of a risky client.

Key developmental aspects of self-identity should be mapped chronologically (Box 5.2). The weighting of weaknesses and strengths (vulnerabilities and compensatory buffers to developmental insult) across these aspects should be discussed with the client. Early signs of behavioural distress are identified and subsequently reframed as compromised management of compounded emotions. Learned coping mechanisms, irrespective of their functionality, are identified. The consequent emerging framework of self-identity facilitates a structured exploration of identifying, generally for the first time, any deviation from a healthy developmental trajectory and likely unaddressed triggers. This process involves validating characteristic overwhelming emotions and dysfunctional behaviour that occur in a crisis. A typical profile is captured in Box 5.3.

Box 5.2 Key aspects of a developmental history

Nature and timing of biological building blocks:

Family history of mental illness, personality disorder and substance misuse
Pregnancy and obstetrics complications
Physical developmental milestones
Head injuries
Chronic childhood illness

Cognitive building blocks:

Signs of early learning difficulties (including speech, reading or language deficits, use of remedial teachers, being kept down in class, non-mainstream schooling)
Neuropsychological function: premorbid/current IQ (including significant differences in verbal versus non-verbal); attention, memory and executive function
Attention deficit disorder
Autism spectrum disorder

Emerging personality development and childhood attachment:

Childhood temperament
History of being bullied
Unstable or chaotic family life
Loss of parents through death or divorce
History of trauma including exposure to verbal, physical, sexual or psychological abuse, domestic violence, emotional neglect, deprivation and abandonment
Low socioeconomic class

Signs of functional distress:

Bed-wetting
Head banging/rocking/temper tantrums
Urinary tract infections
Nightmares/sleepwalking/sleep terrors
Oppositional defiant behaviour

Conduct disorder (including multiple detentions, truancies, early disengagement from school, running away from home, fire-setting, cruelty to animals, lying, cheating, stealing, fighting with peers, bullying)
Early engagement with counsellors, therapists, psychiatric services
Early use of illicit substances (and any recurrent distressing reactions to drugs)
Attention from police/forensic system
Exploitative relationships (as instigator or recipient)
(A structured clinical audit form capturing this is available from the authors)

The therapist should plan to make contact on a routine basis, reinforcing the principle of consistent boundaries and structure. This includes weekly one-hour sessions at the same time and place. Reminder messages should be left by phone, text, email or calling card 24 hours before the next session, and again an hour prior to the planned time. Should contact prove difficult, reminders can be sent via caregivers. In the event that clients avoid initial appointments, public mental health services should maintain this reminder strategy for up to three months. These unsuccessful contacts (with clear evidence of each attempt) that may initially be perceived as disheartening, rejecting or wasteful of resources by the clinician, may represent the only predictable anchor point in a client's otherwise chaotic lifestyle. In this case, avoidance itself becomes structured, paradoxically increasing the likelihood of engagement. For example, in the event of a crisis within this time frame, a predictable pattern of care has been established that reflects service consistency in the face of rejection, maximising the likelihood of the client engaging in session 1.

Box 5.3 Typical profile of the target population

Behavioural or academic problems in primary school (attentional deficits, detentions, fights, bullying or being kept down) and/or oppositional defiant/conduct disorder traits in primary or early high-school;
Early verbal learning deficits in primary school associated with disenfranchisement at early adolescence and triggering early school dropout;
Pre-adolescent disruption to the family unit, domestic violence, experience of abuse/trauma prior to 12 years of age;
Signs of emotional distress (e.g., bedwetting, nightmares) preadolescence;
Early adolescent attempts at self-medicating with alcohol and cannabis;
Ongoing reliance upon cannabis for the purposes of 'chilling out'/detaching from distressing emotions (usually anxiety associated with uncontained anger);

Attracting attention of the police for antisocial behaviour (e.g., supporting a drug habit, or assaults/disregard for societal norms prior to the age of 17) irrespective of whether a formal charge/conviction has occurred;

Neurodevelopmental lag/delay as evidenced by: reaching late adolescence with verbal IQ relative to non-verbal deficits; concrete thinking; poor ability to articulate the impact of their behaviour on others or to imagine how others see them; impulsivity; history reflecting poor emotional regulation, particularly in close relationships; reduced insight; immaturity of social relationships; intervening services take on the character of a justice worker (preparing court reports/advocating or problem-solving issues with the justice system), and;

Previous diagnosis of ODD, conduct disorder, ADHD, substance misuse

The intervention does not preclude normal duty of care and adherence to risk management protocols, including secondary consultation to forensic services where appropriate.

Session 1 – initial engagement, gathering and providing information

A key goal of session 1 is to have the client agree to collaborate on information gathering about who they are and how they came to be in crisis. This creates the opportunity to reflect on this, possibly for the first time.

The therapist's demeanour should demonstrate calm, reasoned verbal and non-verbal communication, reflecting that they feel comfortable to sit with the client's chaos. General engagement techniques for young people are listed in Box 5.4.

Usually the client will begin to articulate their distress with these approaches. In the event they do not, ask the client if they mind telling you what their understanding is of how they came to be in the position they have found themselves in. Should they demur, clarify key current physical, cognitive and emotional difficulties. If all else fails, ask them if they mind completing the 90-item Symptom Checklist (SCL-R 90;[55] see session 2 later).

Box 5.4 General engagement techniques for young people

- Treat the young person as responsible and capable of having a say in decision-making;
- Be calm, reassuring, professional and friendly;
- Express concern for their safety and wellbeing;
- Show genuine interest in the young person and their explanatory model;

- Clarify the young person's expectations and what they want;
- Reduce anxiety by normalising the experience;
- Provide a clear, concise explanation of their illness avoiding jargon;
- Find common ground between what they want and need: tailor goals to the situation;
- Be kind, empathic, open, firm, fair, consistent, non-judgemental and non-authoritarian: be engaging;
- Ensure you have been understood; and
- Do not give up: maintain a consistent approach in the face of rejection.

The delivery of information begins in this session. Material includes emotional intelligence (the ability to perceive, control and evaluate emotions) and the role of emotions. The aim is to affirm and reframe the client's behavioural outbursts as a reflection of their brain's way of releasing built-up emotion. A clear distinction is made between a normal emotional reaction coupled to its function and the destructive consequences of compounded emotions that have been thwarted in achieving their primary aim (see Figure 5.1). Anger is described as a key emotion facilitating basic animal survival. Illustrate what can occur when this energy is thwarted from its primary goal, is repressed or is expressed in a manner that masks its true intent.

At this stage, a simple psychoeducation tool is used. An illustration of the brain is used to outline the limbic system and frontal lobes. The limbic system is described as the 'feeling and reacting brain'. The frontal lobes are described as the 'thinking brain'. Put simply for clients, an overactive emotional system draws energy away from conscious decision-making.

At the end of session 1, the client should have begun to engage in articulating their experience in the context of this framework. The therapist offers five more sessions, planning to work *with* the client to help regain control over their emotional energy store. State that this process involves learning to identify early warning signs of impending release of emotional distress. By recognising and then acting on these signs, it allows early intervention, pre-empting loss of control and preventing a behavioural crisis. Reflect on the distressing consequences of not acting at this stage and being unable to regain control (see Figure 5.1).

State that at the end of session 6, the therapist will write up a summary of the client's developmental history, the findings to date and a management plan. This will be emailed to the client, giving them the chance to modify or delete any information they may choose, facilitating a collaborative approach.

Session 2 – completing SCL-R 90; using questions to characterise patterns of emotional distress; completing key features of developmental history

This session focuses on the task of constructing a personalised account of development with the aim of identifying when key functional trajectories first deviated and the likely cause. The consequent impact of compounded distress is explored with a focus on finding early warning signs of decompensation.

Ask the client what they recall from session 1. This allows the therapist to evaluate the emotional impact of the session and how the client interprets information. It is possible that the previous session stirred up or released repressed emotional material resulting in behavioural change, so it is important to enquire about this. If no material is forthcoming, enquire specifically about interactions with people that may have involved emotions, any other experiences that have been different to usual (such as experiencing anxiety, irritability, poor sleep or outbursts), or whether significant dreams can be recalled. Material is discussed and reframed in the context of the psychoeducation from session 1.

From there, move on to complete a structured symptom assessment, using the 90-item Symptom Checklist – Revised (SCL-R 90).[55] This tool elicits a broad range of psychological problems and symptoms from the preceding week. It allows baseline evaluation and acts as a tool against which to assess treatment effect. By focusing on a tool, rather than direct social interaction with the therapist, the process can be valuable in eliciting unexpressed, highly distressing feelings. Once symptoms have been identified, reframe their emergence in the context of material from session 1, highlighting the excessive build-up of emotion that has led to the client's individual experience of distress.

Remind the client that the process committed to in session 1 was to work together to attain a sense of control. Ask them if they mind going through the first stage of this process, which involves them identifying their signature early warning signs of impending loss of control. Emphasise that by recognising these signs in the future, the client will be in a better position to prevent loss of control. This approach constitutes one of many subtle embedded structures reminding the client that the therapist trusts them to take control.

Devote the remainder of the session to creating an autobiographical history, drawing on material derived from Box 5.2. Encourage the client to identify early examples of being overwhelmed and how they reacted. Explore more adaptive responses the client could employ. By the end of the session it is likely that a logical account of symptom distress, as elicited via the SCL-R 90, is beginning to emerge for the client.

Session 3 – completing cognitive screen; utilising findings to assist the client to construct emerging self-identity

Remind the client of the basic principles of emotional processing outlined in previous sessions. Use the brain image tool to illustrate a common experience that triggers a normal emotional response, for example, parental breakup.

The remainder of the session focuses on assisting the client to identify their strengths and weaknesses in the way they use attention, memory and organisational abilities to make meaning of their world. Explain that this is important as many children may have their verbal abilities clouded by emotional stress, which is interpreted by others (and subsequently themselves) as a trait reduction in intellectual capacity.

Conduct some neuropsychological measures of current and premorbid IQ, attention, verbal and visual memory and executive function. Verbal memory results are also likely to show the client only attends to a fraction of the information given to them. Utilise this finding to examine the likely impact of not having all the available information. For example, social anxiety is a common vulnerability associated with relating to others through inefficient frameworks of understanding, constructed on limited information. Identify the key likely strength in visual relative to verbal information processing and provide examples of how this can buffer verbal vulnerabilities. Elicit likely school experiences of poor verbal engagement and associated feelings of reduced self-efficacy and compromised control leading to vulnerability for behavioural disruption and school disengagement. Reframe these experiences in the context of the likely emotional reaction at the time to any perceived threat. This is a useful time to initiate a non-threatening discussion of illicit drug use, which often commences in response to such distressing feelings.[56] Discuss how the effects of cannabis and other drugs on cognitive function compound that of emotional distress.[57]

Session 4 – gain an organised account of the client's developmental history; utilise findings to date to identify key features of deviation from a healthy developmental trajectory; present MMPI-2 for completion before next session

Complete key aspects of developmental history as listed in Box 5.2. Allow the client to identify the point at which key traumatic events resulted in significant emotional responses. When traumatic or highly emotional events are being described, it is important to affirm to the client that the source of the resulting ineffective emotional response reflected a natural defence against pain. Reframe this in the context of key elements of emotional processing and use it to explain the following:

- The word 'emotion' means to '*e-mote*' or trigger energy that underlies motivated thought, language or behaviour for the purpose of restoring a sense of safety;
- Each individual's emotional experience is as unique to themselves as their fingerprint;
- A build-up of emotion can become distressing if it is not achieving restoration of feeling safe or being 'at rest';
- Such distressing build-up is akin to anxiety;
- If this emotional energy is not released, the brain will find its own way of discharging it, usually resulting in feelings of loss of control or helplessness.

By this time, the client should have begun to identify their own characteristic style of discharge. Reassure them that you are working together in the most efficient way to make meaning of who they are, based upon available information. Distinguish secondary, and likely distracting, emotional distress in response to such behaviour from the underlying primary emotion, which is the key focus of this therapy.

Offer the client the chance to complete the Minnesota Multiphasic Personality Inventory-2 (MMPI-2)[58] before the next session, explaining its rationale and asking them to spend no more than five seconds thinking about the answer to each question. Explain that the results will assist in an objective determination of unconscious emotions, what they are and why they are there.

Provide a stamped addressed envelope to return results before the next session. Remind the client about their next session (same time and place if possible) and of the 24- and one-hour reminder routine.

Session 5 – emotional intelligence; MMPI-2 feedback; provision of Young's schema questionnaire

Illustrate the brain's 'meaning-making' ability. Using a picture of a cloud, have the client partner the therapist in focusing on it intently until they both come up with a word describing what the shape looks like to them. Prior to each articulating the description, explain that people vary in how long it takes them to achieve consciousness of a crystallised word in response to ambiguity and that their word is likely to be different from that selected by others. Ask the client to state the word best describing what comes to mind. The therapist should state their own word. Then illustrate the point that each has been allowed to view the outside world through another's eyes. Make the connection between this process and that of sitting with emotions until language reflecting them is acquired.

Expand this notion by suggesting they engage in this process socially, which will allow them to ascertain whether they are the same, different, or overlap with others in their perception of the world. Explain how this process is a key element in acquiring language of the self, leading to a more crystallised sense of identity. Ask the client how, since puberty, they have made meaning of their emotional energy (similar to the cloud example where emotion is initially regarded as being unstructured and unsaid, hence unpredictable). Now help them reinterpret their experiences. Reframe their likely over-emotional perceptions by drawing upon the analogy that it is not helpful to misjudge the usefulness of fire or water based solely upon experience of bushfires or floods. In other words, anger is a healthy energy when regulated appropriately. Reassure the client that the remaining task is to simply learn to sit with their emotional state until their brain naturally places language (consciousness) around feelings. Illustrate that it does not make sense to judge another's feelings and associated language as being 'better, worse, right, wrong' etc. Illustrate how engaging in this process with any 'other' allows the individual to objectively evaluate the approaches of others to coping with similar challenges. This provides a safe context for having the client decide in a non-threatening manner whether it is feasible, realistic or appropriate to adopt the more functionally adaptive approaches of the 'other'.

Go through the MMPI-2 results as per the report structure provided, referring to the context of the current working framework of self-development as an anchor. Check whether the pattern of findings resonate with the client's personal experience and whether they are reflecting possible early warning signs.

Session 6 – summary of self-development; key vulnerabilities and triggers for deviation from healthy developmental trajectory; ongoing management options

Elicit from the client the impact of the previous five sessions. What has stood out for them? Clarify any outstanding secondary emotional distress from past dysfunctional experiences and the meanings behind them and reinforce the need to learn to listen to the underlying primary emotion in times of crisis. This will reduce the likelihood of secondary distress. Assist the client in listing early warning signs of compounding emotional distress. Remind them that having ready access to this material reflects the means of maintaining control more adaptively. Sequentially review the main lessons learned from each session.

Discuss ongoing treatment options. Agree on key information that can be summarised in a written account for the client's own reference, or for a referral for further treatment if indicated. Inform the client that this summary will provide a management plan for ongoing development. Articulate specific goals for future treatment should the client decide later to engage with another therapist.

Agree on a planned response from mental health services should the client decide to renege on personal responsibility, hence handing control for decision-making over to authorities. Explore appropriate options and assist the client in implementing a structured (daily to weekly) prompt to create space for ongoing maintenance of self-control monitoring. Revisit the extent of support/assistance that the client may like until they feel independent with respect to this. Summarise the key ongoing goals for independent client focus, including likely educational/vocational pursuits.

Arrange follow-up at one and three months via phone call to monitor progress. End with the opportunity for the client to articulate what has impacted them most over the six sessions, what they have noticed has changed and what they would like in terms of support to maintain any functional decisions they have made.

References

1 National Institute for Health and Clinical Excellence (NICE). *Antisocial personality disorder: treatment, management and prevention.* London: NICE; 2013.

2 Sansone RA, Sansone LA. Childhood trauma, personality disorders, and eating disorders. In Sansone RA, Levitt JL (Eds) *Personality disorders and eating disorders: exploring the frontier.* New York: Routledge; 2006. p 59–76.

3 Sousa C, Herrenkohl TI, Moylan CA, Tajima EA, Klika JB, Herrenkohl RC, et al. Longitudinal study on the effects of child abuse and children's exposure to domestic violence, parent-child attachments, and antisocial behavior in adolescence. *Journal of Interpersonal Violence* 2011;26(1):111–36.

4 Pereda N, Jiménez-Padilla R, Gallardo-Pujol D. Personality disorders in child sexual abuse victims. *Actas Españolas de Psiquiatría* 2011;39(2):131–9.
5 Briggs-Gowan MJ, Carter AS, Clark R, Augustyn M, McCarthy KJ, Ford JD. Exposure to potentially traumatic events in early childhood: differential links to emergent psychopathology. *Journal of Child Psychology and Psychiatry* 2010;51(10):1132–40.
6 Greenwald R. The role of trauma in conduct disorder. *Journal of Aggression, Maltreatment, and Trauma* 2002;6(1):5–23.
7 Robins LN, Tipp J, Przybeck T. Antisocial personality. In Robins LN, Regier DA (Eds) *Psychiatric disorders in America.* New York: Free Press; 1991. p 258–90.
8 Moffitt T E, Caspi A, Harrington H, Milne BJ. Males on the life-course persistent and adolescence-limited antisocial pathways follow-up at 26 years. *Development and Psychopathology* 2002;14(1):179–207.
9 Loeber R, Burke JD, Lahey BB. What are the adolescent antecedents to antisocial personality disorder? *Criminal Behaviour and Mental Health* 2002;12(1):24–36.
10 Simonoff E, Elander J, Holmshaw J Pickles A, Murray R, Rutter M. Predictors of antisocial personality disorder. Continuities from childhood to adult life. *British Journal of Psychiatry* 2004;184:118–27.
11 Salekin RT. Psychopathy and recidivism from mid-adolescence to young adulthood: cumulating legal problems and limiting life opportunities. *Journal of Abnormal Psychology* 2008;117(2):386–95.
12 Tyrer P, Mitchard S, Methuen C, Ranger M. Treatment rejecting and treatment seeking personality disorders: type R and type S. *Journal of Personality Disorders* 2003;17(3):263–8.
13 Kernberg O. *Severe personality disorders – psychotherapeutic strategies.* New Haven: Yale University Press; 1984.
14 Linehan MM, Heard HL, Armstrong HE. Naturalistic follow-up of a behavioural treatment for chronically parasuicidal borderline patients. *Archives of General Psychiatry* 1993;50(12):971–4.
15 Ryle A. The contribution of cognitive analytic therapy to the treatment of borderline personality disorder. *Journal of Personality Disorders* 2004;18(1):3–35.
16 Chanen AM, McCutcheon LK, Germano D, Nistico H, Jackson HJ, McGorry PD. The HYPE clinic: an early intervention service for borderline personality disorder. *Journal of Psychiatric Practice* 2009;15(3):163–72.
17 Khalifa N, Duggan C, Stoffers J, Huband N, Völlm BA, Ferriter M, et al. Pharmacological interventions for antisocial personality disorder. *Cochrane Database of Systematic Reviews* 2010;8:CD007667.
18 Gibbon S, Duggan C, Stoffers J, Huband N, Völlm BA, Ferriter M, et al. Psychological interventions for antisocial personality disorder. *Cochrane Database of Systematic Reviews* 2010;6:CD007668.
19 Landenberger NA, Lipsey MW. The positive effects of cognitive behavioural programs for offenders: a meta-analysis of factors associated with effective treatment. *Journal of Experimental Criminology* 2005;1:451–76.
20 Lipsey M W, Landenberger NA, Wilson SJ. Effects of cognitive-behavioural programs for criminal offenders. *Campbell Systematic Reviews* 2007;6:1–27.
21 Lipton DS, Pearson FS, Cleland CM, Yee D. The effectiveness of cognitive-behavioural treatment methods on offender recidivism: meta-analytic outcomes from the CDATE project. In McGuire J (Ed) *Offender rehabilitation and treatment: effective programmes and policies to reduce re-offending.* Chichester: John Wiley & Sons; 2002. p 79–112.
22 Tong LSJ, Farrington DP. How effective is the 'reasoning and rehabilitation' programme in reducing re-offending? A meta-analysis of evaluations in three countries. *Psychology, Crime & Law* 2006;12(1):3–24.

23 Wilson DB, Bouffard LA, Mackenzie DL. A quantitative review of structured, group-oriented, cognitive-behavioural programs for offenders. *Criminal Justice and Behavior* 2005;32(2):172–204.

24 Davidson KM, Tyrer P, Tata P, Cooke D, Gumley A, Ford I, et al. Cognitive behaviour therapy for violent men with antisocial personality disorder in the community: an exploratory randomized controlled trial. *Psychological Medicine* 2009;39(4):569–77.

25 Vannoy SD, Hoyt WT. Evaluation of an anger therapy intervention for incarcerated adult males. *Journal of Offender Rehabilitation* 2004;39(2):39–57.

26 Damasio AR, Grabowski TJ, Bechara A, Damasio H, Ponto LL, Parvizi J, et al. Subcortical and cortical brain activity during the feeling of self-generated emotions. *Nature Neuroscience* 2000;3(10):1049–56.

27 Pantelis C, Stuart GW, Nelson HE, Robbins TW, Barnes TR. Spatial working memory deficits in schizophrenia: relationship with tardive dyskinesia and negative symptoms. *American Journal of Psychiatry* 2001;158(8):1276–85.

28 Pantelis C, Yücel M, Wood SJ, McGorry PD, Velakoulis D. Early and late neurodevelopmental disturbances in schizophrenia and their functional consequences. *Australian and New Zealand Journal of Psychiatry* 2003;37(4):399–406.

29 Pantelis C, Velakoulis D, McGorry PD, Wood SJ, Suckling J, Phillips LJ, et al. Neuroanatomical abnormalities before and after onset of psychosis: a cross-sectional and longitudinal MRI comparison. *Lancet* 2003;361(9354):281–8.

30 Brewer WJ, Wood SJ, DeLuca C, Pantelis C. Models of olfaction for exploring neurodevelopment. In Brewer WJ, Castle D, Pantelis C (Eds) *Olfaction and the brain.* Cambridge: Cambridge University Press; 2006. p 103–18.

31 Anderson V. Assessing executive function in children: biological, physiological and developmental considerations. *Neuropsychological Rehabilitation* 1998;8(3):319–49.

32 Spear LP. The adolescent brain and age-related behavioural manifestation. *Neuroscience and Biobehavioural Reviews* 2000;24(4):417–63.

33 Steinberg L. Cognitive and affective development in adolescence. *Trends in Cognitive Sciences* 2005;9(2):69–74.

34 Barkataki I, Kumari V, Das M, Taylor P, Sharma T. Volumetric structural brain abnormalities in men with schizophrenia or antisocial personality disorder. *Behavioural Brain Research* 2006;169(2):239–47.

35 Yang Y, Raine A, Lencz T, Bihrle S, LaCasse L, Colletti P. Volume reduction in prefrontal gray matter in unsuccessful criminal psychopaths. *Biological Psychiatry* 2005;57(10):1103–8.

36 Yang Y, Raine A, Colletti P, Toga AW, Narr KL. Abnormal temporal and prefrontal cortical gray matter thinning in psychopaths. *Molecular Psychiatry* 2009;14(6):561–2.

37 Huebner T, Vloet TD, Marx I, Konrad K, Fink GR, Herpertz SC, et al. Morphometric brain abnormalities in boys with conduct disorder. *Journal of the American Academy of Child and Adolescent Psychiatry* 2008;47(5):540–7.

38 Yang Y, Raine A, Narr KL, Colletti P, Toga AW. Localization of deformations within the amygdala in individuals with psychopathy. *Archives of General Psychiatry* 2009;66(9):986–94.

39 Anderson SW, Bechara A, Damasio H, Tranel D, Damasio AR. Impairment of social and moral behavior related to early damage in human prefrontal cortex. *Nature Neuroscience* 1999;2(11):1032–7.

40 Glenn AL, Raine A. Psychopathy and instrumental aggression: evolutionary, neurobiological, and legal perspectives. *International Journal of Law and Psychiatry* 2009;32(4):253–8.

41 Blair RJR. Dysfunctions of medial and lateral orbitofrontal cortex in psychopathy. *Annals of the New York Academy of Sciences* 2007;1121:461–79.

42 Blair RJR. The amygdala and ventromedial prefrontal cortex in morality and psychopathy. *Trends in Cognitive Sciences* 2007;11(9):387–92.

43 Reyes AC, Amador AA. Qualitative and quantitative EEG abnormalities in violent offenders with antisocial personality disorder. *Journal of Forensic and Legal Medicine* 2009;16(2):59–63.

44 Völlm B, Richardson P, Stirling J, Elliot R, Dolan M, Chaudhry I, et al. Neurobiological substrates of antisocial and borderline personality disorder: preliminary results of a functional fMRI study. *Criminal Behaviour and Mental Health* 2004;14(1):39–54.

45 Gordon HL, Baird AA, End A. Functional differences among those high and low on a trait measure of psychopathy. *Biological Psychiatry* 2004;56(7):516–21.

46 Intrator J, Hare R, Stritzke P, Brichtswein K, Dorfman D, Harpur T, et al. A brain imaging (single photon emission computerized tomography) study of semantic and affective processing in psychopaths. *Biological Psychiatry* 1997;42(2):96–103.

47 Rilling JK, Glenn AL, Jairam MR, Pagnoni G, Goldsmith DR, Elfenbein HA, et al. Neural correlates of social cooperation and non-cooperation as a function of psychopathy. *Biological Psychiatry* 2007;61(11):1260–71.

48 Kiehl KA, Smith AM, Hare RD, Mendrek A, Forster BB, Brink J, et al. Limbic abnormalities in affective processing by criminal psychopaths as revealed by functional magnetic resonance imaging. *Biological Psychiatry* 2001;50(9):677–84.

49 Glenn AL, Raine A, Schug RA. The neural correlates of moral decision-making in psychopathy. *Molecular Psychiatry* 2009;14(1):5–6.

50 Dolan M, Park I. The neuropsychology of antisocial personality disorder. *Psychological Medicine* 2002;32(3):417–27.

51 Morgan AB, Lilienfeld SO. A meta-analytic review of the relation between antisocial behavior and neuropsychological measures of executive function. *Clinical Psychology Review* 2000;20(1):113–36.

52 Birbaumer N, Veit R, Lotze M, Erb M, Hermann C, Grodd W, et al. Deficient fear conditioning in psychopathy: a functional magnetic resonance imaging study. *Archives of General Psychiatry* 2005;62(7):799–805.

53 McGorry PD, Edwards J, Mihalopoulos C, Harrigan SM, Jackson HJ. EPPIC: an evolving system of early detection and optimal management. *Schizophrenia Bulletin* 1996;22(2):305–26.

54 Brewer WJ, Lambert TJ, Witt K, Dileo J, Duff C, Clrenjak C, et al. Intensive case management for high-risk patients with first-episode psychosis: service model and outcomes. *Lancet Psychiatry* 2015;2(1):29–37.

55 Derogatis LR, Savitz KL. The SCL-90-R and the Brief Symptom Inventory (BSI) in primary care. In Maruish ME (Ed) *Handbook of psychological assessment in primary care settings*. Mahwah, NJ: Lawrence Erlbaum Associates; 2000. p 297–334.

56 Murray DM, Perry CL. The prevention of adolescent drug abuse: implications of etiological, developmental, behavioural, and environmental models. *NIDA Research Monograph* 1985;56:236–56.

57 Yücel M, Lubman DI, Solowij N, Brewer WJ. Understanding drug addiction: a neuropsychological perspective. *Australian and New Zealand Journal of Psychiatry* 2007;41(12):957–68.

58 Butcher JN, Dahlstrom WG, Graham JR, Tellegen A, Kaemmer, B. *The Minnesota Multiphasic Personality Inventory-2 (MMPI-2): manual for administration and scoring*. Minneapolis: University of Minnesota Press; 1989.

6 Youth mental health

The need for new models of care

Paul Patterson

Introduction

There are compelling arguments from the authors of chapters throughout this book on the need for new and specialist models of care that respond to both the growing knowledge base and business case for investing in youth mental health as an urgent and critical priority. Although the next step would logically be to invest in piloting new service models and restructuring current provision to form more appropriate structures capable of matching the high levels of unmet need in young people, there are currently few established and evaluated models to help inform the decision-making process for policy makers and funders. Despite this situation, it is still possible to extrapolate from current knowledge the basic parameters and constituent elements required for any youth service to adhere to. This will need to be coupled with the understanding that local needs and diversity will always make it unlikely that one type of approach will be the best fit for all local circumstances or meet regional needs without an ongoing and iterative process of consultation and implementation in co-production with local stakeholders.

Priorities for new services have been proposed from several sources and are outlined in Box 6.1.[1,2] Although there is a general consensus on the major elements required of a new youth strategy, there are relatively few operating services that could be described as 'fulfilling the brief'. At the time of writing, several new service models have been commissioned in England and other countries, but of those that have attempted a comprehensive approach to youth mental health, most have originated from the examples set by the 'Early Intervention in Psychosis'[3,4] movement of which the Australian EPPIC/Orygen model is the progenitor.

Box 6.1 Key elements of a youth mental health model

- Co-participation with young people at all levels of service design and implementation
- Focus on prevention and early intervention with ethos of recovery and hope
- Elimination of discontinuities at times of greatest need (transitions and age ranges)

- Single point of access across care pathways
- Social inclusion, education, employment and constructive time use as core outcomes
- Inclusion of families and carers in planning and evaluation
- Best practice interventions for a wide range of disorders plus peer support
- Focus on ameliorating emotional distress over diagnostic categorisation
- Effective partnerships with statutory and third sector agencies across health, social care, vocational, educational, housing vulnerable populations and forensic services within regions
- Training in mental health literacy, wellbeing and resilience for all staff working with young people as well as parents and young people in schools and colleges
- Training for black and minority ethnic (BME) community leaders, and young outreach BME staff in youth mental health and engagement
- Specialist youth mental health workforce with the right skills, attitude and training
- Close integration with schools to bring education and mental health together
- Online digital hubs for training, support and education with statutory service support
- One-stop centrally located centres to improve early help-seeking and reduce stigma
- Models of care reflecting the latest understanding of developmental processes and emerging adulthood, emphasising clinical staging
- Proportionate and ring-fenced funding streams reflecting an emerging and vital professional specialism

Examples of current youth models

headspace is a comprehensive enhanced primary care model for youth mental health care from Australia operational since 2006 (https://headspace.org.au). Working across the 12–25 age range it provides multidisciplinary youth-friendly service hubs linking with schools and specialist services to an early intervention model and sits on top of existing primary care services. Importantly, *headspace* integrates physical, sexual and drug disorder services within their mental health hubs. This increases their utility and reduces stigma for users. They have been scaled up through a series of funding rounds, reaching a total of 110 centres in early 2019.[5] *headspace* incorporates an accredited educational and training programme, active youth participation, school support and web-based digital education and interventions (*eheadspace*) alongside a real investment in ongoing research and evaluation (Orygen) with positive evaluation.

Jigsaw (formerly also known as Headstrong) is the innovative model of youth mental health from Ireland (www.jigsaw.ie). It demonstrates the most comprehensive example of meaningful integration of young service users in the development of the service, in response to the high levels of unmet need reported. In the Irish model, young people are consultants and key agents for change in developing drop-in hubs with local, statutory and third sector stakeholder organisations. The process involves generating local awareness and buy-in through a process of education and training to maximise the support and availability of specialist resources for young people aged 12–25 and to improve care pathways.[6] This enables rapid access to appropriate interventions in non-stigmatising centres.

Birmingham (UK) has recently commissioned a new fully integrated mental health service for 0–25-year-olds to ensure a seamless service that will provide early identification and support for a full range of mental health conditions across the age range (www.forwardthinkingbirmingham.org.uk). Launched in 2015, the key targets for this service model include: clear navigation and simple access to the appropriate service, no duplication of services or gaps between services, providers working together effectively in support of individual needs, a range of preventative initiatives including support from universal services that promote emotional resilience, and access to a wide range of targeted and specialist services so that more people can avoid unnecessary hospital admissions by being supported in the community. This unique approach will provide a real opportunity to evaluate how issues of transitioning, information sharing across providers and universal education can be engaged in an evolving comprehensive programme within a demographically diverse urban environment.

In Norfolk (UK) a new service approach to working with 14–25-year-olds has been established with some re-engineering of the current child and adolescent services and recovery teams, targeting those with emerging serious mental illness in an assertive outreach approach.[7] This specialist youth mental health service model emphasises vocational and functional outcomes over a focus on symptoms alone. It is driven by robust research and knowledge transfer and is well integrated with local vocational, educational and third sector youth organisations to enable positive transitions out of service and improved care pathways into the new team. Many other countries are investing in research to identify appropriate strategies for their youth mental health care needs. In 2014, Canada launched the 'ACCESS Canada' project to address youth mental health across the provinces using a nationwide research network and focusing on improving access to evidence-based interventions for the 11–25-year age group, with attention to the needs of its geographically, linguistically and culturally diverse local populations.[8]

In the US there is growing recognition of vulnerability in the young adult population. The Institute of Medicine and National Research Council have recommended that young adults aged 18–26 years are treated as a discrete group, with priority given to improving the transition from paediatric to adult medical and behavioural health care, enhancing preventive care for young adults and developing evidence-based practices.[9] Additionally, in 2014 as part of the Obama administration's response to gun violence, $99 million in new grants was made available to support existing mental health services and schools in promoting improved mental health in young people across a range of projects.

In New Zealand, the Prime Minister's Youth Mental Health Project was launched in 2012 aiming to help prevent the development of mental health issues and improve young people's access to youth mental health services, with up to 26 initiatives phased to deliver improvements for young people. One example is the SPARX e-therapy initiative for 12–19-year-olds for the treatment of depression and low mood, combining Cognitive Behavioural Therapy (CBT) techniques and gamification to engage young people.[10]

The European Union (EU)–funded ADOCARE project investigated the status of adolescent mental health care across ten EU states. The results suggested there is very poor availability of specialist adolescent mental health services, while the services that are available are of a very mixed quality across the countries taking part.[11] International support for a new and comprehensive focus on youth mental health has been demonstrated by the launch of the International Declaration on Youth Mental Health in 2013.[12] This document made reference to 11 basic standards that should be expected from mental health services within a 10-year period. Further recognition that this has become a specialty subject is exemplified by the biennial International Conference on Youth Mental Health, coordinated by the International Association for Youth Mental Health (www.iaymh.org).

Ethos of a new service model

'Prevention and early intervention' has become an encouraging mantra for those working on system change for youth mental health. The epidemiological evidence showing how the majority of mental illness first emerges in youth, alongside better understanding of risk factors and changes occurring in the early stages of illness,[13] allows for a discourse of prevention and an attitude of hope to establish in staff and teams working with younger populations. This builds on the example of public health promotion in physical health care and success of early detection and intervention programmes for mental disorders such as psychosis, alongside better understanding of developmental processes such as attachment and emotional regulation in early childhood and the impact of adversity and trauma on affective and cognitive development.[14,15]

These foundations have allowed for clear intervention targets to emerge with appreciation of applying the right intervention at the right time, avoiding the fostering of both service dependency and institutionalisation on one side or overlong treatment delay with missed opportunities for a 'light-touch' therapeutic tonic at the other. However, incorporating these lessons into new and efficient models of mental health care for young people leads to practical questions. These include consideration of age range to focus on, model parameters and staff expertise, user involvement, partnership working and issues of cost and benefits which have to be discussed in the context of local needs and funding priorities. Although a template of elements of good practice may be possible to develop, it is unlikely that 'one hat' will fit all regional priorities and demographic diversity. What is clear is that strong local leadership and service 'champions' will be required to steer positive and lasting change against the current backdrop of economic uncertainty and competing health priorities. Leaders will need to engage actively with local funders and policy-makers to ensure new approaches are adequately understood and supported. At this point it might be helpful to explore some of the emerging key elements any service providers should be considering as a preliminary to service redesign.

Youth participation

Young service user and carer involvement in service development and redesign is often described as one of the most critical elements. However, this is seldom applied or supported systematically. It remains all too easy to claim user participation off the back of limited or tokenistic consultation exercises rather than real engagement and co-participation with the service customers.

Many models of youth involvement emphasise a linear hierarchy of levels (e.g., Hart's 'Ladder of Involvement')[16] where the direction of travel is to enable young people to take on increasing degrees of responsibility in the projects. These tend not to take account of young people's actual level of interest in being involved at the higher level of participation, nor do they consider the specific needs of young people with mental health difficulties, who may require or prefer to bow in or out of involvement at short notice for periods of time. Such templates are necessary, however, to increase awareness that co-participation should be an essential element of any properly run service that has the function of working with and supporting young people's health needs. One of the more flexible models regarding youth participation that has been adopted by other mental health participation programmes, such as *headspace* in Australia, is 'Westhorp's continuum of youth involvement'.[17] This describes the key principles of involvement alongside recognition of the needs of young people whilst valuing all levels of participation. The Irish Headstrong 'Youth Advisory Panels' and Australian 'Youth Advisory Boards' provide a dynamic voice for young people with mental health problems, and many get involved in both local and national decision-making and political activity on behalf of youth mental health as well as active service development. The Birmingham, UK, 'Youth Board' is an example of a project-driven youth representation group that has been involved in redesign, training and education projects in the local mental health trust as well as in related art and digital media projects. These examples encourage the active empowerment of young people to influence systems of change and provide a strong endorsement of the appropriateness of the services they work with. It is vital that such foundations are encouraged by real investment in training and employment of staff to enable the ongoing progress of youth participation as the first step in any new model provision.

Location

We know that young people are unlikely to actively seek help from health professionals for mental health issues and are more likely to disclose to friends and family if at all. This, alongside the justifiably negative image of many mental health service venues make it particularly unlikely that young people or their family carers will rush to actively seek help from such settings without the impetus of a crisis driven by high levels of distress and concern. Adult inpatient units are often highly inappropriate settings for teenagers experiencing a first or acute episode of disorder, and their family members are often left feeling guilty, angry and helpless in the aftermath. Any youth mental health service that is going to encourage prevention and early intervention needs to be accessible and well designed, ideally co-located with other health and youth services in centralised low-stigma settings staffed by friendly, well-trained professionals who have excellent engagement skills and natural sensitivity and rapport. This is what young people are asking for from mental health services. Since parents are often likely to be the actual help-seeking instigators, it is important that service access points are venues familiar to adults and that there are clear protocols for engaging with family members. Other natural contact points such as schools also need to have defined points of access to timely and appropriate mental health support.

Related to the importance of location is the need to have clear and direct care pathways to support for those seeking help. Single Point of Access (SPA) provides a clear pathway into services through a single route for assessment, triage and signposting for new referrals. Designed for both routine or urgent referrals and enquiries, the single point of access contact centre should ideally be staffed by fully qualified and skilled health care professionals 24 hours a day, seven days a week, 365 days a year, allowing the most appropriate response to meet the level and type of difficulties being referred. SPA teams can provide advice and guidance through a triage process where the urgency of care required is assessed and in situations of mental health crisis, home treatment teams and partner organisations from across the public and private sectors are integrated to allow signposting immediately to the most relevant services to aid their recovery.

Staff training and partnership working

Birmingham, UK, youth mental health services have developed good integration with housing and vocational training organisations, and some attempt has been made to underpin this work with a shared understanding of engagement and working dynamics. The 'Psychologically Informed Environments' (PIE) approach was described in work from the Royal College of Psychiatry[18] and involves improving psychological understanding and ability to reflect on motivations and dynamics of all staff working in an organisation. A partnership between Birmingham and Solihull Mental Health NHS Foundation Trust and St Basils Youth Homeless Service has enabled mental health support to be more accessible for homeless young people who would have otherwise struggled to access clinical services. It has extended informed support and assistance for those who are distressed and clarified the pathway for referrals to statutory youth mental health teams for those who require clinical support. This has contributed to a normalisation of positive mental health by offering understanding and informed support in non-clinical surroundings. Positive impact includes reductions in serious incidents involving young people and decrease in staff sickness with associated economic benefits, as well as improved referrals of young people to statutory services and overall improvements to care pathways.

Jigsaw, working alongside the Headstrong youth mental health programme in Ireland, has an integrative role in supporting young people to find the most appropriate mental health service as well as actively supporting individuals themselves. The Jigsaw service works with all appropriate service providers in a region to enable young people aged 15–25 to access the most appropriate services in as seamless a way as possible, whatever their level of need, through the support of a panel of youth advisors. It is an evidence-based, integrated service designed to strengthen a community's capacity to support young people's mental health. It works on a partnership model aligning existing resources and expertise within communities and is fully integrated with the Headstrong model of education and community education.

Statutory mental health services tend to employ mainly clinical staff with medically focused training and a smaller number of psychology or social care professionals. Psychiatry tends to be at the top of the hierarchical clinical staff pyramid, and whereas there is a clear focus on improving health and reducing emotional distress and negative symptoms, there is often poor integration with vocational training, education and, where necessary, rehabilitation into community life. For young people who are often in danger of slipping off the vocational and social networks ladders at a time when their networks are relatively new and fragile, having some established and consistent working practices and bridges across the mental health and vocational divide is vital to prevent ongoing recovery from turning into chronic patient status and reliance on health and social care systems. Similarly, recovery can be difficult in situations where basic accommodation needs are unmet or where substance use has not been addressed as part of a comprehensive package of care. The needs of young people in care or leaving care are often unrecognised, and the outcomes from these groups suggest that the lack of integrated support in such cases is a factor in the poor outcomes for these groups. Without some common understanding and training for all staff involved in working with young people, inconsistency of approach will continue to be experienced by young people. Along with a potential widening of organisational partnerships to embrace concepts of 'wraparound'[19] and successful vocational and functional outcomes for young people with mental health difficulties, comes a need to improve the understanding of all staff in mental health literacy, engagement and interpersonal dynamics. At a minimum, any staff working with young people should be encouraged to have a basic level of mental health literacy such as that provided by Mental Health First Aid training (see Chapter 8).

A first step towards more systematic professional expertise should be the development of a competencies framework for training, guided by a steering group's expertise and informed by relevant training guidelines. Social care staff who are responsible for supporting 'looked after children' (children in the care of a local authority) and children leaving care, staff working in youth housing and drop-in centres and even general practitioners and physicians often receive negligible training in child mental health, emotional wellbeing and resilience, despite at times working with some of the most emotionally vulnerable young people. Basic elements of a training programme could include modules on:

- Families and the role of attachment and emotional security in the early environment
- Emotional and cognitive development in young people – first 12 years
- Emotional and cognitive development in young people – 12–25 years
- Impact of childhood trauma on emotional development and mental health
- Introduction to common mental disorders in young people
- Engagement and positive conflict resolution for staff working with vulnerable young people
- Reducing stigma, increasing awareness and improving help-seeking in youth mental health
- Reducing risk behaviour and building emotional resilience in young people and families
- Developing Psychologically Informed Environments (PIE) for the workplace
- Transitions: youth mental health, emotional and vocational independence

Widening basic mental health literacy and understanding is vital to both reduce the current levels of stigma that interfere with early help-seeking and improve confidence in engaging with young people and assisting them to find appropriate support at the earliest opportunity.

Transitions – what age range is best?

A major part of the rationale for redesigning mental health services for children and young people involves the current 'split' in services coinciding with what we now know to be the peak ages of vulnerability for emerging mental disorder.[20] Most services have been built around historical notions of what constitutes 'childhood' and 'adulthood' with the majority featuring a handover in provision between the ages of 16–18 years. It is now generally accepted from both scientific and social perspectives that the road from adolescence to adulthood is much longer and more winding than previously assumed, with brain maturation now understood to continue into the mid- to late twenties.

So, what is the ideal age range to focus on for new and emerging youth mental health services? Whichever range is chosen, there will be transition points and a need to pay close attention to issues of clinical information sharing, family/carer involvement, shared care-team meetings, continuity of treatment and shared understanding of developmental and biopsychosocial processes. There would appear to be logic in mirroring the normal transitional age for entry into secondary school education as one parameter, since this period reflects major developmental (puberty) and social changes, and age 25 at the other end as the majority of mental disorders have already emerged by this time point. However, two 'transition' points are created where one existed, and the same issues of optimal handover of clinical information, treatment approaches and staff engagement will require addressing. Research on earlier years is also providing evidence that mental disorder in preschool-aged infants may not be qualitatively different to that in older age groups.[21,22] The prevalence of psychiatric disorders during any one year in adolescence is suggested as 20–25%,[23,24] and evidence suggests that it is the duration of mental health difficulty in adolescence that is critical in influencing whether disorders persist through youth into adulthood,[25] further supporting the need for the early intervention approach.

Working with schools and education – investing in resilience

In 2010 the UK Royal College of Psychiatrists stated that 'School-based mental health promotion programmes are likely the best investment for prevention'[26] summarising the evidence base for promoting mental health education as a preventative strategy. Education has a gatekeeper function to vocational opportunities in life, and the vast majority of young people spend a considerable proportion of their time in mandatory educational settings, generally up to their 16th or 18th year. However, relatively few experience any guidance on mental health literacy and awareness. This appears an incongruous situation, as prevention and early intervention in mental health really only makes sense if educational and statutory health providers are working in close partnership to promote emotional health and wellbeing for all young people. Good mental health has been found to have implications for school environments and academic achievement, whereas its absence contributes to many common concerns of school managers such as bullying, disruptive behaviour, self-harm, drug and alcohol use and teenage pregnancy.[27–29] It is only in more recent years that policy has encouraged a closer union of these natural partners.

Schools, colleges and other educational institutions are the natural settings for proactive education in emotional resilience, mental health and wellbeing. Teachers particularly need training in mental health literacy and to be capable of identifying emerging mental disorder and supporting resilience. New youth services will need to develop ever closer working relationships with these educational institutions if they are to realistically improve the early identification and intervention rates of emerging mental health problems. If we are to truly remove stigma as a barrier to help-seeking, a focus on mental health as a positive attribute, for which we all have personal and collective responsibility, needs to be promoted as a mandatory part of the standard education system, much in the way that education on drug awareness or (less consistently) sexual health is routinely part of the school syllabus.

The National Lottery–funded HeadStart programme aims to explore and test new ways to improve the mental health and wellbeing of young people aged ten to 16 by investing up to £56m in six local partnerships across England between 2016 and 2021.[30] These will seek to facilitate and support (1) the implementation of a locally developed, cross-disciplinary, multi-layered and integrated prevention strategy, with the young person and their needs at its core; (2) the development of the necessary local conditions to enable that strategy to become sustainable in time; and (3) the development of a more robust evidence base around 'what works' in the area of mental wellbeing, to be proactively shared beyond Head-Start with the aim of contributing to the national and local policy debate. This programme intends to build sustainability and represents a substantial investment in the concept of universal wellbeing and emotional resilience as a preventative strategy for young people.

Costs

The World Health Organization (WHO) observes that 'there is a substantial gap between the burden caused by mental disorders and the resources available to treat and prevent them'.[31] Cost is a key factor related to the current interest in prevention of mental illness. This refers not only to the cost of treatment, but also to the financial impact of lost days of work and productivity due to mental ill-health. Prevention as a means to reducing long-term health costs becomes a catalyst for investment in public mental health and finding the best ways of increasing knowledge, awareness and earlier treatments. Only one in three adults and as few as one in four children receive mental health treatment and support when needed. A few high-income countries, such as the UK and Sweden, invest 10% or more of their health budgets on mental health services, but even this amount appears to be insufficient.

A recent Australian report suggests that poor mental health in young people costs Australia at least $6.29 billion per annum, including $1.3 billion in direct health costs and $1.2 billion in unemployment and disability payments.[32] The same report recommends investing in digital technology to support prevention and intervention as a potentially highly cost-efficient method to improve access for the majority who currently are not receiving appropriate interventions.

In England, mental health care spending accounts for approximately 11% of the total NHS budget (and 23% of the total burden of health care).[33] The UK charity YoungMinds has reported that, in total, less than 1% of the total NHS budget (and around 8% of the total mental health budget) is spent on child and adolescent mental health services.[34] As McGorry has stated, 'Our care system is weakest where it should be strongest'.[1] The implications of redesigning services to improve prevention and early intervention possibilities are that either new funding must be found (unlikely in the current financial era) or that funding will need to be redistributed from current adult and primary care teams, with the proportion currently being spent on the 16–25 age group redistributed to child and adolescent services. This will need to be either through workforce reorientation or actual disinvestment/investment procedures. Either way, a great deal of support and careful business case evaluation, with local support of senior clinical and academic leaders to enable robust assessments of local conditions and priorities is required.

Continual research and evaluation

No new service model should be embarked upon without consideration of a robust evaluation and assessment strategy. This is necessary to ensure that the new approach is both acceptable and appropriate to key stakeholders of the service (patients, carers, staff), but also that indices such as waiting times, non-attendance rates and actual symptom improvement are systematically captured and acted upon to improve services in a continual cycle of positive change. Outcome measures should focus beyond individual illness recovery to wider metrics of vocational and social outcomes. Improved 'wellbeing' and resilience has to be an ultimate aim of any new service approach. Health economics are also essential to capture cost returns on investment and are a powerful ally in negotiating ongoing funding and commissioning of innovative approaches. Ideally service redesign should be planned in liaison with academic partners with appropriate funding provided to enable timely and regular reports on efficacy and fidelity to the service protocols as well as highlighting areas that would benefit from improvement. The fundamentals of evidence-based practice are critical to newly emerging paradigms of care, and comprehensive evaluation provides the solid base from which youth mental health can evolve as the future standard.

Summary

Adolescence is a particularly important transition point. It is a distinct developmental stage in its own right and a time of major physical, emotional and neurological change. Youth mental health as an area of specialty is relatively new and under-explored, yet holds promise for enabling some of the most positive changes to service delivery, efficacy and acceptability in recent years. Opportunities to apply active interventions at the earliest opportunity in line with actual patient needs, rather than adhering to exclusive and acute-level diagnostic thresholds, is the equivalent of investing in safety standards and smoke alarms instead of sole reliance on the emergency firefighting skills of an excellent but overwhelmed workforce. Combining earlier staged interventions across developmental stages with a radical investment in youth mental health education, training and school-based emotional resilience support would greatly help to demystify services and reduce stigma – itself a major obstacle to help-seeking and awareness.

Encouraging service user–led youth involvement in the design and ongoing application of new services and educational initiatives from the earliest opportunity would ensure the appropriateness and acceptability of the model. Integrating the clinical services with housing, vocational and training partner specialists would allow for a seamless wraparound support to meet social and developmental needs, reduce the likelihood of early relapse and maintain a healthy transition into mainstream society. Providing trustable online educational support and local signposting and mapping of physical service locations would reduce the unnecessary confusion and helplessness that is often the first experience of members of the public attempting to navigate the mental health system. It would be even better if those services were accessible through a single integrated point of contact with triage expertise and guidance. This really would be a radical and welcome departure from the status quo.

References

1 McGorry P, Bates T, Birchwood M. Designing youth mental health services for the 21st century: examples from Australia, Ireland and the UK. *British Journal of Psychiatry* 2013;54:s30–5.
2 Howe D, Batchelor S, Coates D, Cashman E. Nine key principles to guide youth mental health: development of service models in New South Wales. *Early Intervention in Psychiatry* 2014;8(2):190–7.
3 McGorry PD, Killackey EJ. Early intervention in psychosis: a new evidence based paradigm. *Epidemiologia e Psichiatria Sociale* 2002;11(4):237–47.
4 Birchwood M, Todd P, Jackson C. Early intervention in psychosis. The critical period hypothesis. *British Journal of Psychiatry* 1998;172(33):53–9.
5 McGorry P, Trethowan J, Rickwood D. Creating headspace for integrated youth mental health care. *World Psychiatry* 2019;18(2):140–1.
6 O'Keeffe L, O'Reilly A, O'Brien G, Buckley R, Illback R. Description and outcome evaluation of Jigsaw: an emergent Irish mental health early intervention programme for young people. *Irish Journal of Psychological Medicine* 2015;32(1):71–7.
7 Wilson J, Clarke T, Lower R, Ugochukwu U, Maxwell S, Hodgekins J, et al. Creating an innovative youth mental health service in the United Kingdom: the Norfolk Youth Service. *Early Intervention in Psychiatry* 2018;12(4):740–6.
8 Malla A, Iyer S, Shah J, Joober R, Boksa P, Lal S, et al. Canadian response to need for transformation of youth mental health services: ACCESS Open Minds (Esprits Ouverts). *Early Intervention in Psychiatry* 2019;13(3):697–706.
9 Institute of Medicine and National Research Council. *Investing in the health and well-being of young adults*. Washington, DC: The National Academies Press; 2015.
10 Merry SN, Stasiak K, Shepherd M, Frampton C, Fleming T, Lucassen MFG. The effectiveness of SPARX, a computerised self help intervention for adolescents seeking help for depression: randomised controlled non-inferiority trial. *BMJ* 2012;344:e2598.
11 Coppens E, Vermet I, Knaeps J, De Clerck M, De Schrijver I, Matot JP, et al. *Adolescent mental health care in Europe: state of the art, recommendations, and guidelines by the ADOCARE* network*. Brussels: European Union; 2015.
12 Coughlan H, Cannon M, Shiers D, Power P, Barry C, Bates T, et al. Towards a new paradigm of care: the International Declaration on Youth Mental Health. *Early Intervention in Psychiatry* 2013;7(2):103–8.
13 Kessler RC, Berglund P, Demler O, Jin R, Merikangas KR, Walters EE. Lifetime prevalence and age-of-onset distributions of DSM-IV disorders in the National Comorbidity Survey Replication. *Archives of General Psychiatry* 2005;62(6):593–602.
14 Read J, van Os J, Morrison AP, Ross CA. Childhood trauma, psychosis and schizophrenia: a literature review with theoretical and clinical implications. *Acta Psychiatrica Scandinavica* 2005;112(5):330–50.
15 Cassidy J, Shaver PR. *Handbook of attachment: theory, research, and clinical applications*. New York: Guilford Press; 1999.
16 Hart RA. *Children's participation: from tokenism to citizenship*. Florence: UNICEF International Child Development Centre; 1992.

17 Westhorp G. *Planning for youth participation: a resource kit.* Adelaide: Youth Sector Training Council of South Australia; 1987.
18 Johnson R, Haigh R. Social psychiatry and social policy for the 21st century – new concepts for new needs: the 'psychologically-informed environment'. *Mental Health and Social Inclusion* 2010;14(4):30–5.
19 Burns BJ, Goldman SK. *Promising practices in wraparound for children with serious emotional disturbance and their families.* Washington, DC: Center for Effective Collaboration and Practice, American Institutes for Research; 1998.
20 Singh SP, Paul M, Ford T, Kramer T, Weaver T, McLaren S, et al. Process, outcome and experience of transition from child to adult mental healthcare: multiperspective study. *British Journal of Psychiatry* 2010;197(4):305–12.
21 Wichstrøm L, Berg-Nielsen TS, Angold A, Egger HL, Solheim E, Sveen TH. Prevalence of psychiatric disorders in preschoolers. *Journal of Child Psychology and Psychiatry* 2012;53(6):695–705.
22 Egger HL, Angold A. Common emotional and behavioral disorders in preschool children: presentation, nosology, and epidemiology. *Journal of Child Psychology and Psychiatry* 2006;47(3–4):313–37.
23 Patel V, Flisher AJ, Hetrick S, McGorry P. Mental health of young people: a global public-health challenge. *Lancet* 2007;369(9569):1302–13.
24 Davies SC. *Annual report of the Chief Medical Officer 2013, public mental health priorities: investing in the evidence.* London: Department of Health; 2014.
25 Patton GC, Coffey C, Romaniuk H, Mackinnon A, Carlin JB, Degenhardt L, et al. The prognosis of common mental disorders in adolescents: a 14-year prospective cohort study. *Lancet* 2014;383(9926):1404–11.
26 Royal College of Psychiatrists. *No health without public mental health: the case for action.* London: Royal College of Psychiatrists; 2010.
27 Kim YS, Leventhal B. Bullying and suicide. A review. *International Journal of Adolescent Medicine and Health* 2008;20(2):133–54.
28 Skogen JC, Sivertsen B, Lundervold AJ, Stormark KM, Jakobsen R, Hysing M. Alcohol and drug use among adolescents: and the co-occurrence of mental health problems. Ung@hordaland, a population-based study. *BMJ Open* 2014;4(9):e005357.
29 Vigod SN, Dennis CL, Kurdyak PA, Cairney J, Guttmann A, Taylor VH. Fertility rate trends among adolescent girls with major mental illness: a population-based study. *Pediatrics* 2014;133(3):e585–91.
30 HeadStart. *Improving the wellbeing and mental health of young people.* Retrieved from: www.tnlcommunityfund.org.uk/funding/strategic-investments/headstart
31 World Health Organization. *Investing in mental health.* Geneva: World Health Organization; 2003.
32 Hosie A, Vogl G, Carden J, Hoddinott J, Lim S. *A way forward: equipping Australia's mental health system for the next generation.* Australia: EY and ReachOut Australia; 2015.
33 Naylor C, Parsonage M, McDaid D, Knapp M, Fossey M, Galea A. *Long-term conditions and mental health: the cost of co-morbidities.* London: The King's Fund and Centre for Mental Health; 2012.
34 YoungMinds. *A new era for young people's mental health.* London: YoungMinds; 2018.

7 What makes a good youth mental health service?

Lisa Butterly

Introduction

This chapter is a personal perspective of what makes a good youth mental health service. My own background is evidence for the need for reform of services for young people with mental health issues, in particular, the formation of a separate service for those aged between 12 and 25 years. There are a number of themes discussed throughout including access to education and loss of vocational capacity as a result of illness and service involvement. The discussion emphasises the importance of 'time' in the delivery of services and provides justification for improved access to vocational and/or therapeutic options for young people with mental health difficulties. This chapter also includes a table of recommendations identifying *problems* with current services for young people, *solutions* to those problems and potential *actions*.

Personal experience of mental health services as a young person (16–24 years old)

My mental health difficulties started as a young teenager. In secondary school, I noticed a change in my thought processes. I was not able to think clearly. I started to hear voices. This escalated until I really struggled to think and concentrate. I ended up very confused, constantly distracted and paranoid of others. I did not understand what was happening but I knew it was not right. My schoolwork suffered greatly as my mood spiralled downwards. I was not able to sleep and became isolated. Within six months I had become very depressed and agitated. I attempted suicide and was subsequently taken to the child psychiatric services in my area. I was subsequently admitted to the adolescent unit at a psychiatric hospital in Dublin for observation and assessment.

Five weeks later my parents were called to a meeting to discuss the results. All that was said was that I was showing signs of a 'serious mental illness'. To balance that news my parents were told that there were a number of positive aspects in my case which could be significant in the long term. These included high level of intelligence and creativity as well as personality type. The prognosis depended on how well I coped outside the hospital setting. Returning to school and staying connected with my peer group were identified as key to helping my progress in the years ahead. However, I was unable to return to school from 16 years old due to a lack of resources in the education system, and friendships quickly disappeared within a year of the first hospitalisation. Consequently, I lost educational opportunities and connection to my peer network. For the following two years I was medicated for the symptoms of schizophrenia and regularly attended a child psychiatrist. I was admitted to the hospital in Dublin a number of times in this period.

At 18 years old, I transitioned to the adult mental health services. I had a psychiatrist, luckily a good one. It was a classic bio-medical model of care but, to be fair, that was not my psychiatrist's choice. She did not have the power to employ a psychologist in the local service. She could not provide access to education courses for me. She could not change the culture of discrimination which existed at that time. What she could do was make sure that we tried a lot of medications with the hope that we would find one that helped and had little side effects.

Medication was always troublesome. Side effects ranged from mild to severe. For example, with one medication my joints froze, another impaired my vision; I gained weight, lost weight, became more depressed, lost my balance, slept too much or slept too little. Some medications alleviated the symptoms of the illness, some made no difference whatsoever. The trick was to find a balance between the alleviation of symptoms and side effects. It was a long road to find that balance.

Between 18 and 24 years old, the story repeated each year. I was admitted to the local psychiatric hospital for three or four months, sometimes twice a year. As an outpatient in the adult service, I attended the weekly clinic and continued to take medication.

Comparative perspective (child and adult services)

There was an emotional impact of both the child and adult services but I found the adult system more hostile. I was legally an adult but I was still a child in need of protection. The child service had a more caring and individual approach.

As an inpatient in the child service, I had access to a team of nurses, an occupational therapist, a psychologist and a psychiatrist. I had a daily timetable of activities, but the child service was not perfect. My inpatient care was in Dublin. My outpatient care was in County Louth, over 75 km away. Any progress that was made while I was an inpatient was fruitless because I was discharged into a social, developmental and educational void.

The age range of the adolescent ward was 12 to 18 years old. In the adult hospital I was locked in an environment with an age range of up to 65 years old, which was frightening. I nostalgically refer to those first years in the adult system as the 'David Attenborough era' because I felt like an observer who was given access to a world I did not belong to. Moving to the adult service felt like starting a waiting game: I waited for time to pass or for a day when I would have enough courage to end it all with suicide.

It was an ongoing struggle to hold onto some sense of self-worth when everything around me was telling me to give up and accept the bleak circumstances. I think staff in the adult service would have described me as quiet, helpful, pleasant and compliant. Privately, I was feeling lost, scared, angry, trapped and invisible. At the same time, I was quietly hopeful that the situation would improve. I was clearly consumed with a lot of contradictions which were difficult to make sense of and had nothing to do with the symptoms of an illness. I was simply caught between opposing realities: the memory of the reality before I got ill, which was positive and progressive, and the reality I was stuck in, which was relentless and unforgiving.

As a broad comparison, the child service gave some hope of recovery. The adult service stole that hope and not only made it difficult to recover but difficult to live. The child service recognised my age group between 16 and 18 years old and provided a range of care options and interactions with other young people and practitioners. The adult service ignored my age or age-related requirements and, in doing so, ignored any potential to recover. Nonetheless, I refused to believe that I was a 'lost cause' no matter how much the adult system acted as a reminder to that reality on a daily basis. In fact, I came to a quick conclusion that it was the adult mental health system that was the 'lost cause' rather than the many young people I encountered over the years through service involvement.

There are a number of inconsistencies and contradictions in the messages communicated by the adult mental health system which can have an emotional, developmental and long-term impact on young people. Similarly, recovery is made even more challenging when the system of care and treatment shows little or no awareness of the realities faced by young people outside the care setting. Table 7.1 provides a brief summary of some common challenges experienced by young people who develop a mental illness and have significant service involvement.

Transformation

The chance for some relief from the situation, outlined in Table 7.1, appeared on the horizon with three consecutive changes. I call them my golden triangle. The first was the introduction of olanzapine to the Irish market. I was the first patient in the local service to test the new medication and within a few weeks I was a different person. I had more clarity and consciousness. The side effects were bearable.

Shortly after starting this new medication, I received a series of sessions with a psychology fellow in Dublin. This access to a talking therapy was provided by a neurologist and not, as one might expect, a psychiatrist. In six one-hour sessions I transitioned from being a patient to being a person again. It was a complete liberation and validation of my mind which gave me an unprecedented level of confidence in my ability to recover. Another significant change occurred in 2001. I was accepted onto a short return to education course in an adult education centre in my area due to eventually reaching the age requirement. That course turned the key and unlocked the door to my future, a new and hopeful future in the education system. The waiting game from 16 years old appeared to have an end in sight. I was determined to grab the opportunity.

Table 7.1 Common challenges experienced by young people using mental health services

Problem	*Treatment/Prognosis*	*Reality*
Diagnosed with mental illness	Medicated, hospitalised	**Trauma** Sharp disconnect between life before and life after the onset of mental illness
Stigma of mental illness	Treatment: return to normality as quickly as possible, return to school, maintain peer network Prognosis: much better chance of recovery if everything returns to normal after discharge from hospital	**Alienation/Rejection** School system poorly equipped to support students with a mental illness Loss of peer network Loss of social connections Loss of academic or vocational opportunities
Transition from child to adult services at 18 years old	Medicated, hospitalised, little or no access to talking therapy, 'see how it goes from here' attitude	**Annihilation of selfhood and identity** Apathy for life Self-stigma
Employability and social disability	Find a part-time job or attend a course to rebuild motivation, interest in life, peer network, social and vocational capacity	**Otherness** No educational qualifications means unemployable Limited access to formal education courses Hospitalised annually Life stagnated

I followed the short introductory course with a one-year general studies course (National Certificate Vocational Award) and a one-year Leaving Certificate course. Following the Leaving Certificate results in August 2003, I was accepted by a university to undertake a bachelor of arts degree. I completed the BA degree and then completed a master of arts degree at another university. I have since completed my PhD. I have not been hospitalised since 2001, although I still slightly panic when anyone suggests that I need a 'rest'.

The overall benefits of returning to education were huge. I thrived in a learning environment. I felt connected to the world again. Formal education provided me with the vocabulary and critical thinking skills required to communicate ideas and analyse problems in the hope of finding solutions to those problems. Through education I was able to redefine my experiences in a more positive way. I was able to build a new context for mental illness, challenge negative attitudes and try to highlight the need for better support for young people with an enduring mental health issue across the entire country. I have particular views in terms of service reform, and I am most critical of systematic failures within the adult services which have a negative impact on the lives of young people. For instance, it would be better for young people if they were officially recognised as requiring specific supports with regard to mental health care. I also believe that the transition from the child to the adult services at 18 years old is more damaging than service providers realise because it can mean the difference between recovery and long-term disability.

The establishment of a specific youth mental health service could reduce the isolation and confusion experienced by young people and address relevant life challenges for this age group. There are a number of life challenges which are noteworthy: education, social connections, friendship, identity exploration and discovery, and sexual health.

The transition from child to adult services at such a crucial stage in emotional and intellectual development has the power to influence the future of every young person with a mental health difficulty. Some young people will be lost and forgotten

Table 7.2 Recommendations to enhance youth mental health services

Problem	*Solution*	*Action*
Inadequate service structure and lack of recognition of age group (12–25 years)	Restructuring and recognition	Extend the child service officially beyond 18 years old and build an intermediary system specifically around the needs of young people with mental health issues. At the centre of the service should be full recognition of the experiences of that age group and the transition from childhood to adulthood.
Training of service providers	Rewrite training curricula Offer training to existing staff New model of qualifications for youth mental health	The training curriculum for service providers should mirror the intermediary system. This requires a complete redefinition of 'child and adolescent mental health' to 'youth mental health'.
Geography of resources and inconsistency with care facilities can dictate outcomes in youth mental health	Improve recovery outcomes or chance of recovery by creating synthesis between the delivery of treatment and the location of that treatment	Reorganise facilities or build new ones which can provide both inpatient and outpatient treatment in as many regions as possible Remove the inconsistencies in care provision and reduce the level of disruption experienced by the young person, their families/carers and practitioners
Current system focuses on mental health diagnosis and does not treat vocational or social disabilities in young people	Develop a youth mental health system that can lead to third level education, employment, independence and security in adult life	Establish a dedicated liaison programme as part of the youth mental health service. A dedicated group of people can be employed to act in the health, social and vocational interests of a young person, whether that is to identify care options in each area, identify routes to education and source funding, routes to employment, or assist in welfare support and housing.

in the adult system. Some will lose years of their lives to service involvement. Some will recover but require lifelong support from mental health services. The lucky ones will recover and reach their full potential as adults. I have included a number of practical recommendations for service reform which can give young people a chance to recover and transition safely and securely into adulthood (Table 7.2).

Lessons learned from childhood to adulthood

It is unfair to place the burden and consequences of an inadequate adult mental health service on the shoulders of young people and then expect them to flourish in spite of insurmountable challenges. It is time to reshape mental health services in order to provide the best possible chance of recovery for young people with the most practical delivery of services in order to achieve good life outcomes. Positive recovery stories are not exceptions in a given population, they are blueprints for change.

Conclusion

I am acutely aware that my chances of recovery were greatly reduced as a result of having to transition from the child to adult services at 18 years old. Of course, it is impossible to say what would have happened if there was a more age-appropriate service available at the time. However, it is possible to say that my recovery was the result of a combination of support, a psychiatrist who kept up to date with developments in medicated treatment and a high level of self-determination. Not every young person has the level of support or self-determination required to recover in the adult system. In fact, the odds are stacked against any young person who transitions from the child to the adult services and does not have a network behind them or the determination to pursue their goals and ambitions.

A separate service for youth mental health is a rational solution to an irrational and unnecessary problem which has caused many difficulties for young people, families/carers and practitioners for generations. On a much broader level, what makes a good youth mental health service is one that is established on a countrywide basis, is legally recognised, politically and economically supported, and culturally respected.

Part III

Specialised interventions

8 Using Mental Health First Aid to support young people

Claire M. Kelly, Betty A. Kitchener and Anthony F. Jorm

The concept of Mental Health First Aid

In many countries of the world, first aid programs are available to members of the public, teaching them to assist someone who is injured or otherwise experiencing a physical health crisis before professional medical treatment, if needed, can be obtained. These courses do not generally train members of the public to assist someone who is developing a mental health problem or experiencing a mental health crisis.

Mental Health First Aid (MHFA) training has been developed to address this gap. Just like in conventional first aid, the help is typically rendered not by health professionals, but by people within the social networks of those in need.

The definition of Mental Health First Aid is *the help offered to a person developing a mental health problem, experiencing the worsening of an existing mental health problem or in a mental health crisis. The first aid is given until appropriate professional help is received or until the crisis resolves.*[1]

The place of Mental Health First Aid in the spectrum of interventions

There is a wide range of interventions available to support people with mental illness, ranging from prevention programs to treatments for mental illness and rehabilitation after severe mental illness. The following diagram shows the range of interventions, which might be needed by an individual as they begin to develop a mental illness, seek treatment, and move on to recovery.

Mental Health First Aid can be described as part of early intervention – indeed, it is the earliest stage of early intervention. Mental Health First Aid involves the actions that a member of the public can take to support a person with a mental illness or in a mental health–related crisis and to assist the person to seek appropriate professional help.

Early intervention is particularly important for young people because mental illness can have negative effects on a young person's development. Mental illness can also have a number of other negative effects such as: interference with the transition from secondary school to tertiary studies or employment; problems with

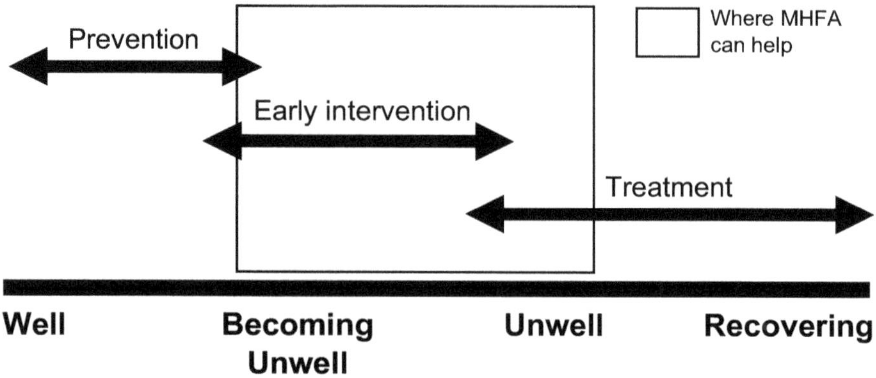

Figure 8.1 Spectrum of mental health interventions from wellness to mental disorders and through to recovery, showing the contribution of Mental Health First Aid

personal relationships; poor health habits (such as substance misuse, sedentary lifestyle and inadequate diet) and problems with the law. There is a lot of evidence that, the longer the delay between the onset of symptoms and the start of treatment, the less likely the young person is to have a good outcome.[2]

Why Mental Health First Aid for supporting young people?

Mental Health First Aid is particularly important for adults living and working with young people for a number of reasons:

- **Mental health problems frequently have their first onset during adolescence or early adulthood.** In the US, the median age of onset for any mental disorder is 18 years, and three-quarters have their first onset by age 25.[3] Similar figures apply in other countries. Adults who have frequent contact with young people will inevitably encounter some of those experiencing their first symptoms, as well as those who already have a significant mental illness.
- **Young people are not generally well informed about mental health problems and how they can be treated.** They usually will not have as much experience as adults in seeking professional help. The significant adults in a young person's life can play an important role in guiding them to help. In order to be able to do this, many adults will need to improve their own knowledge and attitudes regarding mental illness.
- **There is significant stigma and discrimination associated with mental illness, which may prevent young people from seeking help.** The main reasons young people give for not seeking help are embarrassment and concerns about what other people will think, whether friends,

family or health professionals.[4] If adults make a conscious effort to display non-stigmatising attitudes about mental illness, this can help young people to overcome these concerns.

- **Young people with mental health problems may not be aware that they would benefit from help**. This may be a result of the symptoms themselves, which may cloud the young person's thinking and rational decision-making, or the symptoms may cause such distress that the young person cannot take effective action. Adults can help young people to take positive action when young people are unable to do so themselves.
- **Professional help may not be readily available as soon as it is needed**. If professionals are not available, parents and other adults in the young person's network can offer more immediate help. They may also be able to help make the young person aware of a range of effective self-help strategies, online and telephone services.
- **Adolescent development and mental illness have a relationship that is complicated and important**. The changes associated with adolescent development may make it difficult to identify the symptoms of mental illness. The challenges of adolescent development can increase the risk of developing mental health problems. In addition, mental illness can interfere with normal adolescent development, including brain development, particularly when substance misuse occurs. Understanding the relationship between adolescent development and mental illness can help adults, particularly parents, to identify worrying changes and seek help early.

The Mental Health First Aid (MHFA) training and research program

The MHFA program started in 2000 in Canberra, Australia, with the Standard MHFA course on how adults can assist other adults and soon spread across Australia and internationally.[5] Many other countries have arranged to licence the program and adapt it for local conditions. A current list of the countries where MHFA training is available can be found on the MHFA website (https://mhfa.com.au/our-impact/our-global-impact).

In 2007, in response to broad interest and demand, the Youth Mental Health First Aid (YMHFA) program was launched. The YMHFA program is designed for adults assisting adolescents, and targets for training include parents, school staff, youth workers, allied health professionals, those engaged in recreational activities (such as sports coaches and scout leaders) and other adults who work with or care about adolescents. Although the course is designed to help adolescents aged 12–18 or in secondary school, much of the content is relevant for young adults as well. The age of 18 has a number of important social meanings in Australia. It is the age at which young people are considered adults, can vote, complete secondary school and can purchase alcohol legally. In other countries, the target age for YMHFA differs, sometimes incorporating young adults up to the age of 25. Details of the countries currently providing YMHFA courses can also be found on the MHFA website.

In Australia, the 14-hour YMHFA course is conducted by specially selected instructors who undergo a rigorous 5.5-day training process. This course teaches about five categories of mental health problems (depression, anxiety problems, eating disorders, psychosis and substance use problems). Participants do not learn to diagnose or treat these conditions, but learn how to recognise a cluster of symptoms which suggest that help might be needed. They also learn about the risk factors for each mental illness and evidence-based professional and self-help treatments available. Participants also learn the first aid for a range of crisis situations (suicidal thoughts and behaviours, non-suicidal self-injury, panic attacks, traumatic events, medical emergencies from eating disorders, severe psychotic states, severe intoxication and medical emergencies from alcohol and other drug use, and aggressive behaviour).

Development of Mental Health First Aid guidelines

The content of conventional first aid courses is based on internationally developed guidelines for how to help with various medical emergencies. Similarly, the content of the MHFA course is based on a series of guidelines developed through international consensus studies, incorporating the views of mental health professionals (clinicians and researchers), consumers (people who have lived experience of mental illness) and caregivers (family members and close friends who provide day-to-day assistance to a person with mental illness). Only first aid strategies that are agreed by a large majority of all three groups are incorporated into the guidelines.

Given cultural differences in what is considered appropriate Mental Health First Aid, it is not possible to have universal guidelines. While most of the guidelines have been produced for high-income English-speaking countries, some culturally specific guidelines have also been developed. These include guidelines for assisting Aboriginal and Torres Strait Islander people and a number of guidelines for use in Asian countries. All of these guidelines are available for free download from the MHFA website.

Mental Health First Aid guidelines:

Depression
Psychosis
Eating disorders
Substance use problems
Suicidal thoughts and behaviours
Non-suicidal self-injury
Panic attacks
Traumatic events
Communication with adolescents
Assisting an LGBTIQA+ person

Mental Health First Aid for Aboriginal and Torres Strait Islander people:

Communicating with an adolescent
Cultural considerations
Depression
Psychosis
Suicide
Non-suicidal self-injury
Problem drinking
Problem drug use

Mental Health First Aid for Asian countries:

Psychosis
Suicide – Japan
Suicide – the Philippines
Suicide – India
Suicide – Sri Lanka

All of these guidelines, and links to research papers, are available from https://mhfa.com.au/resources/mental-health-first-aid-guidelines

Effects of Mental Health First Aid training

The standard MHFA course has been evaluated in a number of studies including several randomised controlled trials. These trials have consistently shown improvements in knowledge of mental illnesses, increased belief in evidence-based treatments, reduction in stigmatising attitudes and increases in helping behaviour toward people with mental health problems.[6] An e-Learning version of the course has been evaluated and shown similar results.[7] Benefits of MHFA training have been found to be sustained over time.

The youth course has so far undergone a number of evaluations, including two randomised controlled trials, one in schools and one with parents of adolescents.[8,9] Again, the results have been positive, with improvements similar to those found in the Standard MHFA course, and these are also maintained over time.[6] These improvements suggest that Youth MHFA does increase the likelihood that an adult will take action to assist a young person who is developing a mental health problem.

Applying the Mental Health First Aid Action Plan

Participants learn a MHFA Action Plan which prompts them to offer appropriate help. The Action Plan is as follows:

- **A**pproach, assess and assist with any crisis
- **L**isten and communicate non-judgementally

- **G**ive support and information
- **E**ncourage the person to get appropriate professional help
- **E**ncourage other supports

In the MHFA Action Plan, the actions are not sequential. For example, 'L – Listen and communicate non-judgementally' is not something you start doing and stop doing – it is something which, ideally, we would all do all of the time, but at least certainly needs to be foremost in the mind of a mental health first aider whilst trying to assist someone.

The rest of this chapter will focus on applying the MHFA Action Plan. Each action will be described in some detail and then applied to help a fictional student, Molly. The actions will not be applied in strict order.

Case study: Molly

Molly is a 16-year-old girl who is in Grade 11 at the secondary school where you work. She started at the school at the beginning of Grade 7 and you know her quite well. Previous to this year, she has been an above-average student and active in the school community. Last year, she was on the volleyball team and the basketball team. She has never been in any real trouble, although she tends to chat in class and is sometimes asked to be quiet. She has maintained the same group of good friends and at lunch-times she used to spend her time playing ball games with friends. Her home life has appeared to be stable and she has been a caring and kind friend to younger students.

This year, things have been different. She has started to get in trouble for handing assignments in late, and although the standard of the work she hands in is very high, her grades have dropped somewhat due to late submission of work. She is quieter in class. You have seen that her friends are still playing ball games at lunchtime, but she is not often with them. Some investigation reveals that she spends her lunchtimes working in the library.

You are walking to your office during class time and find Molly leaving a bathroom. She appears to have been crying. As your concerns about Molly have been mounting over time, you have decided to use the MHFA Action Plan to help her.

Action 1: approach the young person, assess and assist with any crisis

This is a two-part action. The first part is *Approach the young person,* and the second is *Assess and assist with any crisis.*

How to approach

If you are concerned about a young person you care about, you need to approach them about your concerns. Consideration should be given to how, where and when to approach the young person in order to make them more comfortable and likely to talk about what is happening. If you feel unable to make the approach at all, it is important to ask somebody who can.

- An ideal **place** might be somewhere private, such as an office or an empty classroom. Alternately, it may be somewhere that lies within the young person's comfort zone, such as a café or playing a friendly game of basketball.
- An ideal **time** is one where you are unlikely to be interrupted, and you have enough time to raise your concerns and allow the young person enough time to talk. Asking a young person to stay behind after class is probably not a good idea, as this may single them out in front of their peers.
- **How** you approach the topic is going to depend on your relationship with the young person, your professional responsibilities (if any) and how serious your concerns are. Focusing on your concerns, rather than what they are doing wrong, is important. For example, don't say "Your grades have dropped". Instead, focus on how upset they are, and how it is affecting their life, by saying something like "It seems like you don't have the energy to do the things you usually do".
- **If the young person is resistant to your help**, or doesn't want to talk for any reason, let them know that they can talk to you another time, or help them to identify another person who can help. If they don't follow up, you need to approach them again. Young people may not have the maturity to decide for themselves that they do need help.

Approaching Molly

This may be a good time to approach Molly. She is not in class, and you are not busy right now. This means that you have at least half an hour, which is probably about as long as she will be able to talk to you. You take her to your office and ask a front office worker to tell her classroom teacher that she is with you so that she is not reprimanded later for her absence.

You begin by mentioning the crying and ask her if something happened today to cause her distress. She says no, she's just exhausted and she's been struggling for a while. She tries to apologise for her grades.

You tell her that you are not concerned about the grades, but about the fact that she seems to be isolated from her peers, unhappy, and less involved in school than she used to be. You tell her that you think she may be developing a mental health problem and that you would like to talk to her about what she has been experiencing.

How to assess for a crisis

Sometimes, when approaching a young person, it may be clear that they are in crisis. Other times, indications of an underlying crisis may emerge during the conversation. Possible crises include:

- The young person may harm themselves (e.g., by attempting suicide, by using substances to become intoxicated, by engaging in non-suicidal self-injury or by attempting to achieve extreme weight loss).
- The young person experiences extreme distress (e.g., a panic attack, a severe psychotic state or a reaction to a traumatic event).
- The young person's behaviour is very disturbing to others (e.g., if they become aggressive or lose touch with reality).

> **Assessing Molly for signs of crisis**
>
> Although Molly is sad and upset, you do not think at this stage that she is in crisis. You will be looking for signs of crisis throughout the rest of your conversation.

Action 2: listen and communicate non-judgementally

Listening and communicating non-judgementally is essential to enable the young person to talk about what they are feeling. Engage the young person in conversation. Ask how they are feeling and how long it has been going on for. This can help the young person to feel heard and understood, while not being judged in any way. Young people who are distressed need empathy. This can make it easy for the person to feel comfortable to talk freely about their problems and to ask for help.

Non-judgemental listening and communication involves managing your verbal and non-verbal communication and your attitudes.

Try to portray **attitudes** of **acceptance, genuineness** and **empathy**.

- **Acceptance** means respecting the young person's feelings, values and experiences as valid. You can portray this by avoiding making comments that may be interpreted as critical, judgemental or minimising.
- **Genuineness** means showing the young person that you really accept them as they are. Young people are able to recognise when an adult is trying to 'fake it'. Don't use language, slang or mannerisms than are not familiar to you.
- **Empathy** means being able to imagine what another person might be experiencing. It is not the same as sympathy, which is feeling pity for another person. Avoid the temptation to say "I know just how you are feeling" – you don't. Instead, say "I imagine that this has been really hard for you".
- Portraying negative attitudes about young people, or about mental illness, will prevent the young person from talking openly.

Use **verbal skills** which show that you are listening and paying attention. For example:

- Ask questions, check your understanding and summarise what you have understood.
- Look out for non-verbal cues; their tone of voice and body language will give extra clues about how they are feeling.
- If the young person is struggling to communicate, be patient and use simple prompts such as "I see" and "ah".
- Don't criticise the young person or express frustration at their symptoms.
- Avoid giving glib advice such as "cheer up".
- Do not interrupt the young person when they are speaking.
- Remember that pauses and silences are okay. The young person may need time to think about what has been said, or may be struggling to find the words they need.

Use **non-verbal skills** to reinforce what you are saying. For example:

- Pay close attention to what the young person says.
- Maintain a comfortable level of eye contact and avoid staring.
- Your body should be in a position which portrays openness; ideally, sitting alongside and leaning toward the young person.
- Do not fidget or write notes, as this may indicate that your attention is elsewhere.

Listening to and communicating with Molly

You ask Molly how she has been feeling and how long she's been feeling this way for. She starts to cry again, says that she's feeling very sad and very anxious, and that it has been getting worse since the beginning of the year. She feels that nothing she does is good enough. She spends hours on every assignment and can't bring herself to hand anything in until it is perfect – which is why her homework and assignments are often late.

You ask if something has happened this year to bring about these changes and she says she is very stressed about the idea of the last two years of school and the importance of getting into a good course at a good university.

You find yourself wanting to tell her that worrying about Year 12 results is a waste of time and that she should instead focus on keeping a balance, handing work in on time and just doing her best. You stop yourself just in time, remembering that Year 12 results, while obviously a factor in Molly's distress, are not what you should be focusing on right now. You agree with her that this can be a tough time for students.

You ask if she has spoken to her friends about these concerns. Molly says she has tried to, but they don't seem as concerned. She is not seeing much of them at the moment. They are going out on the weekends and having fun, and while they used to ask her along, they have given up as she always says she has to study.

You ask Molly if she has spoken to her parents about her concerns. She says she hasn't. She is the oldest child in the family and they have their hands full looking after the younger ones. She does her best to hide her feelings at home, because she doesn't want to worry them. They are not pressuring her to do well at school, but are supportive of her hopes to go to university.

Action 3: give support and information

Once a young person with a mental health problem has felt listened to, it can be easier for them to accept support and information from the first aider.

The **support** a first aider offers should be appropriate to the relationship. A parent or caregiver might suggest that the young person do fewer chores for a while until things start to improve. A teacher might help by arranging for a student to take advantage of anything the school has in place to assist students who are struggling. An offer of additional emotional support may also be helpful.

As well as providing support, the first aider should act in a supportive way. If the first aider has realistic expectations for the young person, offers hope for recovery and remains consistently supportive, the young person may feel more able to accept help.

The **information** a first aider gives should be accurate, relevant and tailored to what the young person is able to understand at the time it is being given. A young person who is experiencing symptoms which might hamper comprehension (such as a high level of distress, psychotic symptoms or an inability to concentrate) will not be able to absorb or make use of complex information.

The first aider should treat the young person with respect. Depending on the severity of the problem, there is likely to be a range of options regarding what to do next, and the first aider should allow for an appropriate level of autonomy. However, a young person may not be able to make good decisions in a distressed state, so autonomy should be tempered with a degree of leadership.

The first aider should give the young person relevant fact sheets, pamphlets or websites that explain that mental illnesses are real medical conditions, that help is available and that most people recover. This can be very reassuring for the young person.

What's not supportive

There are a range of things that people tend to say in an effort to help that are not supportive at all. For example, we know that, even if it is untreated, depression tends to get better over time. However, saying "You'll get over it" is not helpful. Instead, saying that "Things will probably get better with time, but they will improve more quickly if we look for someone who can help" provides similar information, but in a more useful and supportive way. Similarly, it can be tempting to try to take over and make decisions on a young person's behalf, but supporting them to make their own decisions is more helpful in the long term.

Giving Molly support and information

Molly is quite distressed, and may not be able to take in a lot of information, so you provide her with a fact sheet from a reputable website and suggest she look at the site in her own time. As a first aider, you are not able to diagnose Molly's problem, but you tell her that she has some symptoms which are consistent with anxiety and depression and encourage her to read further in those areas.

Molly does not seem interested in learning more from the website. She tells you that since you've started talking, she is feeling more and more that she wants to take action.

She tells you that there are things she hasn't told you. She starts crying and rolls up her sleeve, showing you a number of cuts, some of which are in the later stages of healing and some of which seem quite fresh.

Going back to Action 1: assess and assist with any crisis

Even if there are no obvious signs of crisis at the outset of your discussion with a young person, it may be that there is something more serious bubbling under the surface. It is important to be familiar with the signs of mental health–related crises and to know how to explore further when these signs become apparent.

Self-injury may be a suicide attempt. Even if the cuts are superficial and could not have resulted in death, the young person may have intended to die when they injured themselves. In addition, self-injury can be a way to combat suicidal feelings,[10] even if the injury was not intended to cause death – in a sense, a way of preserving life by temporarily relieving the overwhelming feelings which have led to the suicidal thoughts. This means that if someone has injured themselves, it is important to ask if they have been thinking about suicide.

Suicidal thoughts and behaviours

A person might indicate that they are having thoughts of suicide in many different ways, from overtly talking about suicide to expressions of helplessness and hopelessness. A young person may be exploring themes of death and suicide in schoolwork, art and creative writing. Suicide intervention skills can be learned in a number of different courses (including MHFA) and require more attention than can be provided here. However, at its simplest, suicide intervention has three key actions, and in the absence of other training, these three actions may save a person's life.

1) If you suspect that someone is having thoughts of suicide, it is important to ask directly.

This means asking a question such as "Have you been thinking about suicide?" or "Have you been thinking about killing yourself?"

Ambiguous questions such as "Have you been thinking about hurting yourself?" or "You're not suicidal, are you?" may not give the direct response needed.

2) If the person says yes, work together to keep them safe.

If you can stay with the person, do so. If not, it may be that a family member, another trusted adult or a professional helper is available. You may need to take the person to a hospital.

3) Connect them with professional help.

A person with skills in supporting young people at risk of suicide is best. Ideally, help should be sought right away, but this may not be practical – it might be a few days or even longer before there is help available. In the meantime, caring and responsible adults in the young person's life can help to keep them safe.

If the young person is suicidal, it should never be kept a secret. Ideally, their parents or guardians should be aware of what is happening. In the absence of a supportive adult at home, a trusted school professional may be available to provide support. Even if the only person you tell is a mental health professional, it is essential you tell someone.

Non-suicidal self-injury

Even if the young person does not have thoughts of suicide, self-injury indicates that they are in need of help. People injure themselves for a range of different reasons. Common reasons include a need to escape from overwhelming feelings, a form of self-punishment or an attempt to ask for help. The most common injuries are cuts and scratches to the skin, however, burns, bruises, and overdosing can also be forms of non-suicidal self-injury.

If the young person needs emergency medical attention, this is the priority. Regardless of intent, emergency help should be sought if the young person has poisoned themselves, overdosed on any kind of substance or has a severe injury, for example, heavy bleeding or a large burn. When medical treatment is sought for a physical problem, the first aider should ask for a mental health assessment for the young person.

The severity of the injury should not be assumed to reflect the severity of the distress. Even minor, superficial injuries can indicate an urgent need for support. A mental health assessment should be sought even if the injury does not need medical attention.

Assessing and assisting Molly

Molly has indicated that she has been injuring herself. The cuts do appear to be mainly superficial, but you can see that she has been cutting herself for quite some time. There does not appear to be a need for first aid or emergency medical help.

You ask Molly what she's feeling when she cuts herself and she says she doesn't know. You ask her if she has ever tried to kill herself, and she says no. You ask her if she's been thinking about killing herself and she is shocked – she says no, she would never do that. You tell her that if she ever finds herself thinking about suicide, she can talk to you about it.

The fact that self-injury is present does mean that Molly should seek professional help.

Action 4: encourage appropriate professional help

The first aider should make sure that they know about sources of appropriate help that are available locally so that they can talk to the young person about options. Even if you are not sure that the problem is severe enough to warrant professional help, it is better that a skilled clinician makes that decision. Professional help is needed if the symptoms last for more than a few weeks or are interfering with the young person's daily functioning. Appropriate treatment can help the young person to get better more quickly and decrease the chances of future episodes.

If the young person is still an adolescent, or is living with their parents or guardians, it is best to get them involved. If the adolescent is resistant, explore why. It may be that they are trying to protect their parents or don't want to worry them, in which case talking about it might help. However, it may be that they are experiencing abuse or neglect at home, in which case involving their parents may result in increased risk to the young person. Going behind the young person's back is not a good idea. It is better to work out between the two of you who else should be involved.

What if the young person doesn't want help?

If the problem is not severe, you may tell the young person that they should think more about professional help and come back to you if they change their mind. However, discussing the reasons they are reluctant to seek help can be a first step to overcoming these barriers. Sometimes the young person has some inaccurate beliefs about treatment which you can help to correct. You could try seeking advice from a mental health professional about what you can do to help.

If it appears that the young person is not mature enough to make a good decision about help-seeking, you should talk to someone about it (one of their parents or guardians, a senior colleague or a health professional). However, unless the young person is a danger to themselves or others, you should not try to compel them to seek treatment.

Talking to Molly about professional help

You tell Molly that you think professional help is important for her. The fact that she has been injuring herself for some time, and that she is feeling overwhelmed by her feelings, means that there is probably something serious going on that a mental health professional might be able to help her to cope with.

Molly is sick of feeling the way that she does, and agrees that it would be a good idea. She even allows you to call her mother and ask her to come down to the school to talk about what has been happening.

When her mother arrives, she is shocked and says that Molly must be working very hard to conceal her feelings at home. She asks you who you think might be able to help and you give her brochures from a few local youth mental health services. Molly decides she wants to make the appointment herself, with her mother in the room. An appointment is made for the following week.

Action 5: encourage other supports

Other supports can include supportive people as well as self-help strategies.

Supportive people can include family and friends. It can be a good idea for family and friends to learn as much as they can about the problem. If they understand how difficult things can be, they are less likely to put pressure on the young person to do more than they are able to or to expect too much of them.

Self-help groups can also be useful, particularly self-help groups of other young people. If the young person is at school or university, it is a good idea for key people there to know what is going on. It may be possible to make allowances for late submission of assignments or to sit exams at a time when the young person is best able to think clearly; for example, if the young person is depressed, they may function better in the afternoon than they do first thing in the morning.

Self-help strategies can also help. For example, there is some evidence that regular exercise can help adults with depression, and most experts agree that it is probably helpful for adolescents as well. Other effective self-help strategies include getting a massage, light therapy and relaxation therapy.

There are a lot of self-help strategies which do not have any evidence for their effectiveness and some which are potentially harmful. Self-help strategies are generally more effective with the guidance of a clinician and should not be seen as an alternative to professional help. In Australia, Beyond Blue has published a series of free booklets reviewing what works for depression and anxiety, including self-help methods.[11–13]

Encouraging Molly to use other supports

Molly's mother says that she wants to find out as much as she can about what Molly is experiencing so that she and Molly's father can be supportive. Before Molly and her mother leave your office, you ask Molly if she is willing to come back and talk to you about getting some extra support from the school. She agrees.

The following week, she comes back. She has had her first appointment with a psychologist and says that, although she doesn't feel much better, she feels more positive about the idea that she can get better. She says she is interested in finding out more about how the school can help.

You tell her that if she is willing to talk to the student support centre, there are things that the school can do to ensure that her grades are not adversely affected by her mental health problems, and you also tell her that there are people at the school who can provide additional support between her counselling appointments. She agrees to go with you to the student support centre.

You also ask her if the psychologist talked about self-help strategies. Molly says that she has decided to start getting some more exercise and hopes to join the volleyball team again for training sessions. She has also been given a workbook by her psychologist that should help her to put what she learns each week into practice.

Conclusion

Adolescence and young adulthood is the peak age of onset for mental illness, but many young people do not receive help for their problems. If a young person has an adult in their life with the skills and knowledge to recognise when a mental health problem is developing and offer appropriate support, it is more likely that help will be sought. MHFA training can equip adults with these skills.

References

1 Kitchener BA, Jorm AF, Kelly CM. *Mental Health First Aid International manual.* Melbourne: Mental Health First Aid International; 2015.

2 Kelly CM, Kitchener BA, Jorm AF. *Youth Mental Health First Aid: a manual for adults assisting young people.* 4th ed. Melbourne: Mental Health First Aid Australia; 2017.

3 Kessler RC, Berglund P, Demler O, Jin R, Merikangas KR, Walters EE. Lifetime prevalence and age-of-onset distributions of DSM-IV disorders in the National Comorbidity Survey Replication. *Archives of General Psychiatry* 2005;62(6):593–602.

4 Jorm AF, Wright A, Morgan AJ. Where to seek help for a mental disorder? National survey of the beliefs of Australian youth and their parents. *Medical Journal of Australia* 2007;187(10):556–60.

5 Kitchener BA, Jorm AF. Mental Health First Aid: an international programme for early intervention. *Early Intervention in Psychiatry* 2008;2(1):55–61.

6 Morgan AJ, Ross A, Reavley NJ. Systematic review and meta-analysis of Mental Health First Aid training: effects on knowledge, stigma, and helping behaviour. *PLoS One* 2018;13(5):e0197102.
7 Jorm AF, Kitchener BA, Fischer J, Cvetkovski S. Mental Health First Aid training by e-learning: a randomized controlled trial. *Australian and New Zealand Journal of Psychiatry* 2010;44(12):1072–81.
8 Jorm AF, Kitchener BA, Sawyer MG, Scales H, Cvetkovski S. Mental Health First Aid training for high school teachers: a cluster randomized trial. *BMC Psychiatry* 2010;10:51.
9 Morgan AJ, Fischer JA, Hart, Kelly CM, Kitchener BA, Reavley NJ, et al. Does Mental Health First Aid training improve the mental health of aid recipients? The training for parents of teenagers randomised controlled trial. *BMC Psychiatry* 2019;19:99.
10 Klonsky ED, Muehlenkamp JJ. Self-injury: a research review for the practitioner. *Journal of Clinical Psychology* 2007;63(11):1045–56.
11 Purcell R, Ryan S, Scanlan F, Morgan A, Callahan P, Allen NB, et al. *A guide to what works for depression in young people*. 2nd ed. Melbourne: beyondblue; 2013.
12 Jorm AF, Allen NB, Morgan AJ, Ryan S, Purcell R. *A guide to what works for depression*. 2nd ed. Melbourne: beyondblue; 2013.
13 Reavley NJ, Allen NB, Jorm AF, Morgan AJ, Ryan S, Purcell R. *A guide to what works for anxiety*. 2nd ed. Melbourne: beyondblue; 2013.

9 E-mental health for young people

Jack Cotter and Sandra Bucci

The advent of e-Health

The past two decades have seen exponential growth in the use of the internet, with current estimates suggesting there are over three billion users worldwide. Wireless internet connections have become widespread and are now common among households and businesses across the world, while high-speed 4G connections provide many with access to the internet while on the move. This has paved the way for the development of new forms of portable technology such as smartphones and tablet computers, which have revolutionised how we engage with the internet. Software applications ('apps') for these devices are relatively easy to develop and can be made widely available for use. For young people in particular, accessing the internet and using these technologies have become routine aspects of daily life. Many are now 'digital natives' having grown up since childhood using modern computing technology, meaning they quickly adapt to both new hardware and software and rapidly learn to operate it intuitively.

Given this wide scale uptake, clinicians and researchers have begun to question whether the internet and these associated digital technologies could play a beneficial role in various aspects of healthcare. This has been termed 'e-Health' and is an area emerging from its relative infancy, attracting an ever-increasing amount of interest and funding. Internet-enabled devices can provide access to a wide range of healthcare resources, including information about an illness, peer support and real-time web-based consultation with healthcare professionals (often referred to as 'telehealth'). Increasingly, these are also being used to electronically monitor health and wellbeing, while there is a burgeoning literature examining the efficacy of e-Health interventions for the treatment of a wide variety of health issues, ranging from smoking cessation and insomnia, to chronic pain, diabetes management and human immunodeficiency virus (HIV) prevention.[1–5]

The potential application of internet and modern digital technologies to enhance mental healthcare is another area that has received considerable clinical interest. This is known as e-mental health and "encompasses the use of digital technologies and new media for the delivery of screening, health promotion, prevention, early intervention, treatment, or relapse prevention as well as for improvement of health care delivery (e.g., electronic patient files), professional education (e-learning), and online research in the field of mental health".[6] Major consortiums of researchers, clinicians and service-users have publicly recognised the potential for 'digital mental health' and set out priorities and considerations for future research in these areas.[7,8] National health institutions and professional bodies have also begun to adopt these technologies and have published specific guidelines and ethical standards in an effort to ensure quality, safety and patient security remain paramount during their continued development and integration into mainstream clinical services.

Young people are often reluctant to seek professional mental healthcare and are also likely to face inadequate access to resources and treatment, yet this is a group for whom early intervention would likely lead to reduced symptom severity and functional disability in the long term. Perceived stigma and embarrassment, poor understanding and recognition of symptoms, a preference for self-reliance and lack of accessibility have all been identified as key barriers to mental health help-seeking among young people.[9] Given the nature and capabilities of these technologies, coupled with their existing habitual use among young people, e-mental health approaches may be particularly useful in helping to overcome a number of these issues. In this chapter, we will provide an overview of related resources available to young people and consider the key strengths and limitations of these novel methods.

The internet as an information source

The internet has become one of the main routes through which the public access health-related information. A general population survey of 14,956 people conducted in 2007 across seven European countries reported that over 50% of responders had used the internet for health-related purposes.[10] This was a substantial rise from previous years, suggesting current estimates are likely to be much higher. There is evidence that people with mental health problems do not differ from others in the general population in how they engage with and use the internet,[11,12] and it is likely that many individuals, particularly young people, will use it to gather information about any symptoms they are experiencing.[13,14] For many users, the privacy afforded by online resources when seeking mental health-related information is important, reducing the fear of stigma or embarrassment that may be associated with seeing a clinician or discussing psychiatric issues with friends or family. While this should not replace seeking formal clinical advice, these information sources have the potential to improve the recognition of psychiatric symptoms and the awareness of local mental health services that are available. Providing access to resources to inform young people's own decision-making is also likely to be viewed as empowering.

There are a wide range of websites available that provide mental health–related information. Centrally controlled government healthcare agency sites such as those run by the National Health Service in the UK (www.nhs.uk) and the National Institute of Mental Health in the US (www.nimh.nih.gov) provide information about symptoms and treatment as well as local services and ongoing clinical trials. Mental health charities such as Rethink Mental Illness (www.rethink.org), Mind (www.mind.org.uk), SANE Australia (www.sane.org) and the National Alliance on Mental Illness (www.nami.org) have also developed their own websites providing illness-related information, opportunities for support and stories based on personal accounts of lived experience. Following recognition of the importance of engaging young people, online resources specifically tailored towards the needs of this particular group have been developed. ReachOut (au.reachout.com) and *headspace* (www.headspace.org.au) have created websites that cover a range of day-to-day troubles and mental health issues faced by young Australians. Furthermore, *eheadspace*, part of the Australian *headspace* initiative, is a confidential, free and secure site for young people to discuss problems with qualified youth mental health professionals. In the UK, organisations such as YoungMinds (www.youngminds.org.uk) provide online resources specifically targeted at young people. Collectively, these have been designed with the intention to improve mental health literacy, reduce stigma and facilitate help-seeking among young people and families affected by mental health problems.

There has also been a shift from users being passive readers to active contributors to online resources and content. These are known as 'Web 2.0' sources and have been recognised as being increasingly important for providing health-related information. The leading example of this is Wikipedia, which is among the world's most frequently accessed websites. Wikipedia differs from the aforementioned examples in that it allows readers to modify content on its site. While there are potential pitfalls and dangers inherent with this approach, it allows a range of professionals, including researchers and clinicians with a broad spectrum of interests, to provide a diverse and up-to-date overview of topics while also allowing those with personal experience to contribute. Other examples include social media and networking sites such as Facebook, Twitter and YouTube. These have been identified as potentially important sources for providing mental health–related psychoeducation and support to young people, though there is currently a lack of high-quality evidence for their efficacy.[15] The inclusion of both information and individuals' 'recovery stories' on these platforms, for example, may help others to understand and overcome mental health issues they are facing and provide a positive message of hope for the future.

There is a concern that young people who have had no previous contact with clinical services and are seeking information about mental health issues for the first time may have difficulty distinguishing between high- and low-quality sources of information. While it remains a contentious issue, evidence suggests that the quality of mental health information available online is generally improving.[16,17] A team of expert researchers and clinicians from the Orygen Youth Health Research Centre examined the quality of 14 websites commonly used by the general public to access information on schizophrenia and depression.[18] They evaluated the content for key illness-related topics and rated them for accuracy, up-to-dateness, breadth of coverage, referencing and readability. All sources were reported to be reasonably accurate. Wikipedia was rated highest for accuracy, up-to-dateness and references for both schizophrenia and depression, but among the poorest for readability, while ratings suggested many centrally controlled websites failed to keep their information up-to-date. The authors concluded that many of these websites (including Wikipedia) are appropriate to recommend to patients as a general resource for information on schizophrenia and depression.

Using the internet to promote help-seeking among young people

Many hope that online resources and signposting to local clinical services will ultimately help to promote help-seeking among young people experiencing mental health difficulties. In 2013, Kauer and colleagues performed a systematic review investigating the effectiveness of online services in facilitating mental health help-seeking among individuals aged 14–25 years.[19] This included 18 studies that evaluated a range of internet-based interventions, including self-help programmes, psychoeducation and online screening tools. The authors reported that randomised controlled trials found no changes in help-seeking behaviour, though lower-quality studies did report some significant benefits. Subsequent work by Taylor-Rodgers and Batterham evaluated mental health help-seeking among 67 students aged 18–25 years.[20] Participants were randomised to receive either a three-week online psychoeducation intervention providing information about depression, anxiety and suicide or to a control arm providing information about general well-being. Those randomised to receive psychoeducation reported increased help-seeking attitudes and intentions. They also exhibited improved mental health literacy with regards to anxiety but not depression or suicidality, while depression-related stigma also decreased. Recent pilot work has also demonstrated the acceptability and feasibility of an online navigation tool developed specifically for young people that matches their mental health issues, symptom severity and service-type preferences with appropriate youth-friendly services.[21] While some encouraging findings have been noted, these studies collectively suggest that there is still much more to learn and incorporate into online resources in order to enhance their effectiveness in promoting help-seeking among young people experiencing mental health problems.

Using digital interventions to improve clinical outcomes

The potential to enhance treatment accessibility using the internet and associated digital technologies is viewed as an important area for exploration that may help to overcome challenges associated with existing mental health treatment provision. Patients often face lengthy waiting lists with limited, if any, access to psychotherapeutic support. Digital interventions have the potential to provide rapid access to some forms of treatment that would not otherwise be immediately available. In theory, these need not be restricted by time as with traditional face-to-face appointments, and could be available 24 hours a day, seven days a week, 365 days a year, providing people with out of hours help that may otherwise be difficult to obtain. Resources could plausibly be accessed at home, in the community or on the move through a variety of platforms, as and when required. These may also be useful for individuals who live in rural areas, long distances from services or those who cannot afford transport costs, as well as people who may have physical impairments or psychological issues that make it difficult to attend services.

With the ever-increasing demand for services and rising costs associated with mental healthcare, there is also a need for effective, low cost interventions. Online resources and apps can be relatively cheap to develop and maintain and can be made available to a large number of individuals simultaneously. If digital interventions can be shown to be clinically effective then this approach has the potential to provide a cost-effective alternative to face-to-face therapy, capable of easing the burden on more traditional (and expensive) modes of treatment. This has been recognised by healthcare agencies such as the NHS, which has provided a list of endorsed low-intensity intervention apps for mental health–related issues including stress, anxiety and low mood (www.nhs.uk/apps-library). A number of commercial organisations have also identified the opportunities afforded by modern technologies for providing psychotherapy and support for mental health symptoms and have built novel healthcare businesses based on both therapist and artificial intelligence (AI)–driven approaches to real-time, on-demand treatment.

Interventions delivered over the internet or as a smartphone app comprise a diverse and rapidly evolving clinical field. E-mental health–based interventions have been designed for individuals experiencing various mental health problems including depression, eating disorders, anxiety, bipolar disorder and psychosis and have been developed in an effort to improve outcomes including psychiatric symptom severity, social functioning and treatment adherence.[22–26] These interventions may be delivered in isolation or as a precursor, adjunct or following traditional face-to-face therapy and may or may not include therapist contact, the importance of which remains an area of continued debate. Some interventions have been designed to be openly available, while others require referral from a clinician for access.

Much of the research to date has focused on examining the effectiveness of cognitive-behavioural–informed therapies (CBT), particularly for depression, in those with mild to moderately severe forms of illness. These typically consist of a set of modules to be completed, followed by additional homework to be completed between sessions. Users can be provided with questionnaires throughout treatment to monitor symptoms, safety and progress. In a systematic review evaluating online interventions for the treatment of depression in young people aged 12–25 years, Rice and colleagues concluded that those that incorporated cognitive behavioural elements appeared promising for reducing depressive symptoms.[22] Increasingly, apps are now being developed to deliver real-time CBT-based strategies to people who report experiencing an exacerbation in mental health symptoms during ongoing smartphone-based symptom monitoring. For example, a smartphone app designed to improve motivation in young people with a diagnosis of schizophrenia has recently published encouraging results from a 12-week pilot trial. The authors reported that those patients randomised to receive the 'personalized real-time intervention for motivational enhancement' (PRIME) app, which included goal achievement tracking, CBT-based coaching and peer support, exhibited significantly greater improvements in mood and motivation post-treatment compared to waitlist controls.[27] Other digital interventions trialled in young people include treatments for anxiety and obsessive-compulsive disorder, as well as efforts to reduce substance misuse and promote general well-being.[28–31] These early stage studies have all generally reported positive results, in combination with a range of important considerations for future research. As a result of the detrimental impact that mental health problems can have on families, efforts are also currently underway to evaluate online interventions for carers of young people recovering from psychosis.[32]

In addition to these more conventional psychotherapy-based approaches, a number of novel cognitive neuroscience-informed digital interventions are also currently in development. This includes 'Temstem', a smartphone app that uses language games in an effort to reduce distress and improve social functioning in people who experience auditory verbal hallucinations.[33] These games were designed based on neuropsychological studies that suggest that activation of particular areas of the brain during language tasks can help to temporarily suppress auditory verbal hallucinations. Similarly, playing a visuospatial task (Tetris) in the emergency department has been shown in a proof-of-concept trial to prevent the formation of intrusive memories after exposure to a traumatic event.[34] A modified N-back task that uses affective facial stimuli has also reported promising results for reducing mood symptoms in patients with major depressive disorder[35] and is the subject of ongoing commercial development. While these remain in an early stage of development, these novel approaches have the potential, if shown to be effective in more definitive studies, to be integrated into apps for routine use by individuals as an adjunct to standard treatment to enhance their well-being.

The past few decades have also seen rapid advances in virtual reality (VR) technology, leading to interest in its potential use for the purposes of mental health research and treatment. This technology has been used in an effort to explore clinical symptoms and cognitive functioning, as well as a novel method to deliver more ecologically valid forms of interventions, such as social skills training and psychotherapy.[36] Virtual reality environments, in which participants interact with computer-controlled situations or avatars, enable clinicians to expose patients to challenging and stressful scenarios while observing and helping to modify their responses. For example, preliminary evidence suggests that VR may be useful for augmenting standard CBT for those with social anxiety or psychosis experiencing paranoid ideation by providing personalised and graded exposure to stressful social situations.[37] A series of recent studies have also been published based on the use of AVATAR therapy, a system developed to help people experiencing auditory hallucinations to challenge their beliefs about the perceived power and control of the voices they hear. Participants are asked to create an avatar based on the entity that they believe is talking to them. They then engage in a conversation with the avatar of their voice, which is controlled by a therapist who becomes less hostile and concedes power over the course of therapy. Beneficial results have been reported using this intervention, including a reduction in the severity of persistent auditory verbal hallucinations among users.[38,39]

Digital monitoring

Mental health problems are heterogeneous and associated with varied clinical profiles and trajectories. Through the use of daily or weekly monitoring assessments, digital technologies have the potential to facilitate self-management, identify early signs of elevated relapse risk, provide medical staff with more detailed information to inform clinical decision-making and help overcome issues such as non-attendance at scheduled clinical appointments, memory problems and recall biases. Efforts in this emerging area to date have involved both 'active' and 'passive' approaches to digital assessment based on software and sensor data. Active measures (similar to the traditional 'ecological momentary assessment' [EMA] approach) require participants to engage with a specific task, such as answering questions about their symptoms, in response to prompted assessments over a period of time. Passive measures are typically collected 'in the background' based on data derived from smartphones or wearable devices and can include a broad spectrum of information such as typing and scrolling speed, heart rate, location tracking and the number of messages sent to others.

A number of specialist 'early warning system' smartphone apps have been developed that aim to prevent relapse and allow people with mental health difficulties to better monitor and manage their symptoms. Users typically receive prompts at semi-random times and are asked to complete a range of symptom-related questions on their smartphone. This data is wirelessly uploaded to a secure central server which can be accessed by their care team in real time. These also typically alert both the patient and their clinical team to indications of relapse in an effort to enhance early intervention. The symptom data can also be accessed to inform clinical consultations and to allow users to monitor how they have been feeling over time. Examples include a smartphone app recently developed specifically for young people attending early psychosis services.[40] The app prompts users to input information regarding their symptoms and uploads this to a secure web-portal where their care team can remotely monitor their well-being using an online dashboard and receive alerts regarding symptom exacerbations or medication non-adherence. Use of the app has been shown to be feasible and acceptable among service users, with high comparability reported between self- and clinician-rated psychotic and mood symptom assessments. As with several of the other apps currently in development, efforts are underway to demonstrate its effectiveness in clinical practice for detecting relapse and facilitating early intervention.

There has also been a great deal of interest in the potential for harnessing passively collected data from devices themselves in order to inform both our understanding of mental health problems and their clinical management. This has been referred to as digital phenotyping, 'the moment-by-moment quantification of the individual-level human phenotype in situ using data from smartphones and other personal digital devices'.[41] These devices have the potential to provide additional objective and diverse data points to compliment the limited snapshot of information typically provided during clinical or research visits. In addition, these methods have the potential to overcome problems associated with patient self-report measures, such as issues with low literacy, reporting biases, cognitive deficits and motivation.

While this is an area still very much in its infancy, there have been a number of recent small-scale studies that have reported promising results, paving the way for further developments in this field. In a study of 47 young adult students, geospatial activity and sleep duration were associated with daily stress levels. Sensor-derived speech duration, geospatial activity and sleep duration were also associated with changes in depression, and sensor-derived kinaesthetic activity was associated with loneliness.[42] A recent pilot study in people with a diagnosis of schizophrenia demonstrated that a combination of passive and active data collected using a smartphone app could detect patterns of behavioural anomalies (based on geolocation tracking and social behaviour derived from text messaging and call logs) that significantly predicted relapse two weeks prior to occurrence.[43] Other studies have also reported the ability to predict clinical symptom scores based only on passively collected sensor data.[44,45]

Poor data quality due to missing data, loss of internet connectivity or failure to carry or charge a smartphone or wearable device are key concerns in this area, yet this data has also been shown to contain potentially useful information. Torous and colleagues reported that passively collected metadata temporally correlated with symptom measures. For example, individuals reporting more severe negative symptoms and anhedonia took longer to complete EMA-based surveys and exhibited lower completion rates.[46] This suggests that assessing how patients engage with these technologies may also be useful. Other important developments in this field include the publication of statistical recommendations and the creation of open-access research platforms to help with the collection and analysis of these complex and diverse datasets.[47,48]

Considerations for future research

Patient acceptability and engagement

There are a number of important factors to consider in both the design and evaluation of e-mental health resources. Critics have suggested that there is a danger that these technologies are novel and engaging to start with, but that user interest fades over time or when they are no longer incentivised to participate in research studies. High levels of attrition and disengagement remain an important issue in this field, with many who are provided with access to digital resources never or rarely logging in to use them. While disengagement with treatment is far from a problem faced exclusively by interventions delivered online, it remains an important issue to consider in the evaluation of these approaches. It is important in the development, design and delivery of novel healthcare technology to ensure service user, carer, as well as clinician involvement occurs from the outset. Such efforts are likely to improve patient acceptability and engagement, as well as ensure suitable cultural adaptation where relevant.

It is also crucial to consider health-specific issues in the development of e-mental health tools. Intrinsic motivation is required for young people to login and engage with online resources. This may be particularly problematic for people who experience depression or severe negative symptoms associated with a diagnosis of schizophrenia, where an individual might experience a general lack of interest and motivation, as well as problems with concentration. As with traditional face-to-face treatment, evidence suggests e-Health interventions are more effective and well adhered to when they are tailored to the specific needs of the individual. A good example of this is the 'Active Assistance for Psychological Therapy' (Actissist) app, a smartphone application designed for young people with early psychosis. The app was specifically developed with careful consideration of factors such as cognitive impairment, positive and negative psychotic symptoms, and low reading levels, which are all potentially problematic in this group. The resulting app was deemed highly acceptable by users, produced high reported levels of engagement and showed promising effects on symptom reduction.[49]

It seems reasonable to assume that young people are likely to engage with e-Health given the routine use of online resources by this group. However, it is unlikely that all individuals are comfortable, willing or suited to undergoing digital monitoring or treatment. An improved understanding of which individuals are genuinely likely to benefit from a digital health tool is important to optimise developments in this emerging field.

Dangers, security and ethics

The internet has revolutionised how we access information and communicate with others around the world; however, unsupervised online forums, chat rooms and social networking sites hold potential dangers for young people with mental health difficulties. Unmoderated sites could attract adults to interact with potentially vulnerable young people. A growing trend in online abuse and harassment, or 'cyberbullying', has also been reported on social networking sites. This may be particularly problematic among young people with mental health issues who already experience bullying or have a history of being bullied in their daily lives. Social networking and mobile phones provide opportunities for victims to continue to receive abuse at times when they could otherwise escape torment.

Risk of exposure to potentially negative and inaccurate online content also poses a risk to young people. While the overwhelming majority of online health resources are intended to assist people in accessing information and support, there are a small minority of websites that publicise content that is potentially damaging to health and well-being. This includes sites that praise and seek to normalise issues such as eating disorders. For example, 'Pro-ana' sites exist that provide tips on how to avoid eating while hiding it from friends and family, as well as bombarding readers with images of people and celebrities as 'thinspiration' to encourage and promote such behaviours. Similarly, sites and message boards where individuals openly discuss self-harming methods may intensify such issues in vulnerable individuals.

Establishing and maintaining privacy and confidentiality are key in all aspects of healthcare and should remain central in the development of new digital technologies. Important safety considerations for the development and evaluation of e-mental health interventions have been discussed in detail elsewhere.[50] In short, these have often been overlooked. Data should be appropriately handled and stored and should be protected from unauthorised access or modification. Security measures need to be put in place to safeguard users should the device be lost, stolen or hacked. This should include encrypting data and using passwords to access programmes or websites. In addition, care providers have a moral obligation to safeguard young people should they disclose information relating to harm to themselves or others. There is also a danger to the care provider of financial or legal consequences should anything happen to the person following disclosure of relevant information that was not acted on. High frequency assessments using digital monitoring are likely to result in a substantial rise in the number of incidences of suicidal behaviour and self-harm reports, as well as clinical relapse warnings. An important consideration in the ongoing development of these tools will, therefore, be how to manage any risks that may be flagged, who will be responsible for this and how it will be communicated both to the individual and their clinical team.

Research methodology

While there has been a great deal of interest in the potential integration of digital technologies into routine healthcare, the evidence base for these approaches remains at an early stage in its development. Many projects to date have been pilot studies, conducted over short durations with little understanding of their long-term utility. Randomised clinical trials are needed to control for placebo effects seen with digital health products. Much of the work to date has also been conducted in adults with established mental health problems. There is a need for more research examining these novel mental health technologies specifically among young people. Unfortunately, research projects are also typically a slow process. This issue may be particularly problematic for the field of e-Health where rapid technical advances and changes in user behaviour mean that there is a danger that certain technologies and research findings quickly become outdated.[51] There is a need for agile approaches that takes these changes in hardware, software and user preferences into account.

An important consideration for the routine uptake of digital technologies in healthcare systems is how these will integrate within existing processes, such as patients' medical records, and how clinicians will be trained to use this information effectively. Other key issues, such as the impact of replacing face-to-face interventions with digital interventions and understanding at what stage these are most effective in the treatment pathway, are currently unknown. Finally, routine adoption of digital health technologies among healthcare providers will likely require demonstration that these approaches are cost as well as clinically effective.

Conclusions

E-mental health resources have important implications for youth mental health in terms of providing illness-related information, facilitating help-seeking, monitoring symptoms and well-being, and providing clinical support. While the research in this field to date has been encouraging, it has also highlighted that we still have much to learn to optimise e-mental health approaches. Efforts should be made to improve awareness of high-quality digital health resources that are available to both young people and the wider public to improve mental health literacy, especially for recognising symptoms and services that are available. This and other strategies have the potential to play an important role in battling stigma and ultimately improve help-seeking among people of all ages. A range of diverse digital interventions are also currently in the early stages of development which may help to overcome practical issues associated with existing mental health services. While early evidence suggests that these digital interventions do demonstrate clinical potential and appear to be both feasible and acceptable among prospective end users, the research to date is based predominantly on a series of small pilot studies. Larger trials are currently ongoing which should provide more conclusive results. We have also identified a number of important factors that need to be considered prior to the rollout of these technologies for routine healthcare purposes, particularly among vulnerable young people experiencing mental health problems.

References

1 Taylor GMJ, Dalili MN, Semwal M, Civljak M, Sheikh A, Car J. Internet-based interventions for smoking cessation. *Cochrane Database of Systematic Reviews* 2017;9:CD007078.
2 Zachariae R, Lyby MS, Ritterband LM, O'Toole MS. Efficacy of internet-delivered cognitive-behavioral therapy for insomnia – a systematic review and meta-analysis of randomized controlled trials. *Sleep Medicine Reviews* 2016;30:1–10.
3 Fisher E, Law E, Dudeney J, Eccleston C, Palermo TM. Psychological therapies (remotely delivered) for the management of chronic and recurrent pain in children and adolescents. *Cochrane Database of Systematic Reviews* 2019;4:CD011118.
4 Pal K, Eastwood SV, Michie S, Farmer AJ, Barnard ML, Peacock R, et al. Computer-based diabetes self-management interventions for adults with type 2 diabetes mellitus. *Cochrane Database of Systematic Reviews* 2013;3:CD008776.
5 Nguyen LH, Tran BX, Rocha LEC, Nguyen HLT, Yang C, Latkin CA, et al. A systematic review of eHealth interventions addressing HIV/STI prevention among men who have sex with men. *AIDS and Behavior* 2019;23(9):2253–72.
6 Riper H, Andersson G, Christensen H, Cuijpers P, Lange A, Eysenbach G. Theme issue on e-mental health: a growing field in internet research. *Journal of Medical Internet Research* 2010;12(5):e74.
7 Bhugra D, Tasman A, Pathare S, Priebe S, Smith S, Torous J, et al. The WPA-Lancet Psychiatry Commission on the future of psychiatry. *Lancet Psychiatry* 2017;4(10):775–818.
8 Collins PY, Patel V, Joestl SS, March D, Insel TR, Daar AS. Grand challenges in global mental health. *Nature* 2011;475(7354):27–30.
9 Gulliver A, Griffiths KM, Christensen H. Perceived barriers and facilitators to mental health help-seeking in young people: a systematic review. *BMC Psychiatry* 2010;10:113.

10 Kummervold PE, Chronaki CE, Lausen B, Prokosch HU, Rasmussen J, Santana S, et al. eHealth trends in Europe 2005–2007: a population-based survey. *Journal of Medical Internet Research* 2008;10(4):e42.
11 Schrank B, Sibitz I, Unger A, Amering M. How patients with schizophrenia use the internet: qualitative study. *Journal of Medical Internet Research* 2010;12(5):e70.
12 Spinzy Y, Nitzan U, Becker G, Bloch Y, Fennig S. Does the internet offer social opportunities for individuals with schizophrenia? A cross-sectional pilot study. *Psychiatry Research* 2012;198(2):319–20.
13 Conell J, Bauer R, Glenn T, Alda M, Ardau R, Baune BT, et al. Online information seeking by patients with bipolar disorder: results from an international multisite survey. *International Journal of Bipolar Disorders* 2016;4(1):17.
14 Kalckreuth S, Trefflich F, Rummel-Kluge C. Mental health related internet use among psychiatric patients: a cross-sectional analysis. *BMC Psychiatry* 2014;14:368.
15 Ridout B, Campbell A. The use of social networking sites in mental health interventions for young people: systematic review. *Journal of Medical Internet Research* 2018;20(12):e12244.
16 Reavley NJ, Jorm AF. The quality of mental disorder information websites: a review. *Patient Education and Counseling* 2011;85(2):e16–25.
17 Grohol JM, Slimowicz J, Granda R. The quality of mental health information commonly searched for on the internet. *Cyberpsychology, Behavior and Social Networking* 2014;17(4):216–21.
18 Reavley NJ, Mackinnon AJ, Morgan AJ, Alvarez-Jimenez M, Hetrick SE, Killackey E, et al. Quality of information sources about mental disorders: a comparison of Wikipedia with centrally controlled web and printed sources. *Psychological Medicine* 2012;42(8):1753–62.
19 Kauer SD, Mangan C, Sanci L. Do online mental health services improve help-seeking for young people? A systematic review. *Journal of Medical Internet Research* 2014;16(3):e66.
20 Taylor-Rodgers E, Batterham PJ. Evaluation of an online psychoeducation intervention to promote mental health help seeking attitudes and intentions among young adults: randomised controlled trial. *Journal of Affective Disorders* 2014;168:65–71.
21 Kauer SD, Buhagiar K, Blake V, Cotton S, Sanci L. Facilitating mental health help-seeking by young adults with a dedicated online program: a feasibility study of Link. *BMJ Open* 2017;7(7):e015303.
22 Rice SM, Goodall J, Hetrick SE, Parker AG, Gilbertson T, Amminger GP, et al. Online and social networking interventions for the treatment of depression in young people: a systematic review. *Journal of Medical Internet Research* 2014;16(9):e206.
23 Loucas CE, Fairburn CG, Whittington C, Pennant ME, Stockton S, Kendall T. E-therapy in the treatment and prevention of eating disorders: a systematic review and meta-analysis. *Behaviour Research and Therapy* 2014;63:122–31.
24 Firth J, Torous J, Nicholas J, Carney R, Rosenbaum S, Sarris J. Can smartphone mental health interventions reduce symptoms of anxiety? A meta-analysis of randomized controlled trials. *Journal of Affective Disorders* 2017;218:15–22.
25 Hidalgo-Mazzei D, Mateu A, Reinares M, Matic A, Vieta E, Colom F. Internet-based psychological interventions for bipolar disorder: review of the present and insights into the future. *Journal of Affective Disorders* 2015;188:1–13.
26 Alvarez-Jimenez M, Alcazar-Corcoles MA, González-Blanch C, Bendall S, McGorry PD, Gleeson JF. Online, social media and mobile technologies for psychosis treatment: a systematic review on novel user-led interventions. *Schizophrenia Research* 2014;156(1):96–106.

27 Schlosser DA, Campellone TR, Truong B, Etter K, Vergani S, Komaiko K, et al. Efficacy of PRIME, a mobile app intervention designed to improve motivation in young people with schizophrenia. *Schizophrenia Bulletin* 2018;44(5):1010–20.

28 March S, Spence SH, Donovan CL, Kenardy JA. Large-scale dissemination of internet-based cognitive behavioral therapy for youth anxiety: feasibility and acceptability study. *Journal of Medical Internet Research* 2018;20(7):e234.

29 Lenhard F, Andersson E, Mataix-Cols D, Rück C, Vigerland S, Högström J, et al. Therapist-guided, internet-delivered cognitive-behavioral therapy for adolescents with obsessive-compulsive disorder: a randomized controlled trial. *Journal of the American Academy of Child and Adolescent Psychiatry* 2017;56(1):10–19.e2.

30 Dick S, Whelan E, Davoren MP, Dockray S, Heavin C, Linehan C, et al. A systematic review of the effectiveness of digital interventions for illicit substance misuse harm reduction in third-level students. *BMC Public Health* 2019;19(1):1244.

31 Bannink R, Broeren S, Joosten-van Zwanenburg E, van As E, van de Looij-Jansen P, Raat H. Effectiveness of a web-based tailored intervention (E-health4Uth) and consultation to promote adolescents' health: randomized controlled trial. *Journal of Medical Internet Research* 2014;16(5):e143.

32 Gleeson J, Lederman R, Herrman H, Koval P, Eleftheriadis D, Bendall S, et al. Moderated online social therapy for carers of young people recovering from first-episode psychosis: study protocol for a randomised controlled trial. *Trials* 2017;18(1):27.

33 Jongeneel A, Scheffers D, Tromp N, Nuij C, Delespaul P, Riper H, et al. Reducing distress and improving social functioning in daily life in people with auditory verbal hallucinations: study protocol for the 'Temstem' randomised controlled trial. *BMJ Open* 2018;8(3):e020537.

34 Iyadurai L, Blackwell SE, Meiser-Stedman R, Watson PC, Bonsall MB, Geddes JR, et al. Preventing intrusive memories after trauma via a brief intervention involving Tetris computer game play in the emergency department: a proof-of-concept randomized controlled trial. *Molecular Psychiatry* 2018;23(3):674–82.

35 Iacoviello BM, Murrough JW, Hoch MM, Huryk KM, Collins KA, Cutter GR, et al. A randomized, controlled pilot trial of the emotional faces memory task: a digital therapeutic for depression. *NPJ Digital Medicine* 2018;1:21.

36 Rus-Calafell M, Garety P, Sason E, Craig TJK, Valmaggia LR. Virtual reality in the assessment and treatment of psychosis: a systematic review of its utility, acceptability and effectiveness. *Psychological Medicine* 2018;48(3):362–91.

37 Pot-Kolder RMCA, Geraets CNW, Veling W, van Beilen M, Staring ABP, Gijsman HJ, et al. Virtual-reality-based cognitive behavioural therapy versus waiting list control for paranoid ideation and social avoidance in patients with psychotic disorders: a single-blind randomised controlled trial. *Lancet Psychiatry* 2018;5(3):217–26.

38 Craig TK, Rus-Calafell M, Ward T, Leff JP, Huckvale M, Howarth E, et al. AVATAR therapy for auditory verbal hallucinations in people with psychosis: a single-blind, randomised controlled trial. *Lancet Psychiatry* 2018;5(1):31–40.

39 du Sert OP, Potvin S, Lipp O, Dellazizzo L, Laurelli M, Breton R, et al. Virtual reality therapy for refractory auditory verbal hallucinations in schizophrenia: a pilot clinical trial. *Schizophrenia Research* 2018;197:176–81.

40 Niendam TA, Tully LM, Iosif AM, Kumar D, Nye KE, Denton JC, et al. Enhancing early psychosis treatment using smartphone technology: a longitudinal feasibility and validity study. *Journal of Psychiatric Research* 2018;96:239–46.

41 Onnela JP, Rauch SL. Harnessing smartphone-based digital phenotyping to enhance behavioral and mental health. *Neuropsychopharmacology* 2016;41(7):1691–6.

42 Ben-Zeev D, Scherer EA, Wang R, Xie H, Campbell AT. Next-generation psychiatric assessment: using smartphone sensors to monitor behavior and mental health. *Psychiatric Rehabilitation Journal* 2015;38(3):218–26.
43 Barnett I, Torous J, Staples P, Sandoval L, Keshavan M, Onnela JP. Relapse prediction in schizophrenia through digital phenotyping: a pilot study. *Neuropsychopharmacology* 2018;43(8):1660–6.
44 Stange JP, Zulueta J, Langenecker SA, Ryan KA, Piscitello A, Duffecy J, et al. Let your fingers do the talking: passive typing instability predicts future mood outcomes. *Bipolar Disorders* 2018;20(3):285–8.
45 Wang R, Wang W, Aung MSH, Ben-Zeev D, Brian R, Campbell AT, et al. Predicting symptom trajectories of schizophrenia using mobile sensing. *Proceedings of the ACM on Interactive, Mobile, Wearable and Ubiquitous Technologies* 2017;1(3):110.
46 Torous J, Staples P, Barnett I, Sandoval LR, Keshavan M, Onnela JP. Characterizing the clinical relevance of digital phenotyping data quality with applications to a cohort with schizophrenia. *NPJ Digital Medicine* 2018;1:15.
47 Barnett I, Torous J, Staples P, Keshavan M, Onnela JP. Beyond smartphones and sensors: choosing appropriate statistical methods for the analysis of longitudinal data. *Journal of the American Medical Informatics Association* 2018;25(12):1669–74.
48 Torous J, Kiang MV, Lorme J, Onnela JP. New tools for new research in psychiatry: a scalable and customizable platform to empower data driven smartphone research. *JMIR Mental Health* 2016;3(2):e16.
49 Bucci S, Barrowclough C, Ainsworth J, Machin M, Morris R, Berry K, et al. Actissist: proof-of-concept trial of a theory-driven digital intervention for psychosis. *Schizophrenia Bulletin* 2018;44(5):1070–80.
50 Bennett K, Bennett AJ, Griffiths KM. Security considerations for e-mental health interventions. *Journal of Medical Internet Research* 2010;12(5):e61.
51 Bucci S, Lewis S, Ainsworth J, Haddock G, Machin M, Berry K, et al. Digital interventions in severe mental health problems: lessons from the Actissist development and trial. *World Psychiatry* 2018;17(2):230–1.

10 Broad-spectrum interventions for early or emerging depression and anxiety in young people

Alexandra G. Parker and Rosemary Purcell

Introduction

Given that the majority of mental disorders have their onset in adolescence and early adulthood,[1,2] there is a clear imperative to effectively treat these disorders in a timely manner to prevent both functional disability (e.g., social, educational and vocational abilities and opportunities) as well as relapse and the potential persistence of illness. The phenomenology of mental disorders in young people is often complicated, however, with comorbidity or mixed symptom patterns common.[3] This likely reflects the early manifestation of these conditions being of an undifferentiated 'subsyndromal' nature, preceding the emergence of any clear-cut, differentiated diagnosable disorder.

The clinical staging model proposes that mental disorders develop from initial non-specific symptoms and syndromes.[4–6] Within this model, the natural history of adult-type mental disorders, such as psychotic illness, mood and anxiety disorders, and eating and substance use disorders, is hypothesised to consist of transitions from being asymptomatic and non-help-seeking (Stage 0), through a stage of undifferentiated general symptoms such as anxiety, depressive and somatic symptoms (Stage 1a), to a worsening of existing symptoms (or acquisition of new symptoms) whereby the person appears to have an attenuated form of a distinguishable mental disorder (Stage 1b). This progression may continue (at least for some individuals) until a 'threshold diagnosis' is reached, such as severe major depressive disorder, bipolar disorder or schizophreniform disorder (Stage 2).

The differentiation of early and milder clinical phenomena from those that accompany illness progression and chronicity lies at the heart of the clinical staging framework. This makes it potentially useful in the treatment of young people as it enables clinicians to select interventions not only relevant to earlier stages, but which may also be both more effective and arguably safer than treatments delivered later in the course (such as medications). Most importantly, this model provides a heuristic framework for the testing of *preventively oriented treatments*. In this context, simple and relatively broad-spectrum interventions could be effective if delivered during the emerging or early stages of symptom manifestation, such as Stages 1a and 1b in the aforementioned model. In the case of major depression, research demonstrates that intervening during these earlier stages is clinically warranted given the considerable impairment associated with 'subthreshold' depression, which is equally, if not more, prevalent than the diagnosable disorder.[7–9]

Given the high prevalence and associated disability of subthreshold and early stage mental disorders, interventions that target the early phases are especially warranted in order to meet the high level of need.[10] Most of this need is unmet however, with young people more likely than other age groups to experience inadequate resources and treatment, despite having the highest prevalence of illness.[11,12] Interventions during the early phases of the illness may be successful in not only reducing symptomatology, but also psychosocial and functional burden, and in preventing recurrence of symptoms or illness progression.[11,13]

It is possible that less complex interventions, often used as control conditions in prevention and intervention studies, may be effective in individuals experiencing emerging or subthreshold mental disorders. For example, mild, yet potentially serious disorders in an *early stage* may respond to relatively simple interventions such as psychosocial support (including befriending), self-help strategies and psychoeducation, which can be delivered by a range of allied health professionals in community and primary care settings. This approach is also likely to address the prevalence of these subthreshold or earlier stage presentations, potentially reducing the incidence of new cases or the progression to later and more serious stages of illness. In adult populations, evidence indicates that broad-spectrum interventions such as problem-solving therapy,[14,15] physical activity,[16–19] rest and relaxation,[20] and brief interventions that provide psychoeducation without mental state monitoring[21,22] are effective in reducing depression and anxiety symptoms.

The extent to which such broad-spectrum interventions are likely to be effective in young people is less researched, although the evidence base for psychosocial interventions in this age group is expanding. Indeed, several clinical practice guidelines for the management of depression recommend watchful waiting, psycho-education, guided self-help (e.g., online interventions), non-directive support and lifestyle advice (e.g., physical activity, sleep, healthy diet) for young people with mild symptoms of depression. These approaches can also be used in conjunction with psychological and/or pharmacological treatments for young people with more severe symptoms of major depressive disorder.[23]

This chapter reviews the evidence for such interventions, ranging from broad-spectrum self-help interventions to low-intensity interventions that are guided or delivered by professionals. The interventions have the capacity to be delivered or guided by a range of allied health professionals in community-based or primary care settings, thereby targeting high-prevalence disorders such as depression and anxiety. The assumption in this approach is that many of those who are experiencing subthreshold or early stages of high-prevalence disorders will respond to broad-spectrum interventions and will not require more intensive treatments.

Bibliotherapy

Bibliotherapy is a form of self-help that involves reading books or other written material, mostly in terms of how to use Cognitive Behaviour Therapy (CBT) on themselves. The books provide information and homework exercises that the readers work through on their own. It can be used alone, or guided by a health professional, who may assess the person to both identify their mental health needs and recommend the most appropriate self-help book.

Bibliotherapy with young people

A recent review of randomised controlled trials (RCTs) conducted in children and adolescents (aged 18 years or below) reported that bibliotherapy appears to be beneficial in treating depression but shows less robust effects for anxiety.[24] However, the authors also flagged the limited number of trials of bibliotherapy that have been conducted in young people, highlighting the need for further research in this area.

Bibliotherapy with adults

A meta-analysis of 17 trials comparing bibliotherapy to no treatment in individuals with mild to moderate depressive symptoms found bibliotherapy more effective in reducing symptoms than the control condition.[25] However, in all these studies, the participants were in contact with professionals (e.g., the bibliotherapy was 'guided'). As the book *Feeling Good* by David Burns is a common bibliographic resource,[26] another meta-analysis compared reading this book with no treatment and again reported positive results for the active intervention.[27] While an early meta-analysis indicated that guided bibliotherapy may be *as effective* as individual psychotherapy, this review included only four small trials.[28]

The effectiveness of bibliotherapy for the treatment of anxiety in adults has also been assessed in a number of RCTs. For example, CBT-oriented bibliotherapy has been found to be superior to no treatment for generalised anxiety disorder,[29] post-traumatic stress disorder (PTSD),[30] obsessive compulsive disorder (OCD)[31] and specific phobias.[32,33]

Summary of bibliotherapy

Bibliotherapy is effective in the short term for reducing symptoms of depression and anxiety in adults; however, there is far less evidence of its effectiveness compared to best-practice treatments recommended in clinical practice guidelines, such as CBT (and exposure therapy for anxiety). There is less evidence of its effectiveness among young people, particularly in terms of managing anxiety symptoms.

Physical activity interventions

Physical activity interventions for those with psychological difficulties, such as depression and/or anxiety, are proposed to improve mood by interrupting or distracting the person from dysfunctional or negative thoughts and by the release of endorphins via strenuous exercise.[34] Current Australian guidelines provided by the

Department of Health differ between children and adults. Those aged 5–17 years should be engaging in 60 minutes of moderate to vigorous physical activity per day that can be built throughout the day from shorter bouts of activity, including moderate activities such as brisk walking, bike riding and skateboarding, through to vigorous activities such as football, netball or sports training.[35] The guidelines also recommend at least three days per week of strengthening activities and focusing on reducing sedentary behaviours such as screen time. Those aged 18 years and over should be engaging in moderate-intensity physical activity on most, but preferably all, days, to build a total of 2.5–5 hours of moderate activity or 1.25–2.5 hours of vigorous activity per week.[36] Again, the guidelines recommend strengthening activities on two days per week and reducing sedentary behaviours.

Evidence for physical activity interventions in young people

A recent systematic review of physical activity interventions for depression in adolescents and young adults included 17 trials that were mainly based in schools or universities.[37] Although the quality of the included studies was variable, the meta-analysis showed a large beneficial effect in favour of the physical activity interventions, compared with control or comparison conditions. The authors concluded that supervised, aerobic-based activity of moderate-to-vigorous intensity, engaged in multiple times per week over eight or more weeks appeared to be the most effective approach for reducing symptoms of depression.[37] Biddle and Asare conducted a review of systematic reviews for physical activity interventions in children and adolescents across a range of mental health outcomes, including depression, anxiety and self-esteem.[38] Overall, the evidence from these studies supports an association between increased physical activity and improved mental health outcomes, although it should be noted that the quality of included studies was also variable and often involved non-clinical samples. This review did report, however, that consistent evidence supports the *reverse* relationship: that is, there is a strong association between increased sedentary activity (e.g., computer screen time) and poorer mental health.[38] There is also emerging evidence that other physical activities such as yoga may have beneficial effects on anxiety and depression symptoms in young people;[39] however, further, methodologically rigorous trials are needed to establish the benefit of these interventions.

Evidence of physical activity interventions in adults

A number of recent systematic reviews and meta-analyses of RCTs have reported that exercise interventions are effective at reducing both depression and anxiety symptoms in adults, resulting in small- to medium-sized beneficial treatment effects.[16–19]

Summary of physical activity interventions

There is an emerging evidence base supporting the effectiveness of physical activity interventions in reducing symptoms of depression and anxiety in young people; however, more high-quality trials are needed.

Problem-solving therapy

Problem-solving therapy (PST) aims to assist a person in learning to cope more effectively with their current difficulties as well as developing skills that can be used in other settings and times in their life.[15] The approach aims to identify current problems that are presumed to be related to psychological distress and to work towards future goals, rather than exploring past problems and mistakes.[40] PST was originally developed as a medium-length therapy, on average 8–16 sessions of 1.5–2 hours duration, but has more recently been applied over shorter time frames of six sessions of 30–60-minute durations.[15] Its recent applications progressively work through the following steps:[15,40,41] (1) identifying the problem/s, (2) selecting one or two key problems, (3) identifying goals, (4) generating solutions, (5) choosing a solution, (6) creating a SMART (specific, measurable, achievable, relevant, time-limited) plan and (7) reviewing progress / evaluating the plan. PST has been delivered by a range of mental health professionals and paraprofessionals such as psychologists,[42] trainee psychologists,[41,43] GPs and general practice nurses.[15]

Evidence of problem-solving therapy with young people

The effectiveness of this approach has been assessed in a number of RCTs, delivered either face-to-face or online. This includes a trial that randomly assigned high school and college students with major depression to six sessions of PST (lasting on average 40 minutes) or a wait-list control group.[41] PST was found to be more effective than the wait-list control group in reducing depression symptoms and suicidal ideation as well as increasing assertiveness and self-esteem. These changes were maintained at the 12-month follow-up assessment. In an earlier and smaller trial, PST was delivered in a group format over ten sessions lasting 90 minutes and was compared with supportive psychotherapy in 18–24-year-olds who had suicidal ideation and self-reported depressive symptoms.[43] PST was more effective than supportive therapy in reducing depressive disorder symptoms and hopelessness, but suicidal ideation decreased by a similar amount in both treatment groups. PST has also been delivered as an internet-based guided self-help intervention. Hoek et al. randomised 45 participants to PST or a wait-list control group.[44] Those in the PST arm received one online lesson per week for five weeks, progressively working through the steps of PST to generate a solution and evaluate the effectiveness of this. At the end of the 5-week intervention period and again at four months post-treatment, no group differences were found in depression and anxiety symptoms; however, only six participants completed the whole PST course and around 60% provided post-treatment and follow-up data. Although none of these trials compared PST to a treatment with a stronger evidence base, such as CBT, these studies provide initial support for PST as an intervention with younger age groups, in particular young people with depressive symptoms, though the way this is delivered may be important.

Evidence of problem-solving therapy with adults

A meta-analysis of 13 RCTs in adults with depression demonstrated that PST is an effective treatment for depression, compared to a wait-list control, treatment as usual (TAU), pill placebo and psychological placebo interventions.[14] A further meta-analysis of 31 studies which included interventions for mental and physical health problems found that PST was more effective than no treatment, TAU and attention placebo, and showed similar effectiveness as other interventions, such as CBT or pharmacotherapy.[42] An additional meta-analysis of 21 studies showed PST was as effective in reducing depression as other psychosocial interventions and pharmacotherapy and significantly more effective than no treatment or attention control groups.[45] Component analyses revealed that PST was most effective when the complete package was delivered, involving training in problem orientation and problem-solving skills to generate and implement solutions.

Summary of problem-solving therapy

PST appears to have face validity in its use with young people, focusing on current problems, working within a therapeutic partnership to generate alternative solutions and implement a testable strategy for change. The initial evidence appears to provide support for its effectiveness in improving outcomes in young people with depression symptoms. There is, however, a need for further evidence for its application to anxiety disorders.

Psychoeducation

Psychoeducation aims to help people understand the nature and aetiology of their mental health problems and how they can better deal with their symptoms (including triggers of a depressive or anxious episode, what exacerbates and what improves their mental health). As well as providing information, a therapist also works to support the person's strengths, resources and coping skills in order to avert relapses and to generally assist the person to manage their mental health in the long term. In clinical practice, psychoeducation tends to be used as an adjunct to other treatments such as CBT or supportive counselling rather than on its own. It can be delivered on an individual or group basis (the latter often including family members).

Psychoeducation with young people

A recent systematic review of psychoeducational interventions for adolescent depression reported that the limited number of studies, heterogeneity in delivery format (ranging from 'one-to-one' to multi-group and family approaches, completed at school, in a clinical service or online), and inconsistent approach to defining psychoeducational interventions make it difficult to compare programmes and measure overall effectiveness.[46] However, the authors concluded that these interventions may help to prevent and manage adolescent depression, as a first-line or adjunctive approach, with studies reporting beneficial effects both for young people and their families.

Psychoeducation with adults

A meta-analysis of four RCTs comparing psychoeducation to no treatment for adults with symptoms of depression (n = 3 studies) or general psychological distress (n = 1) found psychoeducation to be more effective than the control condition for reducing depressive symptoms, but not general distress.[47] In one of the included trials, the benefits were still present at 12-month follow-up.

Summary of psychoeducation

The limited evidence to date suggests that psychoeducation is effective in reducing depressive symptoms in both adults and young people, although further evidence is needed regarding its effects on anxiety symptoms. The evidence of its effectiveness is also comparatively weak when compared to best-practice treatments such as CBT. Further research evaluating psychoeducation for young people – with and without family involvement – is required before firm conclusions can be drawn.

Relaxation training

Relaxation training is most commonly used as a treatment for anxiety; however, as anxiety and depression are frequently comorbid, it has been suggested as an intervention for depression as well. This form of training helps to relax muscles, which are often tense in anxious individuals. There are several different types of relaxation training, the most common being 'progressive muscle relaxation', which teaches a person to relax by tensing and subsequently relaxing specific muscle groups. Relaxation training can be learned from a professional or utilised as self-help.

Relaxation with young people

Several RCTs have compared relaxation to other treatments among depressed adolescents. In one study, 32 depressed adolescent mothers were randomised to either ten sessions of massage therapy or relaxation.[48] Participants in the relaxation condition reported a significant improvement in anxiety, but not depressive symptoms. A second study randomised 48 adolescents with major depression to 5–8 sessions of either CBT or relaxation.[49] Relaxation reduced depressive symptoms by the end of the study but was less effective than CBT. At 6-month follow-up, however, there were few differences in depression levels between the two groups. Another study compared light therapy to relaxation in nine adolescents, five of whom were diagnosed with Seasonal Affective Disorder (SAD) and four with non-seasonal depression.[50] Relaxation therapy was more effective than light therapy for those with non-seasonal depression but had no benefit for the group with SAD.

Relaxation with adults

A systematic review of relaxation for depression reported mixed findings.[51] Meta-analysis of five RCTs showed that relaxation training was superior to no or minimal treatment in reducing depressive symptoms. However, data from an additional nine trials demonstrated that relaxation training was less effective when compared head-to-head with CBT.

Mixed results are also evident from RCTs of relaxation in adults with anxiety disorders. For example, meta-analysis indicates that relaxation training is more effective than no or minimal treatment, and that it has *equivalent outcomes* to CBT in individuals with generalised anxiety disorder.[52] However, relaxation training is less effective than CBT or behavioural interventions (e.g., exposure) for managing PTSD, OCD and social phobia.[53–56]

Summary of relaxation

There is evidence that relaxation training is effective for reducing depressive and anxious symptoms (and disorders) in both young people and adults, although often this intervention is less effective than CBT, particularly for more complex anxiety disorders. While further empirical evidence of the benefits of relaxation among young people would be desirable (including larger sample sizes), this intervention has promise within a stepped-care model for those with emerging symptoms or in the early stages of depression and/or anxiety.

Self-guided psychological interventions

Self-guided psychological interventions refer to those whereby the individuals undertaking the treatment do not have any contact with a therapist or coach. These are predominantly internet-based variants of traditional face-to-face therapies, such as CBT. Individuals are guided through programs that provide interactive behavioural and cognitive therapy tutorials to assist in managing or overcoming their problems with depression. Purely self-guided interventions have been argued to have the advantage of increased cost effectiveness and ease of dissemination.

Self-guided interventions with young people

A number of recent reviews of RCTs have reported that both guided and unguided (predominantly computerised) self-help interventions are effective in reducing symptoms of anxiety and depression in young people compared to no treatment, though these may not be as effective as face-to-face treatments.[57–59] The authors suggest that these findings, coupled with the relatively low costs, ease of accessibility and patient acceptability of these forms of treatment indicate that self-help interventions could be a viable option within a stepped-care model of treatment for common mental health disorders, although they also stressed the need for more methodologically rigorous trials.

Self-guided interventions with adults

A meta-analysis of seven RCTs showed that self-guided interventions, which were based on cognitive behavioural techniques, were effective in reducing depressive symptoms compared to control conditions of treatment as usual, wait-list control groups and advising participants to see their general practitioner.[60] Six of the seven studies were internet-based and one used self-help books.

Summary of self-guided psychological interventions

There is emerging evidence that self-guided psychological interventions may be effective in reducing depression and anxiety in young people. Self-guided internet-based CBT interventions have promise within a stepped-care model for those with early or mild mental health symptoms.

Supportive counselling

Supportive counselling (SC) aims to offer non-directive emotional support by establishing a therapeutic alliance based on empathic listening[61] so that the client feels as though their concerns have been heard, that someone cares and that it might be useful to return.[62]

Evidence of supportive counselling with young people

In an RCT of adolescents with major depressive disorder receiving 12–16 weeks of either individual CBT, family therapy or individual non-directive SC, the long-term outcomes over two years showed no differences between the groups with regards to recovery, recurrence or level of functioning, with the majority of participants recovering during this time frame.[63] Non-directive SC was equivalent in terms of treatment outcomes over two years when compared to an evidence-based intervention such as CBT. However, CBT was the superior treatment in the shorter-term outcomes of symptom reduction, with the possible implication that it would be the treatment of choice for young people who, due perhaps to illness duration and intensity, may require a treatment that produces more rapid improvements.[64] There is insufficient evidence for the application of SC to anxiety disorders in young people to enable a determination of its effectiveness.[65]

Evidence of supportive counselling with adults

In a systematic review of studies in adult populations, SC in primary care for psychological problems was superior to usual care by a GP (which may or may not have involved the prescribing of antidepressant medication) in short-term reduction of symptoms; however, long-term benefits were not established.[66] SC was also associated with greater satisfaction with care.

Summary of supportive counselling

Although there is a lack of evidence to support the use of supportive counselling over alternative psychotherapies, such as CBT, bodies such as the United Kingdom's National Institute for Health and Care Excellence (NICE) have recommended a stepped-care approach in their current guidelines for treating children and young people with depression.[23] The guidelines recommend that those with mild depression be initially offered group-based treatments, including non-directive supportive therapy, followed by individual CBT if no improvement in symptoms occurs within 2–3 months. This stepped-care approach acknowledges that milder forms of depression may respond to less intensive interventions such as psychoeducation and mental state monitoring, if offered within an empathic and supportive framework. This was demonstrated in an RCT comparing antidepressant medication with or without additional CBT (the 'ADAPT' study),[67] where a substantial proportion (21%) of children and adolescent participants with moderate to severe major depression responded to a brief intervention offering supportive monitoring of their mental state.

Conclusion

There is an emerging evidence base that broad-spectrum, low-intensity interventions are effective in reducing depression- and anxiety-related symptoms in young people, although there is more evidence of their effectiveness in adults (based on a large volume of research in this age group). The appeal of broad-spectrum interventions for subthreshold or early stages of high prevalence disorders is the possibility of preventing the incidence of new cases or the progression of early stages of illness to later and more serious forms of disorder. These interventions also have the advantage of ease of dissemination that can involve moderate, minimal or no therapist contribution. When therapist contribution is required, these types of interventions can be delivered by a range of professionals, from GPs, mental health nurses, youth workers or allied health professionals (e.g., social workers) and in a range of community and primary care settings. Given the high unmet need and burden of high-prevalence mental health problems in young people, the implementation of broad-spectrum interventions has a potentially significant public health benefit. The interventions reviewed in this chapter can conceivably be integrated in stepped-care models for depression and anxiety, providing low-intensity interventions that have been shown to lead to significant mental health gains.

References

1 Kessler RC, Berglund P, Demler O, Jin R, Merikangas KR, Walters EE. Lifetime prevalence and age-of-onset distributions of DSM-IV disorders in the National Comorbidity Survey Replication. *Archives of General Psychiatry* 2005;62(6):593–602.

2 Kessler RC, Amminger GP, Aguilar-Gaxiola S, Alonso J, Lee S, Ustün TB. Age of onset of mental disorders: a review of recent literature. *Current Opinion in Psychiatry* 2007;20(4):359–64.

3 Australian Institute of Health and Welfare. *Young Australians: their health and wellbeing 2007*. Canberra: Australian Institute of Health and Welfare; 2007.

4 McGorry PD, Hickie IB, Yung AR, Pantelis C, Jackson HJ. Clinical staging of psychiatric disorders: a heuristic framework for choosing earlier, safer and more effective interventions. *Australian and New Zealand Journal of Psychiatry* 2006;40(8):616–22.

5 McGorry PD. Issues for DSM-V: clinical staging: a heuristic pathway to valid nosology and safer, more effective treatment in psychiatry. *American Journal of Psychiatry* 2007;164(6):859–60.

6 McGorry PD, Purcell R, Hickie IB, Yung AR, Pantelis C, Jackson HJ. Clinical staging: a heuristic model for psychiatry and youth mental health. *Medical Journal of Australia* 2007;187(S7):S40–2.

7 Judd LL, Paulus MP, Wells KB, Rapaport MH. Socioeconomic burden of subsyndromal depressive symptoms and major depression in a sample of the general population. *American Journal of Psychiatry* 1996;153(11):1411–7.

8 Judd LL, Akiskal HS, Paulus MP. The role and clinical significance of subsyndromal depressive symptoms (SSD) in unipolar major depressive disorder. *Journal of Affective Disorders* 1997;45(1–2):5–17.

9 Rivas-Vazquez RA, Saffa-Biller D, Ruiz I, Blais MA, Rivas-Vaquez A. Current issues in anxiety and depression: comorbid, mixed, and subthreshold disorders. *Professional Psychology: Research and Practice* 2004;35(1):74–83.

10 Cross SP, Hermens DF, Hickie IB. Treatment patterns and short-term outcomes in an early intervention youth mental health service. *Early Intervention in Psychiatry* 2016;10(1):88–97.

11 McGorry PD, Goldstone SD, Parker AG, Rickwood DJ, Hickie IB. Cultures for mental health care of young people: an Australian blueprint for reform. *Lancet Psychiatry* 2014;1(7):559–68.

12 Cosgrave EM, Yung AR, Killackey EJ, Buckby JA, Godfrey KA, Stanford CA, et al. Met and unmet need in youth mental health. *Journal of Mental Health* 2008;17(6):618–28.

13 Wells K, Sherbourne C, Duan N, Unützer J, Miranda J, Schoenbaum M, et al. Quality improvement for depression in primary care: do patients with subthreshold depression benefit in the long run? *American Journal of Psychiatry* 2005;162(6):1149–57.

14 Cuijpers P, van Straten A, Warmerdam L. Problem solving therapies for depression: a meta-analysis. *European Psychiatry* 2007;22(1):9–15.

15 Mynors-Wallis LM, Gath DH, Day A, Baker F. Randomised controlled trial of problem solving treatment, antidepressant medication, and combined treatment for major depression in primary care. *BMJ* 2000;320(7226):26–30.

16 Cooney GM, Dwan K, Greig CA, Lawlor DA, Rimer J, Waugh FR, et al. Exercise for depression. *Cochrane Database of Systematic Reviews* 2013;9:CD004366.

17 Morres ID, Hatzigeorgiadis A, Stathi A, Comoutos N, Arpin-Cribbie C, Krommidas C, et al. Aerobic exercise for adult patients with major depressive disorder in mental health services: a systematic review and meta-analysis. *Depression and Anxiety* 2019;36(1):39–53.

18 Aylett E, Small N, Bower P. Exercise in the treatment of clinical anxiety in general practice – a systematic review and meta-analysis. *BMC Health Services Research* 2018;18:559.

19 Gordon BR, McDowell CP, Lyons M, Herring MP. The effects of resistance exercise training on anxiety: a meta-analysis and meta-regression analysis of randomized controlled trials. *Sports Medicine* 2017;47(12):2521–32.

20 Kim HS, Kim EJ. Effects of relaxation therapy on anxiety disorders: a systematic review and meta-analysis. *Archives of Psychiatric Nursing* 2018;32(2):278–84.

21 Christensen H, Griffiths KM, Jorm AF. Delivering interventions for depression by using the internet: randomised controlled trial. *BMJ* 2004;328(7434):265.

22 Dowrick C, Dunn G, Ayuso-Mateos JL, Dalgard OS, Page H, Lehtinen V, et al. Problem solving treatment and group psychoeducation for depression: multicentre randomised controlled trial. Outcomes of Depression International Network (ODIN) Group. *BMJ* 2000;321(7274):1450–4.
23 National Institute for Health and Care Excellence (NICE). *Depression in children and young people: identification and management.* London: NICE; 2019.
24 Yuan S, Zhou X, Zhang Y, Zhang H, Pu J, Yang L, et al. Comparative efficacy and acceptability of bibliotherapy for depression and anxiety disorders in children and adolescents: a meta-analysis of randomized clinical trials. *Neuropsychiatric Disease and Treatment* 2018;14:353–65.
25 Gregory RJ, Schwer Canning S, Lee TW, Wise JC. Cognitive bibliotherapy for depression: a meta-analysis. *Professional Psychology: Research and Practice* 2004;35(3):275–80.
26 Burns DD. *Feeling good: the new mood therapy*. 2nd ed. New York: Harper; 2000.
27 Anderson L, Lewis G, Araya R, Elgie R, Harrison G, Proudfoot J, et al. Self-help books for depression: how can practitioners and patients make the right choice? *British Journal of General Practice* 2005;55(514):387–92.
28 Cuijpers P. Bibliotherapy in unipolar depression: a meta-analysis. *Journal of Behavior Therapy and Experimental Psychiatry* 1997;28(2):139–47.
29 Bowman D, Scogin F, Floyd M, Patton E, Gist L. Efficacy of self-examination therapy in the treatment of generalized anxiety disorder. *Journal of Counseling Psychology* 1997;44(3):267–73.
30 Ehlers A, Clark DM, Hackmann A, McManus F, Fennell M, Herbert C, et al. A randomized controlled trial of cognitive therapy, a self-help booklet, and repeated assessments as early interventions for posttraumatic stress disorder. *Archives of General Psychiatry* 2003;60(10):1024–32.
31 Tolin DF, Hannan S, Maltby N, Diefenbach GJ, Worhunsky P, Brady RE. A randomized controlled trial of self-directed versus therapist-directed cognitive-behavioral therapy for obsessive-compulsive disorder patients with prior medication trials. *Behavior Therapy* 2007;38(2):179–91.
32 Scogin F, Bynum J, Stephens G, Calhoon S. Efficacy of self-administered treatment programs: meta-analytic review. *Professional Psychology: Research and Practice* 1990;21(1):42–7.
33 Marrs RW. A meta-analysis of bibliotherapy studies. *American Journal of Community Psychology* 1995;23(6):843–70.
34 Jorm AF, Christensen H, Griffiths KM, Rodgers B. Effectiveness of complementary and self-help treatments for depression. *Medical Journal of Australia* 2002;176(10):S84–96.
35 Department of Health. *Australian 24-hour movement guidelines for children and young people (5 to 17 years).* Canberra: Commonwealth of Australia; 2019.
36 Department of Health. *Australia's physical activity and sedentary behaviour guidelines: adults (18–64 years).* Canberra: Commonwealth of Australia; 2014.
37 Bailey AP, Hetrick SE, Rosenbaum S, Purcell R, Parker AG. Treating depression with physical activity in adolescents and young adults: a systematic review and meta-analysis of randomised controlled trials. *Psychological Medicine* 2018;48(7):1068–83.
38 Biddle SJ, Asare M. Physical activity and mental health in children and adolescents: a review of reviews. *British Journal of Sports Medicine* 2011;45(11):886–95.
39 James-Palmer A, Anderson EZ, Zucker L, Kofman Y, Daneault JF. Yoga as an intervention for the reduction of symptoms of anxiety and depression in children and adolescents: a systematic review. *Frontiers in Pediatrics* 2020;8:78.
40 Mynors-Wallis L. *Problem-solving treatment for anxiety and depression: a practical guide.* Oxford: Oxford University Press; 2005.

41 Eskin M, Ertekin K, Demir H. Efficacy of a problem-solving therapy for depression and suicide potential in adolescents and young adults. *Cognitive Therapy and Research* 2008;32:227–45.
42 Malouff JM, Thorsteinsson EB, Schutte NS. The efficacy of problem solving therapy in reducing mental and physical health problems: a meta-analysis. *Clinical Psychology Review* 2007;27(1):46–57.
43 Lerner MS, Clum GA. Treatment of suicidal ideators: a problem-solving approach. *Behavior Therapy* 1990;21(4):403–11.
44 Hoek W, Schuurmans J, Koot HM, Cuijpers P. Effects of internet-based guided self-help problem-solving therapy for adolescents with depression and anxiety: a randomized controlled trial. *PLoS One* 2012;7(8):e43485.
45 Bell AC, D'Zurilla TJ. Problem-solving therapy for depression: a meta-analysis. *Clinical Psychology Review* 2009;29(4):348–53.
46 Jones RB, Thapar A, Stone Z, Thapar A, Jones I, Smith D, et al. Psychoeducational interventions in adolescent depression: a systematic review. *Patient Education and Counseling* 2018;101(5):804–16.
47 Donker T, Griffiths KM, Cuijpers P, Christensen H. Psychoeducation for depression, anxiety and psychological distress: a meta-analysis. *BMC Medicine* 2009;7:79.
48 Field T, Grizzle N, Scafidi F, Schanberg S. Massage and relaxation therapies' effects on depressed adolescent mothers. *Adolescence* 1996;31(124):903–11.
49 Wood A, Harrington R, Moore A. Controlled trial of a brief cognitive-behavioural intervention in adolescent patients with depressive disorders. *Journal of Child Psychology and Psychiatry* 1996;37(6):737–46.
50 Sonis WA, Yellin AM, Garfinkel BD, Hoberman HH. The antidepressant effect of light in seasonal affective disorder of childhood and adolescence. *Psychopharmacology Bulletin* 1987;23(3):360–3.
51 Jorm AF, Morgan AJ, Hetrick SE. Relaxation for depression. *Cochrane Database of Systematic Reviews* 2008;4:CD007142.
52 Siev J, Chambless DL. Specificity of treatment effects: cognitive therapy and relaxation for generalized anxiety and panic disorders. *Journal of Consulting and Clinical Psychology* 2007;75(4):513–22.
53 Jorm AF, Christensen H, Griffiths KM, Parslow RA, Rodgers B, Blewitt KA. Effectiveness of complementary and self-help treatments for anxiety disorders. *Medical Journal of Australia* 2004;181(S7):S29–46.
54 Bögels SM. Task concentration training versus applied relaxation, in combination with cognitive therapy, for social phobia patients with fear of blushing, trembling, and sweating. *Behaviour Research and Therapy* 2006;44(8):1199–210.
55 Clark DM, Ehlers A, Hackmann A, McManus F, Fennell M, Grey N, et al. Cognitive therapy versus exposure and applied relaxation in social phobia: a randomized controlled trial. *Journal of Consulting and Clinical Psychology* 2006;74(3):568–78.
56 Manzoni GM, Pagnini F, Castelnuovo G, Molinari E. Relaxation training for anxiety: a ten-years systematic review with meta-analysis. *BMC Psychiatry* 2008;8:41.
57 Bennett SD, Cuijpers P, Ebert DD, Smith MM, Coughtrey AE, Heyman I, et al. Practitioner review: unguided and guided self-help interventions for common mental health disorders in children and adolescents: a systematic review and meta-analysis. *Journal of Child Psychology and Psychiatry* 2019;60(8):828–47.
58 Pennant ME, Loucas CE, Whittington C, Creswell C, Fonagy P, Fuggle P, et al. Computerised therapies for anxiety and depression in children and young people: a systematic review and meta-analysis. *Behaviour Research and Therapy* 2015;67:1–18.

59 Lattie EG, Adkins EC, Winquist N, Stiles-Shields C, Wafford QE, Graham AK. Digital mental health interventions for depression, anxiety, and enhancement of psychological well-being among college students: systematic review. *Journal of Medical Internet Research* 2019;21(7):e12869.
60 Cuijpers P, Donker T, Johansson R, Mohr DC, van Straten A, Andersson G. Self-guided psychological treatment for depressive symptoms: a meta-analysis. *PloS One* 2011;6(6):e21274.
61 King M, Sibbald B, Ward E, Bower P, Lloyd M, Gabbay M, et al. Randomised controlled trial of non-directive counselling, cognitive-behaviour therapy and usual general practitioner care in the management of depression as well as mixed anxiety and depression in primary care. *Health Technology Assessment* 2000;4(19):1–83.
62 Geldard K, Geldard D. *Counselling adolescents*. 2nd ed. London: Sage Publications; 2004.
63 Birmaher B, Brent DA, Kolko D, Baugher M, Bridge J, Holder D, et al. Clinical outcome after short-term psychotherapy for adolescents with major depressive disorder. *Archives of General Psychiatry* 2000;57(1):29–36.
64 Brent DA, Holder D, Kolko D, Birmaher B, Baugher M, Roth C, et al. A clinical psychotherapy trial for adolescent depression comparing cognitive, family, and supportive therapy. *Archives of General Psychiatry* 1997;54(9):877–85.
65 Reavley NJ, Allen NB, Jorm AF, Morgan AJ, Purcell R. *A guide to what works for anxiety disorders*. Melbourne: beyondblue; 2010.
66 Bower P, Rowland N. Effectiveness and cost effectiveness of counselling in primary care. *Cochrane Database of Systematic Reviews* 2006;3:CD001025.
67 Goodyer I, Dubicka B, Wilkinson P, Kelvin R, Roberts C, Byford S, et al. Selective serotonin reuptake inhibitors (SSRIs) and routine specialist care with and without cognitive behaviour therapy in adolescents with major depression: randomised controlled trial. *BMJ* 2007;335(7611):142.

11 Interventions for substance misuse in young people

Grant I. G. Christie, Amanda L. Baker and Dan I. Lubman

Introduction

Although the use and misuse of alcohol, tobacco or illicit drugs typically begins during adolescence, most published treatment studies have tended to focus on adults with substance use disorders. Nevertheless, there is a growing body of literature examining interventions for alcohol and other drug (AOD) misuse (including abuse and dependence) among young people,[1,2] and this chapter describes how such interventions can be implemented within standard treatment settings.

The nature of substance misuse varies greatly over this period of development, particularly when we compare substance use during the early teens to that in the mid-twenties. Individual differences in cognitive, emotional and social maturity, combined with environmental factors, necessitate a flexible approach to treatment with young people. Any treatment plan should be designed specifically for each young person, taking into account coexisting problems, developmental issues and treatment challenges. Many young people with substance misuse present with a broad range of coexisting issues, including homelessness, limited educational background and training opportunities, offending behaviour, family dysfunction, deliberate self-harm and mental health problems, such as depression, anxiety and psychosis.[3] While these issues clearly need to be addressed within treatment, it is important that the opportunity to address substance misuse is taken (especially if the young person is primarily seeking help for another problem), particularly as such use is likely to be exacerbating any other presenting problems.

The treatment plan should take into account differences between presentations for substance misuse in adults and young people. Compared to adults, adolescents tend to present for treatment most frequently for cannabis misuse; have higher rates of binge and opportunistic substance use, lower problem recognition and higher rates of mental health problems; are more susceptible to peer influence and are at a vulnerable developmental stage in terms of forming their own identity.[4] Additional treatment challenges include the fact that young people are more likely than adults to enter treatment due to external pressures (e.g., family or legal)[5] and are more likely to only stay in treatment for a short period.[6] An important consideration in treating young people is to be wary of the potential for interventions to increase harm; for example, treatment programs which aggregate young people with antisocial behaviour can escalate problems.[7] Regular evaluation of progress and modifying and improving the treatment plan across time is recommended.[8]

Harms associated with substance use in young people

Almost all young people will be exposed to alcohol and drugs on numerous occasions throughout their development and will experiment with substances in some way. Persisting and severe disorder (or addiction) almost always begins with experimental use in adolescence and rapidly develops in terms of frequency of use, as well as the type of substances used.[9] Alcohol, tobacco and inhalants are usually misused first, however increasingly cannabis is used first by adolescents. Males use more than females although differences between genders have been lessening. The highest rates of substance misuse are seen in those aged between 18 and 25 years, with alcohol and cannabis being the most problematic substances (excluding tobacco). It is important to note that many young people are polysubstance users, in that they use whatever substance is available rather than settling on a preferred substance as adults do.

Tobacco

Tobacco is the most frequently used drug among young people and is the leading cause of death and hospitalisation among Australians.[10] Young smokers tend to have poorer general health, with more physical health complaints such as headaches, fatigue, respiratory symptoms and infections, and also take more sick days.[11] Taking up smoking in adolescence is associated with a lower probability of cessation in adulthood as well as maintenance of higher levels of tobacco intake.[12]

Early smoking is predictive of later problems with tobacco dependence, alcohol and illicit drugs.[13] There is a strong association with smoking and mental health problems, including depression, anxiety, low self-esteem and eating disorders. For example, in a study of 2,525 young people aged between 12 and 18, subjects reporting high levels of depression and anxiety were twice as likely to be smokers.[14]

Smoking among users of mental health services is very common. Cardiovascular disease is the leading cause of death among people using mental health services in Australia.[15] Lifestyle factors, of which smoking is considered to be the most important, interact to radically increase risk of cardiovascular disease among this group.

Alcohol

Compared to illicit drugs and tobacco combined, alcohol causes the most deaths and hospitalisations among children and young people, primarily due to either intentional or unintentional injuries (e.g., traffic accidents, assaults, falls).[13] Other physical harms associated with intoxication are unexpected pregnancy and/or sexually transmitted diseases associated with sexual exploitation.[16] Of particular concern is that between 1999 and 2006, hospitalisations for alcohol-related causes among Australians aged 18–24 years more than doubled, suggesting that more young people are drinking at high-risk levels.[17]

Adolescents who misuse alcohol have higher rates of mental health disorders, including depression (and attempted suicide), conduct disorder, attention-deficit/hyperactivity disorder, post-traumatic stress disorder and social phobia.[18] Alcohol misuse can predispose young people to develop mental health problems; however, established mental health problems also precipitate alcohol misuse in many cases and/or other underlying factors, such as socio-economic status, can contribute to the development of both disorders.

Alcohol and energy drinks

Consumption of alcohol in combination with caffeine-rich energy drinks (such as Red Bull) is becoming increasingly popular among young people, particularly in licensed venues.[19,20] This includes both pre-packaged alcoholic energy drinks as well as combining energy drinks with vodka or Jägermeister (known as 'Jäger-bombs'). Although limited research has been conducted examining the harms associated with this form of drinking, the combination of alcohol with energy drinks can mask the signs of alcohol intoxication, resulting in dehydration, more severe and prolonged hangovers, and even alcohol poisoning. Intoxication-related behavioural harms such as drink driving and violence are also likely to be associated with consumption of these drinks. In addition, regular consumption of alcoholic energy drinks significantly increases the risk of alcohol and other substance misuse.[21]

Cannabis

Regular cannabis use in young people is associated with educational under-achievement, employment instability, reduced life opportunities and increased use of other illicit drugs.[22] Whether these are direct effects of cannabis or relate to other causal pathways (e.g., shared personal characteristics or environments) remains undetermined. Among young people with psychotic disorders, chronic cannabis use impacts negatively on the course and treatment of psychosis and is associated with poor medication compliance, more severe psychotic symptoms, and earlier and more frequent psychotic relapses.[23,24] A number of large prospective studies have demonstrated that early onset cannabis use is associated with greater risk of developing a later psychotic disorder, conferring a twofold increase in relative risk.[25] There are increasing reports of higher levels of depression among young cannabis users; for example, Patton and colleagues reported that early-onset weekly cannabis use in adolescence predicts a twofold increase in rates of depression among young women, with daily use increasing the risk fourfold,[26] while more recent evidence has suggested that this association is causal.[27]

Smokable synthetic cannabinoid products have been available for some years now and have similar psychoactive effects to cannabis, despite having a different chemical structure. These products tend to be more potent and shorter acting than cannabis and are more addictive than cannabis as well as much more harmful.[28] Reports of physical harm including seizures and death associated with the use of these products are now commonplace.[29]

Illicit drugs other than cannabis

The main health-related harm associated with illicit drugs other than cannabis is injection, which can be associated with overdose in opioid use and the spread of blood-borne viruses when injecting equipment is shared.[13] Young people tend to use some drug types fairly commonly and these are briefly overviewed next.

Methamphetamine

Methamphetamine use is associated with a wide range of harms. In addition to problems associated with injection, methamphetamine use is associated with mental health problems (including psychotic symptoms, depression, anxiety), aggression and violence, social problems and sexual risk-taking behaviour.[30,31] Methamphetamine is usually used in conjunction with other drugs, potentially compounding these harms.

Ecstasy

As with methamphetamine users, most users of ecstasy are polydrug users.[32] A range of adverse effects related to ecstasy have been reported by users, including physical harms, such as non-fatal overdose, dehydration and memory impairment, and psychological harms, such as depression and anxiety.

Inhalants

Although only a small proportion of young people use inhalants on a regular basis, they are included here because of their high potential for harm and the fact they are typically one of the first drugs that young people misuse as they are cheap, legal, readily accessible and provide a rapid 'high'.[33] The effects of inhalant intoxication are similar to alcohol, although hallucinations and ataxia may occur at higher doses and further central nervous system depression can result in seizures, coma and cardiopulmonary arrest. Fatal ventricular arrhythmias or 'sudden sniffing death' can occur especially if the user is agitated or suddenly startled.[34] Toxic effects associated with chronic use include neurological, renal, hepatic and pulmonary damage. While severe encephalopathy associated with petrol (especially leaded) sniffing can occur following acute intoxication, most cases occur following prolonged patterns of use.[34] A history of inhalant use is consistently associated with later mental health and substance use disorders as well as injecting drug use, suggesting that early inhalant use may be a potential vulnerability marker for the development of these disorders.

Prevention strategies

Addressing substance use among young people requires a multifaceted approach, incorporating a range of strategies that focus on (i) delaying the age of first experimentation with substances, (ii) reducing the number of young people who transition to regular or problem use and (iii) encouraging current users to reduce risk-taking and use.[35] While preventative approaches that target all young people in the community regardless of their level of risk are clearly critical in this regard, a review of such approaches is beyond the scope of this chapter.

Nevertheless, a range of universal prevention approaches have been found to be effective[35] and include economic measures (such as increasing the price) and specific legislation (such as delaying the age that licit drugs can be legally purchased). Parents also have an important influence on adolescent drinking, and parenting factors that can reduce young people's alcohol consumption include parental modeling, limiting availability of alcohol to the child, disapproval of adolescent drinking, parental monitoring, parent-child relationship quality, parental involvement, general discipline and overall communication.[36]

Service qualities, engagement and treatment retention

As discussed in other parts of this book, young people with mental health and substance use concerns have varied means of help-seeking and difficulty accessing services. In general, young people are less likely to seek help for alcohol or drug problems than for mood or anxiety disorders,[37] and only a small proportion of people with substance-related problems attend treatment programs.[38]

Therefore, one of the key challenges to providers of youth services is simply getting young people to attend.[39] Designing AOD services that are equipped to provide better access and actively engage young people is essential, particularly as young people are generally ambivalent about the need for AOD treatment and those with most need are often the least likely to access help.

Thus the service environment is almost as important as the quality of interventions available, and services need to be attractive and accessible to young people. Young people are more likely to engage with a service if it is interesting, responsive and confidential, respectful, trustworthy and staffed by caring, committed and optimistic professionals.[40,41] Factors related to engaging and retaining young people in treatment are discussed elsewhere[42] and include service flexibility and responsiveness, development of a good therapeutic alliance and family involvement in treatment. Realistic goal-setting with young people is also important, as is offering practical support and semi-formal contact (case management-like activities). Provision of aftercare and assistance when transitioning between services is also recommended.[43] Finally, regular program evaluations and monitoring of treatment outcomes are very important so that services can adapt to changes in their communities and evolve with the advent of new treatments.

Effectiveness of AOD treatment interventions

AOD interventions have been shown to improve outcomes in young people in both research and naturalistic settings and are effective in reducing substance misuse in the short to medium term (6–12 months).[44–47] Such interventions also have a number of secondary positive outcomes, which include reducing criminal activity and problem behaviour; increasing positive activities; improving academic attainment, mental health and family relationships; and attendance at school and college.[48] Treatment effectiveness has been demonstrated in a variety of settings from residential to outpatient, using a variety of therapeutic techniques. Comparative trials show little difference in effectiveness between treatments, although it is clear that sticking to an intervention model increases retention, which in turn is key in improving outcomes.[44,46]

Brief interventions have empirical support not only in adults but also in adolescents and are an efficacious and low-cost means to minimise substance-related harm.[49–55] They not only reduce substance use and substance-related harm in the short term, but also increase engagement into AOD treatment. While few studies addressing smoking or illicit drug use have been conducted among adolescents, it is likely that a similar approach is beneficial.

There is a strong evidence base for motivational enhancement therapy in adults with substance use problems[53,55–57] and a growing literature supporting its use in young people.[54] Cognitive behavioural therapy (CBT) has been found to be an effective treatment for problematic substance use among young people,[58] however it should be tailored to the young person's developmental stage. CBT is more likely to be effective in older adolescents and when combined with social and coping skills[59] and can be provided both individually or in groups. There is also growing evidence for the effectiveness of integrated CBT (i.e., both disorders targeted simultaneously) among young people with co-occurring mental health and substance use disorders.[60]

Finally, there is good evidence for the use of family and systemic therapies in the treatment of adolescent substance misuse, such as multidimensional family therapy, multisystemic therapy and functional family therapy.[61–63] While these have varied theoretical approaches, most programs incorporate a number of common components, such as psychoeducation, parent management training and enhancing communication skills.[64] These therapies have been shown to produce good outcomes in young offenders and young people with conduct disorder and other mental health problems. Such treatments also decrease criminal activity and improve family cohesion.[48,64]

The following parts discuss these interventions in more detail and suggest practical strategies for implementing such approaches.

AOD assessment and interventions

Screening and assessment

In order to be effectively implemented within an existing service, screening and assessment practices cannot be burdensome (e.g., brief screens) and should capitalise on existing relationships (e.g., between the young person and their case manager).[65] Development of rapport and engagement with the service will be enhanced by a non-judgemental and empathic approach. The topic of substance use can be opened up in a non-threatening manner by beginning the interview with general questions about use of legal substances, such as caffeine, alcohol and tobacco, and of prescribed medications.[66] Use of a screening tool can be helpful in eliciting a history of substance use and include:

- The Substances and Choices Scale (SACS)[67] is a screening and outcome measurement instrument for adolescents (up to age 18) with excellent psychometric properties that is highly acceptable to young people and AOD clinicians. The SACS can be used as the starting point for a brief intervention, and a manual guiding clinicians through the steps of a brief intervention is available at *www.sacsinfo.com.*
- The Alcohol, Smoking and Substance Involvement Screening Test (ASSIST)[68] is an eight-item interviewer-administered screen for all types of substance use, accompanied by guidelines for feedback and brief intervention. This can be useful for young people as it provides a brief overview of substance use involvement with tailored advice. It has a section on injecting drug use.
- The Fagerström Test for Nicotine Dependence (FTND)[69] consists of six items measuring aspects of nicotine dependence. It is important to include tobacco in all screening, assessment and interventions for young people.
- The Alcohol Use Disorders Identification Test (AUDIT)[70] screens for problematic alcohol consumption and consists of ten items. The AUDIT-C (first three items)[71] is a quick measure of alcohol consumption, including binge drinking, and may be especially useful if time is limited.
- The Cannabis Use Disorders Identification Test-Revised (CUDIT-R)[72] screens for problematic cannabis use and consists of eight items, two each from the domains of consumption, cannabis problems (abuse), dependence, and psychological features.

A screener for mental health problems should always be given along with those for substance use. These are discussed elsewhere in this book. The Kessler Psychological Distress Scale (K10),[73] a ten-item measure of psychological distress which takes about two minutes to complete, provides a good indication for whether the young person is likely to have a problem with depression or anxiety. It has been recommended for use in a broad range of environments.[74,75]

Brief interventions and motivational interviewing

Young people often attend treatment for only short time periods. Brief interventions thus provide an opportunity to help engage the young person in future treatment as well as reducing their substance use. Brief interventions are often linked to screening processes and incorporate strategies that can be readily applied within many health care settings to encourage more moderate patterns of substance use among young people. Brief interventions involve providing personalised AOD advice and education in an opportunistic way. They usually incorporate motivational interviewing techniques to encourage self-reflection and facilitate change in behaviour. An integrated approach is taken, whereby mental health, substance use and other problems are raised and linked, with the aim of working with client ambivalence to elicit self-motivational statements and behaviour change. Screening, brief interventions and motivational interviewing can be delivered by health workers who may otherwise have limited alcohol and other drug training or expertise.[56,76]

Young people with mental health issues are a particularly important at-risk population, given the high rates of co-occurring substance misuse,[77,78] as well as the impact of substance use on clinical and functional outcomes.[79] It is therefore critical that these young people are provided with information regarding the link between mental illness and substance use, as well as brief interventions that discourage regular use. Brief interventions are effective in reducing substance use among people with mental health problems,[80] as well as improving engagement with and adherence to treatment delivered by psychiatric outpatient services.[81]

Box 11.1 Management of substance use and associated mental health or other problems

1. Screen for substance use and associated mental health and other problems
2. Identify stage of change regarding substance use with readiness ruler
3. Use decisional balance (good things / less good things about substance use)
4. Ask about possible link between substance use and presenting mental health symptoms and other problems
5. Seek permission to provide information
6. Assess confidence to reduce substance use with confidence ruler
7. Explore options for change
8. Negotiate a change plan: "what's the next step?"
9. Provide or refer on for pharmacological treatment and/or psychological intervention
10. Regularly monitor substance use and mental health and other problems over time to prevent or address relapse

Box 11.1 provides a summary that can serve as a session outline, while Box 11.2 illustrates an example of a brief intervention.

Box 11.2 Brief intervention with Jack

Jack was a 17-year-old who was referred to a mental health service for young people at ultra-high risk of psychosis. He lived with his mother, father and younger sister, had left school and was working part-time. He spent most days sleeping, watching television and smoking cannabis and spent his evenings smoking cannabis with friends. At the time of presentation, he was smoking eight cones of cannabis per day. He complained of feeling 'unhappy' and 'paranoid'. Following assessment, he was offered an initial six sessions of counselling, with the aim of reducing his unhappiness and paranoid thoughts. At the first session he was given feedback from his assessment and motivational interviewing around his cannabis use, similar to that outlined in Box 11.1. He readily identified a possible link between his cannabis use and his mental health symptoms and he suggested reducing his cannabis use. At session 2 (some weeks later) he presented with his mother who was keen to receive some information about cannabis and mental health symptoms and how to improve communication with her son. Communication strategies (such as decreasing critical comments and increasing praise) were discussed. Also discussed was the helpfulness of matching communication about cannabis use to her son's stage of change. Jack was also seen alone in session 2. He reported a large reduction in cannabis use with the intent to reduce even further, to less than half of his previous level of use, limiting use to social occasions only. At session 3 he reported that he had achieved this and had been successful in obtaining a full-time job at his workplace. Further reduction in cannabis use was planned and he refused further follow-up.

This vignette illustrates a brief intervention with a harm-reduction focus, with a clinically significant outcome for substance use and an improvement in the young person's functioning. Parental strategies were also employed.

Cognitive behaviour therapy

Cognitive behavioural interventions generally involve self-monitoring, increasing activities not associated with substance use and enhancing awareness of permissive thoughts about substance use and changing them. Given many young people do not attend therapy for very long, it is wise to contract the young person to a stepped-care approach, evaluating the outcome of an initial few sessions and then re-contracting for a further five or six sessions, the duration of which has been shown to be as effective as longer interventions.[44] There is increasing interest in incorporating exercise and physical activity into interventions for young people, and if this can be woven into a behavioural activation approach, it can be very helpful in reducing substance use and increasing self-efficacy.

Motivational interviewing is usually delivered throughout CBT, as client motivation shifts with treatment progress. Homework can be a challenge to implement, and it is recommended that some time be spent on discussing what between-session tasks the young person is willing to work on. Affirming attendance at sessions and any attempts to change is helpful, while remaining positive and available in the face of lapses and relapses is important for engagement.

Baker and colleagues have outlined an integrated CBT approach to coexisting mental health and substance use problems.[82] It is usually helpful to start with more behaviourally focused interventions and progress to more cognitive strategies:

- Self-monitoring: monitoring fluctuations in mental health symptoms and substance cravings and use helps the person to recognise problematic behaviours, situations and thoughts. Monitoring should include examples of triggers and thoughts associated with mental health symptoms and substance use or cravings that are independent of one another and those that are linked (e.g., drinking in response to feeling anxious).
- Goal setting: goals should be established for mental health and drug and alcohol problems, with an emphasis on small, measurable, achievable, realistic targets.
- Increasing activity levels (behavioural activation) and avoiding high-risk situations: here the focus is on situations with a high risk for experiencing mental health symptoms and experiencing cravings/urges to use substances.[83]
- Communication training: role-playing assertiveness regarding refusal of substances; assisting parents to increase praise and decrease criticism and to match communication style with the young person's stage of change regarding their substance use and insight into their mental health problems.
- Integrated cognitive therapy: this involves orientation to the cognitive model,[84] with examples of antecedents (A), beliefs (B) and consequences (C) for mental health symptoms and substance use, separately and linked. Thought-challenging addresses negative or distressing thoughts and also positive expectations and permissive thoughts about substance use. Mindfulness can be helpful in distancing oneself from thoughts,[85] and the young person works toward generating more helpful thoughts and beliefs.
- Addressing underlying core beliefs: working from overt thoughts to underlying beliefs involves employing techniques like vertical arrow questioning – "If that thought were true, what would it mean about you?" – and is associated with high levels of affective arousal.[86]
- Integrated relapse prevention: prevention of relapse to both mental health and substance use problems is addressed toward the end of therapy.[87,88] Avoidance of high-risk situations and management of these situations through the use of coping skills is covered and practised before the client is discharged. The aim is to prepare the young person so that lapses are avoided or prevented from becoming fully blown relapses.
- Computer-delivered CBT for alcohol problems among young people has been shown to be effective,[89] as well as for coexisting depression and alcohol/cannabis use.[90] These may be attractive to young people who have difficulties accessing treatment or who prefer not to attend face-to-face services.

Family-based interventions

Family involvement is key to engaging and retaining young people in treatment, and it is important to develop this from the outset of treatment if possible. Even minor levels of involvement are usually better than none. Family involvement not only secures early changes in substance use and behaviour, but assists with enhancing engagement in treatment later.[91]

Family work and therapy enhances treatment across a range of levels. Including parents improves treatment for young people as well as increasing parental support.[92] Providing a little more in terms of support, information and parenting advice improves parents' ability to cope (with distress and the young person's behaviour) and reduces substance misuse in both parents and children.[93] Family and systemic therapies with the best evidence base incorporate a combination of evidence-based interventions such as CBT and strategic family therapy. They tend to be solution focused and concentrate on several parts of the family and wider system, including individual work, family functioning and parenting. 'Functional' and 'multi-dimensional' family therapies and multisystemic therapy have the best evidence of effectiveness and in many ways could be regarded as 'gold standard' treatment for youth with conduct and substance problems. Interestingly, these latter therapies incorporate both individual and family work.

Residential treatment

Residential treatment has been shown to be as effective as community-based therapies;[44,46,94] however, as this kind of treatment is significantly more expensive, it should be reserved for those unsuited to community treatment. A residential treatment program is more likely to be effective if it is delivered in small units that are close to the youth's community, involves families and has phased and supported reintegration planning. Flexible (and shorter) residential programs need to be promoted, as extended treatment periods of up to a year can be a barrier to access and can lead to many young people missing out on what they require. Shorter programs mean that more young people have access to residential treatment. Family involvement needs to be a key part of such programs, especially for those young people returning to a family environment following discharge. Therapeutic community models with strong hierarchies and punitive models are not recommended for young people.[95]

Pharmacological interventions

The evidence base for pharmacological treatment is based on adult subjects, and there are few efficacy or safety studies in adolescent populations. Although young people suffer very high levels of morbidity and problems related to substance misuse, psychological and social therapies alone are likely to be effective with young people, and adding pharmacological treatment is seldom required.

There is some role for medications in withdrawal management (see the following part) and promoting abstinence in alcohol-dependent young people (e.g., acamprosate and naltrexone). However, such pharmacotherapies should not be utilised in isolation, but rather to augment ongoing psychological therapies.

Opiate substitution therapy with methadone or buprenorphine is usually recommended for the management of opiate addiction in view of the significant morbidity and mortality associated with injecting heroin. Although services can often be reluctant to provide opiate substitution therapy for adolescents, if there is no change in high-risk behaviours following an adequate trial of other treatment modalities (i.e., detoxification and supported abstinence), then this should be considered early in association with specialist addiction services.

Psychiatric or other medications may be required to manage any coexisting mental or physical health problems. It is important that substance misuse is not viewed as a contraindication for treatment, particularly as optimal management of the mental health problem may also lead to a reduction in the young person's substance use. Professionals with competence in both substance use and mental health treatment should ideally be involved, but if this is not possible, then a multidisciplinary approach is recommended.

When prescribing medications, services need to be aware of the risks associated with prescription drug misuse, and clinicians should consider adopting certain precautions if indicated. This may include prescribing for limited periods of time, frequent dispensing (e.g., weekly), a single identified pharmacy and trials of medication linked to clearly defined outcomes.

Young people who use substances are also likely to smoke cigarettes. Nicotine replacement should be offered to young people at every opportunity, but especially within non-smoking environments.

Substance withdrawal (stopping using substances safely)

Young people who have developed dependence (or addiction) to a substance may have an unpleasant 'withdrawal syndrome' in the days after stopping the drug. A withdrawal syndrome usually lasts 7–10 days, although this differs depending on the substance. As a rule, symptoms of withdrawal are typically at their worst between 2–4 days after stopping a substance, and then gradually decrease in severity from that point.

Common symptoms of withdrawal from alcohol and/or drugs include psychological symptoms such as agitation, low mood, irritability, mood swings, anxiety, restlessness, insomnia, difficulty concentrating, tiredness, craving or strong urges to use. Physical symptoms include sweating, goosebumps, feeling hot or cold, cold or flu-like symptoms (e.g., runny nose and sneezing), loss of appetite, nausea and vomiting, stomach cramps, aches and pains, shivering, increased heart rate and headaches. Young people in withdrawal will complain of psychological symptoms more often than physical symptoms.

Most adolescents who misuse substances are able to stop using without medical support. Withdrawal from cannabis, amphetamine and opiates, although unpleasant and difficult, very seldom presents as a significant health risk, even in heavily addicted adults. Withdrawal from alcohol and other sedatives is potentially more problematic and can be a health risk. That said, alcohol use needs to be heavy and sustained in the long term (some years) for significant neuroadaptation (changes in the brain) to occur and increase the risk of a serious physical withdrawal syndrome.

Young people at higher risk of problems during substance withdrawal include:

- Those with heavy long-term daily use of alcohol or other sedatives like benzodiazepines
- Those with an established opiate addiction
- Those with established medical or psychiatric problems, such as epilepsy, diabetes, schizophrenia or bipolar affective disorder
- Pregnant users

Very rarely, a young person may suffer a seizure while in withdrawal. If this occurs, it is important to put the young person in the recovery position and to call an ambulance as soon as possible.

Management of withdrawal

Most adolescents will be able to safely stop using substances with support from their family and friends. Usually the biggest barrier to a successful detoxification is finding a drug-free environment. Nevertheless, some young people may require input from a primary health care provider (GP, nurse or health worker), and a few will need more specialist assistance (via a mental health or AOD service).

The most important aspect of managing a young person who is experiencing withdrawal is a calm and supportive environment. Having an understanding of which physical and psychological symptoms may occur and helping the young person cope with these is important.

In general, the following environmental strategies are useful:

- Ensure the environment is free from substances and will not be visited by people who have or use substances
- Ensure the environment is free from 'cues' or reminders about using substances. For example, pictures of drugs make it harder for people to resist cravings. Visits from drug-using associates will be counterproductive
- Have activities readily available to help alleviate boredom and distract the young person at times they are craving (i.e., DVDs, books, games)
- If possible provide access to a quiet room, separate from other people that the young person can go to be alone if required
- A comfortable ambient temperature, neither too hot nor too cold
- Ensure there are plenty of fluids and a variety of healthy foods available
- Over-the-counter medications (e.g., paracetamol) are usually enough to manage physical symptoms
- An understanding of withdrawal symptoms and difficulties associated with coping with withdrawal and cravings is helpful
- Relaxation exercises can be helpful if anxiety is present (e.g., deep breathing, muscle relaxation and relaxation music)
- A holiday or time away from their usual environment and social sphere is likely to be useful
- Ensure carers/family know how to access medical support if required, especially after hours

In medical settings (i.e., a hospital ward), monitoring of heart rate, respiration, temperature and blood pressure can be done to assess the severity of the withdrawal syndrome. Standardised withdrawal rating scales, such as the Clinical Institute Withdrawal Assessment for Alcohol *Revised* (CIWA-Ar)[96] or the Short Opiate Withdrawal Scale (SOWS),[97] may be useful in inpatient settings where trained nursing staff are available.

Conclusions

Services seeing young people with substance misuse need to be flexible and accessible. Even the slightest barrier to entry will discourage those most needing treatment. Nimble and responsive systems are required, and waiting lists or periods between assessment and entry into services need to be avoided. An emphasis on relationship building in the early stages of entry into services is important, and although comprehensive assessment is the foundation of effective AOD treatment, engagement is arguably more important as there is little point in assessing young people who do not turn up for treatment.

The evidence suggests that AOD treatment is effective for young people and that one type of treatment or service is not significantly more advantageous than another. Providing a range of services and treatment modalities is preferable to meet their variable needs. As community treatment is equivalent in efficacy to other more intensive and expensive treatments (e.g., residential treatment), these latter therapies should be reserved for young people who will not engage in outpatient treatment (or for whom outpatient treatment has not worked), or who require residential/systemic modalities for other reasons.

Outpatient services need to offer a variety of treatment modalities, with flexibility to move between these to suit the young person and their family. Treatment approaches on offer should include individual interventions (such as motivational interviewing and CBT, including family involvement if possible), withdrawal management and effective treatment of any coexisting mental health disorder and risk. Family interventions are also important, particularly for younger adolescents, and the balance of individual to family interventions should increase as the young person develops and becomes more independent. In the near future, it is anticipated that effective digital interventions aimed at supporting young people with addiction, either alone or in conjunction with face-to-face therapies, will be readily available to complement more established therapies.

References

1 Winters KC, Tanner-Smith EE, Bresani E, Meyers K. Current advances in the treatment of adolescent drug use. *Adolescent Health, Medicine and Therapeutics* 2014;5:199–210.
2 Tanner-Smith EE, Lipsey MW. Brief alcohol interventions for adolescents and young adults: a systematic review and meta-analysis. *Journal of Substance Abuse Treatment* 2015;51:1–18.
3 Crome IB. Treatment interventions: looking towards the millennium. *Drug and Alcohol Dependence* 1999;55(3):247–63.

4 Mark TL, Song X, Vandivort R, Duffy S, Butler J, Coffey R, et al. Characterizing substance abuse programs that treat adolescents. *Journal of Substance Abuse Treatment* 2006;31(1):59–65.

5 Melnick G, De Leon G, Hawke J, Jainchill N, Kressel D. Motivation and readiness for therapeutic community treatment among adolescents and adult substance abusers. *American Journal of Drug and Alcohol Abuse* 1997;23(4):485–506.

6 Hser YI, Grella CE, Hubbard RL, Hsieh SC, Fletcher BW, Brown BS, et al. An evaluation of drug treatments for adolescents in 4 US cities. *Archives of General Psychiatry* 2001;58(7):689–95.

7 Dishion TJ, McCord J, Poulin F. When interventions harm: peer groups and problem behavior. *American Psychologist* 1999;54(9):755–64.

8 Rhule DM. Take care to do no harm: harmful interventions for youth problem behavior. *Professional Psychology: Research and Practice* 2005;36(6):618–25.

9 Kandel DB, Yamaguchi K, Chen K. Stages of progression in drug involvement from adolescence to adulthood: further evidence for the gateway theory. *Journal of Studies on Alcohol and Drugs* 1992;53(5):447–57.

10 Australian Institute of Health and Welfare. *Australia's health 2008*. Canberra: Australian Institute of Health and Welfare; 2008.

11 Woodhouse K. Young people and smoking. In Crome L, Ghodse H, Gilvarry E, McArdle P (Eds) *Young people and substance misuse*. London: Royal College of Psychiatrists; 2004. p 114–28.

12 Chen J, Millar WJ. Age of smoking initiation: implications for quitting. *Health Reports* 1998;9(4):39–46.

13 Loxley W. *The prevention of substance use, risk and harm in Australia: a review of the evidence.* Canberra: Department of Health and Ageing; 2004.

14 Patton GC, Hibbert M, Rosier MJ, Carlin JB, Caust J, Bowes G. Is smoking associated with depression and anxiety in teenagers? *American Journal of Public Health* 1996;86(2):225–30.

15 Jablensky A, McGrath J, Herrman H, Castle D, Gureje O, Morgan V, et al. *People with psychotic illnesses: an Australian study 1997–98*. Canberra: Commonwealth Department of Health and Aged Care; 1999.

16 Hingson RW, Heeren T, Zakocs RC, Kopstein A, Wechsler H. Magnitude of alcohol-related mortality and morbidity among U.S. college students ages 18–24. *Journal of Studies on Alcohol* 2002;63(2):136–44.

17 Livingston M, Laslett AM, Dietze P. Individual and community correlates of young people's high-risk drinking in Victoria, Australia. *Drug and Alcohol Dependence* 2008;98(3):241–8.

18 Dawes MA, Johnson BA. Pharmacotherapeutic trials in adolescent alcohol use disorders: opportunities and challenges. *Alcohol and Alcoholism* 2004;39(3):166–77.

19 Pennay A, Lubman D, Miller P. Combining energy drinks and alcohol: a recipe for trouble? *Australian Family Physician* 2011;40(3):104–7.

20 Breda JJ, Whiting SH, Encarnação R, Norberg S, Jones R, Reinap M, et al. Energy drink consumption in Europe: a review of the risks, adverse health effects, and policy options to respond. *Frontiers in Public Health* 2014;2:134.

21 Arria AM, Caldeira KM, Kasperski SJ, Vincent KB, Griffiths RR, O'Grady KE. Energy drink consumption and increased risk for alcohol dependence. *Alcoholism: Clinical and Experimental Research* 2011;35(2):365–75.

22 Hall WD. Cannabis use and the mental health of young people. *Australian and New Zealand Journal of Psychiatry* 2006;40(2):105–13.

23 Lambert M, Conus P, Lubman DI, Wade D, Yuen H, Moritz S, et al. The impact of substance use disorders on clinical outcome in 643 patients with first-episode psychosis. *Acta Psychiatrica Scandinavica* 2005;112(2):141–8.
24 Lubman DI, King JA, Castle DJ. Treating comorbid substance use disorders in schizophrenia. *International Review of Psychiatry* 2010;22(2):191–201.
25 Arseneault L, Cannon M, Witton J, Murray RM. Causal association between cannabis and psychosis: examination of the evidence. *British Journal of Psychiatry* 2004;184(2):110–7.
26 Patton GC, Coffey C, Carlin JB, Degenhardt L, Lynskey M, Hall W. Cannabis use and mental health in young people: cohort study. *British Medical Journal* 2002;325(7374):1195–8.
27 Gobbi G, Atkin T, Zytynski T, Wang S, Askari S, Boruff J, et al. Association of cannabis use in adolescence and risk of depression, anxiety, and suicidality in young adulthood: a systematic review and meta-analysis. *JAMA Psychiatry* 2019;76(4):426–34.
28 Macfarlane V, Christie G. Synthetic cannabinoid withdrawal: a new demand on detoxification services. *Drug and Alcohol Review* 2015;34(2):147–53.
29 Wilkins C, Rychert M. Responding to a new wave of high potency synthetic cannabinoids. *New Zealand Medical Journal* 2018;131(1482):6–9.
30 Darke S, Kaye S, McKetin R, Duflou J. The major physical and psychological harms of methamphetamine use. *Drug and Alcohol Review* 2008;27(3):253–62.
31 Marshall BD, Werb D. Health outcomes associated with methamphetamine use among young people: a systematic review. *Addiction* 2010;105(6):991–1002.
32 Degenhardt L, Dunn M. Ecstasy. In Ross J (Ed) *Illicit drug use in Australia: epidemiology, use patterns and associated harms. National Drug Strategy Monograph Series No. 63.* 2nd ed. Canberra: Department of Health and Ageing; 2007. p 37–44.
33 Lubman D, Hides L, Yucel M. Inhalant misuse in youth: time for a coordinated response. *Medical Journal of Australia* 2006;185(6):327–30.
34 Kurtzman TL, Otsuka KN, Wahl RA. Inhalant abuse by adolescents. *Journal of Adolescent Health* 2001;28(3):170–80.
35 Lubman DI, Hides L, Yücel M, Toumbourou JW. Intervening early to reduce developmentally harmful substance use among youth populations. *Medical Journal of Australia* 2007;187(7):S22–5.
36 Ryan SM, Jorm AF, Lubman DI. Parenting factors associated with reduced adolescent alcohol use: a systematic review of longitudinal studies. *Australian and New Zealand Journal of Psychiatry* 2010;44(9):774–83.
37 Reavley NJ, Cvetkovski S, Jorm AF, Lubman DI. Help-seeking for substance use, anxiety and affective disorders among young people: results from the 2007 Australian National Survey of Mental Health and Wellbeing. *Australian and New Zealand Journal of Psychiatry* 2010;44(8):729–35.
38 Teesson M, Baillie A, Lynskey M, Manor B, Degenhardt L. Substance use, dependence and treatment seeking in the United States and Australia: a cross national comparison. *Drug and Alcohol Dependence* 2006;81(2):149–55.
39 Wu P, Hoven CW, Tiet Q, Kovalenko P, Wicks J. Factors associated with adolescent utilization of alcohol treatment services. *American Journal of Drug and Alcohol Abuse* 2002;28(2):353–69.
40 Duroy TH, Schmidt SL, Perry PD. Adolescents' and young adults' perspectives on a continuum of care in a three year drug treatment program. *Journal of Drug Issues* 2003;34(4):801–32.
41 Schroder R, Sellman D, Frampton C, Deering D. Youth retention: factors associated with treatment drop-out from youth alcohol and other drug treatment. *Drug and Alcohol Review* 2009;28(6):663–8.

42 Britton J. *Young people's specialist substance misuse treatment: exploring the evidence*. London: National Treatment Agency for Substance Misuse; 2009.
43 National Treatment Agency for Substance Misuse. *Young people's substance misuse treatment services: essential elements*. London: National Treatment Agency; 2005.
44 Dennis M, Godley SH, Diamond G, Tims FM, Babor T, Donaldson J, et al. The Cannabis Youth Treatment (CYT) study: main findings from two randomised trials. *Journal of Substance Abuse Treatment* 2004;27(3):197–213.
45 Farabee D, Shen H, Hser Y, Grella CE, Anglin MD. The effect of drug treatment on criminal behaviour among adolescents in DATOS-A. *Journal of Adolescent Research* 2001;16(6):679–96.
46 Morral AR, McCaffrey DF, Rigeway G, Mukherji A, Beighley C. *The relative effectiveness of 10 adolescent substance abuse treatment programs in the United States*. Santa Monica, CA: RAND Corporation, Drug Policy Research Centre; 2006.
47 Williams RJ, Chang SY. A comprehensive and comparative review of adolescent substance abuse treatment outcome. *Clinical Psychology Science and Practice* 2000;7(2):138–66.
48 Liddle HA, Rowe CL, Dakof GA, Ungaro RA, Henderson CE. Early intervention for adolescent substance abuse: pretreatment to posttreatment outcomes of a randomized clinical trial comparing multidimensional family therapy and peer group treatment. *Journal of Psychoactive Drugs* 2004;36(1):49–63.
49 Bien TH, Miller WR, Tonigan JS. Brief interventions for alcohol problems: a review. *Addiction* 1993;88(3):315–35.
50 Heather N. Effectiveness of brief interventions proved beyond reasonable doubt. *Addiction* 2002;97(3):293–4.
51 Moyer A, Finney JW, Swearingen CE, Vergun P. Brief interventions for alcohol problems: a meta-analytic review of controlled investigations in treatment seeking and non-treatment seeking populations. *Addiction* 2002;97(3):279–92.
52 Liddle HA, Rowe CL. *Adolescent substance abuse*. New York: Cambridge University Press; 2006.
53 McCambridge J, Strang J. The efficacy of single-session motivational interviewing in reducing drug consumption and perceptions of drug related risk and harm among young people: results from a multi-site cluster randomised trial. *Addiction* 2004;99(1):39–52.
54 Tait RJ, Hulse GK. A systematic review of the effectiveness of brief interventions with substance using adolescents by type of drug. *Drug and Alcohol Review* 2003;22(3):337–46.
55 Tevyaw TO, Monti PM. Motivational enhancement and other brief interventions for adolescent substance abuse: foundations, applications and evaluations. *Addiction* 2004;99(2):63–75.
56 Miller WR, Rollnick S. *Motivational interviewing*. 2nd ed. New York: Guilford Press; 2002.
57 Project MATCH Research Group. Matching alcoholism treatments to client heterogeneity: project MATCH posttreatment drinking outcomes. *Journal of Studies on Alcohol* 1997;58(1):7–29.
58 Waldron HB, Kaminer Y. On the learning curve: the emerging evidence supporting cognitive-behavioral therapies for adolescent substance abuse. *Addiction* 2004;99(2):93–105.
59 Kaminer Y, Burleson JA, Goldberger R. Cognitive-behavioural coping skills and psychoeducation therapies for adolescent substance abuse. *Journal of Nervous and Mental Disease* 2002;190(11):737–45.
60 Hides L, Samet S, Lubman DI. Cognitive behaviour therapy (CBT) for the treatment of co-occurring depression and substance use: current evidence and directions for future research. *Drug and Alcohol Review* 2010;29(5):508–17.

61 Liddle HA, Dakof GA, Parker K, Diamond GS, Barrett K, Tejda M. Multidimensional family therapy for adolescent drug abuse: results of a randomized clinical trial. *American Journal of Drug and Alcohol Abuse* 2001;27(4):651–88.
62 Henggeler SW, Clingempeel WG, Brondino MJ, Pickrel SG. Four year follow-up of multisystemic therapy with substance abusing and substance dependent juvenile offenders. *Journal of the American Academy of Child and Adolescent Psychiatry* 2002;41(7):868–74.
63 Sexton T, Turner CW. The effectiveness of functional family therapy for youth with behavioral problems in a community practice setting. *Journal of Family Psychology* 2010;24(3):339–48.
64 Liddle HA. Family-based therapies for adolescent alcohol and drug use: research contributions and future research needs. *Addiction* 2004;99(2):76–9.
65 Anthony EK, Taylor SA, Raffo Z. Early intervention for substance abuse among youth and young adults with mental health conditions: an exploration of community mental health practices. *Administration and Policy in Mental Health and Mental Health Services Research* 2011;38(3):131–41.
66 Velleman R. Co-existing problems: from conceptualization to case formulation. In Baker A, Velleman R (Eds) *Clinical handbook of co-existing mental health and drug and alcohol problems*. London: Routledge; 2007. p 20–38.
67 Christie G, Marsh R, Sheridan J, Wheeler A, Suaalii-Sauni T, Black S, et al. The Substances and Choices Scale (SACS): the development and testing of a new alcohol and other drug screening and outcome measurement instrument for young people. *Addiction* 2007;102(9):1390–8.
68 WHO ASSIST Working Group. *The Alcohol, Smoking and Substance Involvement Screening Test (ASSIST): manual for use in primary care*. Geneva: World Health Organisation; 2010.
69 Heatherton TF, Kozlowski LT, Frecker RC, Fagerström KO. The Fagerström Test for Nicotine Dependence: a revision of the Fagerström Tolerance Questionnaire. *British Journal of Addiction* 1991;86(9):1119–27.
70 Saunders JB, Aasland OG, Babor TF, de la Fuente JR, Grant M. Development of the Alcohol Use Disorders Identification Test (AUDIT): WHO collaborative project on early detection of persons with harmful alcohol consumption. *Addiction* 1993;88(6):791–804.
71 Dawson DA, Grant BF, Stinson FS, Zhou Y. Effectiveness of the derived Alcohol Use Disorders Identification Test (AUDIT-C) in screening for alcohol use disorders and risk drinking in the US general population. *Alcoholism: Clinical and Experimental Research* 2005;29(5):844–54.
72 Adamson SJ, Kay-Lambkin FJ, Baker AL, Lewin TJ, Thornton L, Kelly BJ, et al. An improved brief measure of cannabis misuse: the Cannabis Use Disorders Identification Test – Revised (CUDIT-R). *Drug and Alcohol Dependence* 2010;110(1–2):137–43.
73 Kessler R, Mroczek D. *Kessler Psychological Distress Scale (K10)*. Ann Arbor, MI: Survey Research Center of the Institute for Social Research, University of Michigan; 1994.
74 Aitken C, Wain D, Lubman DI, Hides L, Hellard M. Mental health screening among IDUs outside traditional treatment settings – implications for research and health services. *Mental Health and Substance Use: Dual Diagnosis* 2008;1:99–103.
75 Lubman D, Hides L, Scaffidi A, Elkins K, Stevens M, Marks R. Implementing mental health screening within a youth alcohol and other drugs service. *Mental Health and Substance Use* 2008;1(3):254–61.
76 Babor TF, Higgins-Biddle JC. *Brief intervention for hazardous and harmful drinking: a manual for use in primary care*. Geneva: World Health Organisation; 2001.
77 King RD, Gaines LS, Lambert EW, Summerfelt WT, Bickman L. The co-occurrence of psychiatric and substance use diagnoses in adolescent in different services systems:

frequency, recognition, cost, and outcomes. *Journal of Behavioral Health Services and Research* 2000;27(4):417–30.

78 Turner WC, Muck RD, Muck RJ, Stephens RL, Sukumar B. Co-occurring disorders in the adolescent mental health and substance abuse treatment systems. *Journal of Psychoactive Drugs* 2004;36(4):455–62.

79 Tomlinson KL, Brown SA, Abrantes A. Psychiatric comorbidity and substance use treatment outcomes of adolescents. *Psychology of Addictive Behaviours* 2004;18(2):160–9.

80 Baker A, Kay-Lambkin FJ, Lewin TJ. Co-existing mental health and drug and alcohol problems: steps towards better treatment. In Baker A, Velleman R (Eds) *Clinical handbook of co-existing mental health and drug and alcohol problems.* London: Routledge; 2007. p 1–19.

81 Daley DC, Salloum IM, Zuckoff A, Kirisci L, Thase ME. Increasing treatment adherence among outpatients with depression and cocaine dependence: results of a pilot study. *American Journal of Psychiatry* 1998;155(11):1611–3.

82 Baker A, Bucci S, Kay-Lambkin F, Hides L. Cognitive-behaviour therapy for people with co-existing mental health and drug and alcohol problems. In Baker A, Velleman R (Eds) *Clinical handbook of co-existing mental health and drug and alcohol problems.* London: Routledge; 2007. p 55–73.

83 Westmeyer H. On the structure of case formulations. *European Journal of Psychological Assessment* 2003;19(3):210–6.

84 Beck AT, Rush AJ, Shaw BF, Emery G. *Cognitive therapy for depression.* New York: Guilford; 1979.

85 Segal Z, Teasdale J, Williams M. *Mindfulness-based cognitive therapy for depression.* New York: Guilford Press; 2002.

86 Free M. *Cognitive therapy in groups: guidelines and resources for practice.* 2nd ed. West Sussex: Wiley; 2007.

87 Graham HL. Implementing integrated treatment for co-existing substance use and severe mental health problems in assertive outreach teams: training issues. *Drug and Alcohol Review* 2004;23(4):463–70.

88 Marlatt GA, Gordon JR. *Relapse prevention: maintenance strategies in the treatment of addictive behaviors.* New York: Guilford Press; 1985.

89 Tait RJ, Christensen H. Internet-based interventions for young people with problematic substance use: a systematic review. *Medical Journal of Australia* 2010;192(11): S15–21.

90 Kay-Lambkin FJ, Baker AL, Lewin TJ, Carr VJ. Computer-based psychological treatment for comorbid depression and substance use problems: a randomised controlled trial of clinical efficacy. *Addiction* 2009;104(3):378–88.

91 Dakof GA, Tejeda M, Liddle HA. Predictors of engagement in adolescent drug abuse treatment. *Journal of the American Academy of Child and Adolescent Psychiatry* 2001;40(3): 274–81.

92 McIntosh J, MacAskill S, Eadie D, Curtice J, McKeganey N, Hastings G, et al. *Evaluation and description of drug projects working with young people and families funded by Lloyds TSB Foundation Partnership Drugs Initiative.* Edinburgh: Substance Misuse Research Scottish Executive; 2006.

93 McGillicuddy NB, Rychtarik RG, Duquette JA, Morsheimer ET. Development of a skill training program for parents of substance-abusing adolescents. *Journal of Substance Abuse Treatment* 2001;20(1):59–68.

94 Spooner C, Mattick RP, Noffs W. Outcomes of a comprehensive treatment program for adolescents with a substance-use disorder. *Journal of Substance Abuse Treatment* 2001;20(3):205–13.

95 Jainchill N, Hawke J, Messina M. Post-treatment outcomes among adjudicated adolescent males and females in modified therapeutic community treatment. *Substance Use and Misuse* 2005;40(7):975–96.
96 Sullivan JT, Sykora K, Schneiderman J, Naranjo CA, Sellers EM. Assessment of alcohol withdrawal: the revised Clinical Institute Withdrawal Assessment for Alcohol scale (CIWA-Ar). *British Journal of Addiction* 1989;84(11):1353–7.
97 Gossop M. The development of a Short Opiate Withdrawal Scale (SOWS). *Addictive Behaviours* 1990;15(5):487–90.

12 Social disability in young people

The need to improve time use

David Fowler, Paul French, Jo Hodgekins and Jon Wilson

Introduction

It is now widely recognised that most chronic and severe mental health problems begin in adolescence. Seventy-five percent of all mental illnesses emerge between the ages of 15 and 25.[1,2] Mental health problems are common in adolescence affecting up to one in five. However, only a minority become chronic, with an estimate of between 3% and 5% of young people with mental ill-health developing persistent and complex problems.

Those most at risk of long-term disability are those with early social decline combined with non-specific psychopathology, such as depression and social anxiety. This combination of factors seems to be a key indicator of long-term functional outcome and complex emotional dysfunction across a range of disorders, such as depression, bipolar disorder and schizophrenia.

Given that early social decline has such a potentially destructive impact on future mental health, it is an important target for intervention. This could increase our understanding of socially disabling severe mental illness and even prevent it in some cases. The best approach may be to directly examine the factors that lead to the maintenance of social disability at an early stage. Developing a model of the factors which underpin social disability associated with severe mental illness may provide a basis for new approaches to intervention.

A first stage in developing such a preventive approach is the detection of young people at risk of early social disability or those with early signs of social disability. This is not as straightforward as it seems. Many current widely used scales for assessment of social disability, such as the Global Assessment of Functioning (GAF)[3] and the Quality of Life Scale (QLS),[4] are actually highly confounded with symptoms. We suggest, therefore, that it may be best to define early signs of social disability as consistent patterns of low activity or time use.

Defining early signs of social disability in terms of low activity

Social disability can be defined in terms of the number of hours per week engaged in structured activity. This includes time spent in both constructive economic activity such as work, education and childcare, and in structured activity, for example, chores, sports, voluntary work and other structured social activity, such as playing music. Defining social outcome based on hours in activity overcomes the problem of confounding symptom assessments (particularly of emotional disorder and negative symptoms) with social outcome. It provides an assessment with direct face validity to users, clinicians, service managers and policy makers. Direct assessment of hours in constructive economic activity or structured activity is readily understandable by all, valid, sensitive to small but important changes in functioning, and able to be reliably assessed. Time spent in activity can be measured using an instrument such as the Time Use Survey.[5] This is the standard time use interview as used in the Office of National Statistics UK Time Use Survey.

The time use interview assessment is well established and is derived from extensive research on time use in the UK and internationally. It has good concurrent validity with other well-known scales of quality of life and social functioning but is less confounded with symptoms.[6] Focus groups of clinicians and service users have reached a consensus agreement that for this population a four-hour gain in structured activity represents a minimum clinically significant gain.

Poor time use in young people with mental health problems

It has long been known that time spent doing nothing may be a critical driver of poor mental health in schizophrenia.[7] There are various factors that may contribute to social disability in schizophrenia and thus impede social recovery (see Box 12.1). We know little about how these different factors interact to influence activity.

Box 12.1 Factors that contribute to social disability

Persistent positive symptoms (delusions and hallucinations)
Negative symptoms (anhedonia, amotivation, diminished ability to express emotions)
Cognitive deficits and disorganisation
Depression, demoralisation and hopelessness
Social anxiety
Negative beliefs about self, others and the future
Stigma, discrimination and self-stigma
Disuse atrophy of the brain
Side effects of medication such as movement disorders and obesity

Some of the patterns of low activity and social withdrawal which characterise social disability may be usefully characterised as functional behavioural patterns of avoidance. One reason for such avoidance may derive from self-regulation of the experience of early symptoms of psychosis themselves, such as anomalous

Table 12.1 Comparison of constructive economic and structured time use across studies – mean hours per week (SD)

	Constructive economic	*Structured (without hobbies)*
Young people with ultra-high risk symptoms (*n* = 288)	25.11 (27.05)	30.67 (27.81)
Young people with first episode psychosis (*n* = 1027)	17.23 (23.80)	25.44 (27.10)
Young people with chronic psychotic disorder and social impairment (*n* = 77)	12.43 (17.05)	19.66 (17.54)
Aged matched young people in the normal population (*n* = 6000)	50.93 (25.40)	64.18 (27.22)

Note: Constructive economic activity = work, education, voluntary work, childcare and chores. Structured activity = constructive economic activity plus leisure and sports activities

experiences, confusion and information overload. Also, early negative symptoms such as low motivation, avolition, and anhedonia may be characterised as arising at least in part as cognitive and emotional experiential avoidance. Avoidant behaviour and withdrawal can therefore often be regarded as safety behaviours to manage anxiety and psychotic symptoms.

The extent of social disability in young people with mental ill-health has been shown in a series of recent studies in different populations.[8] The Time Use Survey was used to provide data from (1) a group at high risk of psychosis, (2) a group with early psychosis, (3) a group with chronic psychotic disorder and (4) normative data from young people in the non-clinical population (see Table 12.1).

It is striking that many young people are already stuck in patterns of activity doing almost nothing at all. The danger is that these lifestyle patterns become lifelong and result in further hopelessness, lack of motivation, loss of peer networks, depression, negative symptoms and physical ill-health.

Our analyses suggest that a useful cut-off for detecting a socially disabled group using the time use interview is at a level of less than 30 hours per week total structured activity. As can be seen in Table 12.1, this is less than half the mean level of functioning of young people in the normal population. It is likely that many of these factors influencing inactivity may also operate in young people with other mental health problems.

Interventions to improve time use in young people with severe mental illness

A key feature of studies in this area is a focus on social recovery as the primary outcome, with this being operationally defined as an improvement in time engaged in structured activity. The focus may be as much on improvements in structured social and leisure activity and household tasks as on work and education. This is particularly salient in the current economic climate, with high unemployment rates and jobs difficult to find for many people.

The main aim of social recovery interventions is to assist the person in managing ongoing problems (which may include vulnerability to psychotic symptoms, emotional disorder and cognitive deficits) so that they can improve the amount of time they spend engaged in meaningful activity.

A cognitive behavioural formulation of low activity in psychosis as avoidance

As noted earlier, poor time use and lack of social activity in people with psychotic disorders can be thought of as avoidance behaviour used to manage anxiety and psychotic symptoms. A cognitive behavioural approach can provide a useful analysis of how avoidance may be central to understanding psychotic problems and especially for understanding and treating low levels of activity which characterise social disability. Cognitive behavioural analysis can provide a way of understanding how such primary avoidance may occur as a direct result of the way vulnerability to psychosis may be manifested in the context of day-to-day stressors. Individuals may need to be helped to gradually explore the world while learning to manage anomalous experiences and to cope with feelings of information overload. Strategies which help the person normalise and de-catastrophise the experience of anomalies and confusion may also be important (as described by French and Morrison, 2004).[9]

It is also important to recognise that there may be patterns of secondary avoidance arising from processes in depression and social anxiety. These are typically comorbid with symptoms of psychosis or may occur independently as a syndrome of severe and complex comorbid mental health problems. Hopelessness and extreme negative beliefs about self, others, and the world may lead to behavioural patterns of withdrawal typical of chronic depression. Furthermore, social anxiety is often comorbid with early symptoms of psychosis and may need to be targeted directly. In many cases, both social anxiety and depression may have existed for long periods premorbid to psychotic problems. These problems need to be overcome and strategies learnt that could help individuals to adapt and deal with anomalies in ways that enable them to lead meaningful and purposeful lives. The types of procedures useful in overcoming avoidance in depression and social anxiety may then be relevant in psychosis, and cognitive strategies developed for psychotic disorders may be applicable to non-psychotic illness such as depression and social anxiety.

Cognitive behaviour therapy (CBT) has an extensive repertoire of problems to manage and overcome avoidance while encouraging behavioural activation and behavioural experiments. The key is a cognitive behavioural formulation, which assesses presenting problems and, in particular, the problems an individual has in undertaking activity. The nature of the avoidance can then be identified and tackled in a systematic manner. Sometimes these techniques alone may be successful. For example, classic CBT for social anxiety in the form of guided self-help may be effective. However, many patients have complex, comorbid mental health problems confounded with other types of symptoms such as depression or clearer psychotic symptoms and social disadvantage, and these problems may require a multisystemic intervention.

Specific characteristics of a multisystemic, cognitive behavioural approach: the need to weave in systemic and assertive case management practice in delivering cognitive behavioural techniques to promote social recovery

Young people with social disability problems frequently feel hopeless and can be difficult to engage. They tend to present with a range of complex mental health problems and are often stuck in a lifestyle of social withdrawal. This lifestyle may be both maintained and compounded by social disadvantage and the negative attitudes of others. To effectively address these problems, therapists need to be prepared to work in a flexible way that integrates CBT with an awareness of multisystemic formulation and interventions. This may involve addressing the attitudes of others, such as family members or other professionals. A multidisciplinary approach and assertive case management practice may be required. CBT can help people to improve activity while not becoming overloaded with symptoms. Therapists need to be thoroughly grounded in techniques to manage depression, social anxiety and paranoia, as these are frequently the primary targets of intervention. Techniques of promoting hope, motivation and behavioural activation are also important. However, our experience is that the traditional mode of working as a clinic-based cognitive behavioural therapist is not sufficient to create change amongst young people who are at the highest risk of severe social disability.

We have observed that real gains in terms of changing hope and promoting a sense of agency and positive beliefs about self and others in young people occur as a result of the person achieving meaningful changes to their lives or working toward them, including relationships with others, work, education and valued social activities. To achieve this against a background of often years of social withdrawal and social disadvantage means that cognitive behaviour therapists have to be prepared to adopt practices more typically associated with case management, including assertive community treatment, supported education and work, and multisystemic working, and integrate this with cognitive behavioural practice. Systemic and positioning approaches can effectively complement CBT, particularly when the client is part of a complex system. For instance, family members may sometimes encourage withdrawal as a result of their fears of relapse. In such cases, some family meetings to address such attitudes may be important in creating a context for change to happen. It is also the case that sometimes the attitudes of professionals can create a barrier to the person's motivation to improve. In particular, conservatism over the need to avoid stress for fear of relapse can be an issue. Sedation and dysphoria due to over-medication may also be a factor. Here, again, discussions with other professionals may be needed to ensure a consistent message of change and hope is provided. Similarly, the attitudes of education providers, work colleagues and employers can present social barriers to the opportunities available to people. Here, meetings or phone calls to assist the creation of opportunity or to support the employer or education provider may be enough to keep a social opportunity open.

To be effective in promoting social recovery it is therefore important that cognitive behaviour therapists focusing on social recovery are able to formulate these types of barriers and make steps to overcome them. Taking a systemic or positional approach can help the therapist/worker adopt strategies with regard to the client's wider systems that can facilitate the progress of the CBT or therapy of choice. It is therefore useful for the therapist to be a person who is confident to work in people's homes and liaise with families, other professionals, employers and education providers.

Working in the context of a multidisciplinary team that provides back-up to the therapist also assists this work. Adopting a case management or supported employment approach may mean visiting the person at home and liaising with employers or education providers to create a social opportunity. Meanwhile, the cognitive behavioural symptom management techniques may then focus on overcoming symptoms and assisting the person to maintain hope and motivation. Done well, this integration of different styles of working is seamless and automatic and provides a strong basis for a person to recover socially and engage in more meaningful use of time.

Multisystemic social recovery cognitive behavioural therapy (SRCBT)

We have developed an intervention that combines all the elements previously mentioned. It uses a focused subset of specific therapeutic procedures (see Box 12.2 for summary). Predominant amongst the specific therapeutic procedures are (1) assessment procedures to identify meaningful personal goals and key presenting problems, symptoms and a formulation of avoidance patterns and (2) techniques to address negative evaluations of self and others, address self-regulation of psychotic symptoms (including training of coping strategies) and improve social activity. (3) The approach also draws on behavioural experimental approaches to manage social anxiety and depression.[10,11] (4) The work involves a primary focus on social recovery – treating symptoms where they represent barriers to recovery but not as primary targets – and combining the therapist role with case management roles. For example, therapists are asked to adopt an assertive, outreach worker–style of contact, most frequently visiting people at home or in the workplace to carry out behavioural experiments. Therapists are also encouraged to adopt a pragmatic and problem-solving approach to assist people to overcome work-related problems using techniques associated with individual placement support vocational interventions.[12] This often involves setting up interviews with education and work placements and discussing problems in joint interviews with employment and education providers and the client. Participants receive up to 20 sessions of SRCBT over a 9-month period. A trial of SRCBT in young people with established chronic and severe social disability problems some years after first episode psychosis demonstrated gains in structured activity and hope as well as reductions in symptoms.[6] Clear indications of health economic benefits were also demonstrated.[13] We have subsequently applied this type of approach in clinical practice, widening our selection criteria to include all young people presenting with severe and complex mental health problems at risk of social disability. A trial is currently underway in this group (recruitment began in 2013) and will report in the near future.[14]

Box 12.2 Key elements of social recovery cognitive behavioural therapy (SRCBT)

1. Assessment of goals, problems and formulation of avoidance patterns, including barriers, threats and difficulties
2. A focus on promoting hope for social recovery
3. Combining the therapist role with case management roles to provide opportunities for social recovery and address barriers to increasing activity
4. Promoting a sense of agency, consolidating a positive identity and addressing feelings of stigma and negative beliefs about self and others
5. Active promotion of social activity, work, education and leisure linked to meaningful goals
6. Identifying specific pathways to meaningful new activities, e.g., referral to vocational agencies, education providers
7. Specific cognitive behavioural work managing symptoms using behavioural experiments, e.g., reducing safety-seeking behaviours

Conclusion

Social disability and particularly time spent doing nothing may be critical drivers of outcome in a range of mental health problems. A more integrated approach to this issue in complex youth mental health cases is needed. Better outcomes on social disability and hopelessness can be obtained from a more targeted intervention specifically focused on improving social disability amongst those who have low functioning. We have developed a multisystemic form of CBT called social recovery cognitive behavioural therapy, which targets social disability and aims to improve constructive time use.

References

1 Kessler RC, Berglund P, Demler O, Jin R, Merikangas KR, Walters EE. Lifetime prevalence and age-of-onset distributions of DSM-IV disorders in the National Comorbidity Survey Replication. *Archives of General Psychiatry* 2005;62(6):593–602.
2 Kim-Cohen J, Caspi A, Moffitt TE, Harrington H, Milne BJ, Poulton R. Prior juvenile diagnoses in adults with mental disorder: developmental follow-back of a prospective-longitudinal cohort. *Archives of General Psychiatry* 2003;60(7):709–17.
3 Hall RC. Global assessment of functioning. A modified scale. *Psychosomatics* 1995;36(3): 267–75.

4 Heinrichs DW, Hanlon TE, Carpenter WT Jr. The Quality of Life Scale: an instrument for rating the schizophrenic deficit syndrome. *Schizophrenia Bulletin* 1984;10(3):388–98.
5 Lader D, Short S, Gershuny J. *The Time Use Survey, 2005: how we spend our time*. London: Office for National Statistics; 2006.
6 Fowler D, Hodgekins J, Painter M, Reilly T, Crane C, Macmillan I, et al. Cognitive behaviour therapy for improving social recovery in psychosis: a report from the ISREP MRC Trial Platform Study (Improving Social Recovery in Early Psychosis). *Psychological Medicine* 2009;39(10):1627–36.
7 Wing JK, Brown GW. *Institutionalism and schizophrenia*. London: Cambridge University Press; 1970.
8 Hodgekins J, French P, Birchwood M, Mugford M, Christopher R, Marshall M, et al. Comparing time use in individuals at different stages of psychosis and a non-clinical comparison group. *Schizophrenia Research* 2015;161(2–3):188–93.
9 French P, Morrison AP. *Early detection and cognitive therapy for people at high risk of developing psychosis*. London: Wiley; 2004.
10 Butler G. *Overcoming social anxiety and shyness*. New York: Basic Books; 2008.
11 Beck AT, Rush J, Shaw BF, Emery G. *Cognitive therapy of depression*. New York: Guilford; 1979.
12 Killackey E, Allott K. Utilising individual placement and support to address unemployment and low education rates among individuals with psychotic disorders. *Australian and New Zealand Journal of Psychiatry* 2013;47(6):521–3.
13 Barton GR, Hodgekins J, Mugford M, Jones PB, Croudace T, Fowler D. Cognitive behaviour therapy for improving social recovery in psychosis: cost-effectiveness analysis. *Schizophrenia Research* 2009;112(1–3):158–63.
14 Fowler D, French P, Banerjee R, Barton G, Berry C, Byrne R, et al. Prevention and treatment of long-term social disability amongst young people with emerging severe mental illness with social recovery therapy (The PRODIGY Trial): study protocol for a randomised controlled trial. *Trials* 2017;18(1):315.

13 Vocational recovery in young people with mental health problems

Progress and directions

Eóin Killackey

Introduction

In Western societies, a key contributor to the construct of identity is role. While there are many 'roles' drawn on in the construction of an individual's identity and sense of self, such as role in the family and in the community, one of the most important is vocational role. Not only is this role important in contributing to identity, but having a positive vocational role is associated with a wide range of good health outcomes.

People with mental illness tend not to do well in the domain of vocational functioning. It is known that people with psychotic illnesses such as schizophrenia have an unemployment rate of 50% at the onset of illness, which quickly rises to 90% if illness progresses.[1,2] For those with other illnesses such as depression, the vocational issues are about both employment and when employed, the ability to perform optimally.

This chapter will examine the background to vocational functioning in young people with mental illness. It will look at rates of educational attainment and employment. It will present evidence that shows that there are means to address this area of functioning and an argument for why it is important to do so. Finally, it will examine what research, practice and policy in this area need to develop in order to work towards the goal of reducing the gap between the vocational functioning of those with a mental illness and those without. Most of the work in this area has been conducted in the area of psychotic illness, so that will be the main focus of this chapter. However, there are important points relevant to other disorders, and where that is the case, it will be pointed out.

The problem: educational and employment attainment among those with mental illness

In order to understand the importance of this issue, it is instructive to first understand the scale of the problem. It is also important to understand that there are factors extrinsic to the illness that contribute to the difficulties that this population have with employment.

At the outset of psychotic illness, studies have shown a wide range of employment levels. Most of the large variation in these figures is accounted for by the nature of the economies in which the studies occurred. In developing economies for instance, there are many roles which no longer exist in developed economies and which are often a means of employing people who might otherwise not be employed. In most developed economies the unemployment rate is approximately 50% for those presenting for the first time.[1] But in isolation it is hard to understand the meaning of this figure. To add some context, most developed economies today have unemployment rates between 5% and 10%, and this is unusually high due to the after-effects of the global financial crisis. One of the arguments that is sometimes given is that because mental illness is disproportionately an illness of young people, discussions about unemployment should look at youth unemployment, which is typically higher than general unemployment. This is true. However, while youth unemployment is higher (usually two to three times higher) there are two caveats. The first is that this still does not explain the higher rate found among those with psychosis. Secondly, when youth unemployment is broken into two age ranges (15–19 and 20–25) it is found that it is only the 15–19 age range that is generally well above the population rate. By the time people are in their 20s they tend to be no more likely to be unemployed than the general population.

When data for those who develop chronic illness is examined, up to 95% of people are unemployed.[3] This tends to persist so that even when people with illness have made symptomatic recoveries, or have well-managed symptoms, they tend not to enter or re-enter the workforce. So, the question that needs to be asked is, what are the barriers to employment for this group?

Barriers to employment

There are a number of barriers that act against the employment prospects of the young person with psychosis. The main ones, however, are lack of education, stigma, the effect of welfare benefits, mismanifested care and the inappropriate design of employment systems for this group.

Education

One of the key problems that contributes to high unemployment is the level of education possessed by people with mental illness. In developed economies, the level of education required for entry to even more menial jobs has become higher.[3] This is both because of the need for more training in higher-level jobs and the general increase in education leading to more competition for lower-level jobs. As shown in previous chapters, mental illness has its onset at the phase of life that is most associated with the completion of secondary education and the commencement of further training or employment. The onset of illness at this time is extremely disruptive and in many cases acts to completely derail this process.[4] It is well established in the general population that further education is associated with higher pay and lower unemployment.

Some data may illustrate this. In a survey of nearly 400 patients at an early intervention service in Melbourne, Australia, 25% were enrolled in education.

In a more detailed study carried out in that service it was found that less than a quarter had completed secondary school and more than half had less than a Year 10 education. By comparison, state data show that 84% of same-age peers achieve a secondary qualification and that the retention rate at school until the final year is 79% (with some completing the secondary qualification by alternate means).[5] This illustrates the competitive disadvantage that people with mental illness start out with because of educations that were disrupted by the onset of illness. While well known that completion of secondary school is a predictor of vocational success in the general population, the same has been found for people with schizophrenia, such that irrespective of course of illness, those who complete secondary school are much more likely to be employed than those who do not.[6]

Stigma

Stigma operates at two key levels with respect to employment. The first is stigma that comes from society and potential employers. Despite efforts in a number of countries in recent years, the stigma surrounding mental illness stubbornly persists. It contributes to erroneous ideas such as work not being suitable for people with mental illness or that people with mental illness do not want to work. The other form of stigma is more insidious. This is the type of stigma that is directed by the person with mental illness at themselves. This possibly comes about by the individual 'buying-in' to the surrounding societal beliefs about mental illness.

System design

Many people with mental illness, particularly the young, do not identify as having a disability. Despite this, in many countries if a person with a mental illness wants to access the employment services, they are directed to disability employment services. These are often set up to provide services for people with physical disabilities, and the results for people with mental illness are not good. In Australia in 2002, a government report noted that people with mental illness were the largest disability group accessing disability support services and were also the group that received the least benefit from those services. This situation has not changed, despite reform of the disability employment sector.

Benefits

While benefits are a necessary safety net for people with mental illness, providing them a degree of dignity in their life, they are also associated with not returning to work. The reasons for this are complex and vary from country to country with the rules of various schemes. In general though, in many systems returning to work involves gambling a safe pension against an uncertain wage. Additionally, because pensions often include concessions on utility bills and transport, there can be a punitive effect whilst transitioning from welfare to work.

Well-intentioned but limiting care

One of the most important areas affecting return to work is the attitude of carers, clinicians and workers. Where these important figures believe in the potential of the person with mental illness to work, and where they act in accord with this belief, they are a powerful source of motivation for the individual. All too often though these potential supporters discourage the person with mental illness from pursuing their potential. This is often motivated by good intentions such as not wanting to expose the person to the stress of working. However, they neglect both that being unemployed is stressful in itself and that there is great reinforcement for recovery and self-respect in work.

These barriers are in many ways the key reasons underlying the poor work participation of young people with psychosis. They result in a status quo situation where there is often little belief in work being a part of the future of someone with mental illness, and consequently, little assistance is provided to young people with mental illness who would like to work. Were it not for the fact that young people with mental illness have the right to and want to work, that it is monumentally costly for them not to and that employment may be a shortcut to recovery in a wide range of other functional domains, there would be good reason for not doing anything.

Four good reasons for employment

Despite stereotypical images of all work associated with the asylum era as being the exploitation of people who had mental illness, or in many cases were just poor, the fact is that this was not always the case. Contemporary descriptions of the place of employment and training within the New York asylums suggest that in the 1840s it was educative and rehabilitative in nature. The stereotypical images are perhaps more recent, with commentary from 1918 noting that the pedagogical and self-improvement nature of the earlier approach had been lost.

While there is no doubt debate about the conditions of, and intentions behind, work and education in the asylum era, since deinstitutionalisation, people with mental illness have done more poorly than just about any other group on a wide range of functional domains. People with mental illness have done more poorly in terms of their physical health, being in a relationship, being a parent, being socially excluded, having unstable accommodation, being a victim of crime and being in jail. Interestingly, just about the only other condition that predisposes to poor outcome in these areas is unemployment, with those who experience unemployment more likely to do worse than the general population in these domains.

Coincidentally or not, people with mental illness experience more unemployment and less help with employment than any other disability group. The first reason for paying attention to the vocational functioning of people with a mental illness is that employment may be a shortcut to improving functioning in a range of areas. Work participation has a positive influence on health, daily structure, development of coping strategies and meaning of life.[7] It offers opportunities for leisure and socialising, as well as providing financial gain.[8]

The second reason is that the right to work is a fundamental human right enshrined in Article 23 of the United Nations Declaration of Human Rights. Not only is it a human right to be allowed to work, but, contrary to common opinion, people with a mental illness overwhelmingly want to work. A number of studies over more than 20 years and in very different settings have all revealed the same thing: the number one goal of people with a mental illness is to become employed in the open labour market – that is, get a job that anyone with the right qualifications could have applied for.[9,10] It would be surprising to many that this desire to work even ranks ahead of being symptom free. And it is this fierce desire to work that is the third reason that more attention needs to be given to people with a mental illness being assisted to return to, or enter, the workforce.

Finally, unemployment among those with mental illness is enormously expensive. In Australia, where the total cost of schizophrenia is approximately $2 billion Australian dollars per annum, costs associated with unemployment accounted for just over half of this.[11] In comparison, direct treatment costs were about $600 million Australian dollars. In the USA, where the total costs of schizophrenia were US$61 billon, costs associated with unemployment of people with schizophrenia were US$32 billion.[12] Data which show a similar ratio of costs are also available for Europe.[13] The potential savings that could be achieved through an effective approach to vocational rehabilitation for people with mental illness are significant. In the Australian context, it has been estimated that making only a 10% difference in the number of people with schizophrenia in employment would lead to savings of over AUS$140 million.[14]

Box 13.1 Four good reasons for employment

1) Being in work improves functioning in a range of domains
2) Work is a human right
3) People with mental illnesses generally want to work
4) Increasing employment rates benefits the economy

Young people are particularly important to work with around their vocational issues. This is because the 'disability' associated with long-term unemployment has not set in. Young people are more likely to be physically well, have no forensic history and are in a phase of their life where vocational development and exploration is normal. It is also much easier as an 18- or 20-year-old to get a job having no or little work history than it is as a person in their 30s who may have no work history.[15]

Thus far we have considered the barriers to employment in young people with mental illness and reasons why vocational recovery should be a priority for this group. If it is accepted that it should be a priority, the next question is, what can be done about vocational recovery for those with mental illness?

Employment interventions

Over the last 100 years, and particularly in the last 60 years, different methods of vocational intervention have been developed. Only one of the three methods that belong to the modern era of psychiatry has been developed chiefly by mental health professionals. This says a lot about the place of vocational rehabilitation in the priorities of health systems. The interventions that have been developed are industrial therapy, social firms, Clubhouse model (transitional employment, train and place) and supported employment.

Industrial therapy

Industrial or work therapy refers to the wide range of chores and jobs given to residents of the old institutions in the times before deinstitutionalisation.[16–18] In re-examining these programs now, it can be seen that while they did provide an occupation and in some cases might have helped teach new skills, these programs were inadequate in three key ways. First, the skills taught may not have generalised to other employment situations. Second, the tasks may not have been well suited to the occupational interests of the individual. Third, these jobs often did not offer remuneration that would have been equivalent to that earned in a similar job in the community, if indeed any financial remuneration was offered at all.

As part of the deinstitutionalisation process, it was recognised that formerly institutionalised people needed to develop working skills in order to reintegrate into the social and economic life of the general community. This led to the development of two different approaches. In Europe, particularly in Italy, the concept of the social firm was developed.[19] In the USA, the Clubhouse model of vocational rehabilitation expanded.[20]

Social firms

Social firms are a particular kind of social enterprise.[21] They are not-for-profit businesses that are set up to provide a product or service to the public and in doing so create employment for people who may ordinarily be excluded from the labour market due to illness or disability. The criteria required of social firms include: that at least 25% of employees face major barriers to work (e.g., due to mental illness); that at least 50% of the turnover comes from the market activity of the company; and that in these positions people are paid at least the national minimum wage, given real responsibilities and have the potential to progress through the business.[22,23] While it may also be envisaged that skills learned in a social firm would eventually be used to find competitive employment, this is often not an aim of the people or organisation running the business, who are more likely to see themselves as investing in the training of an individual with the target of developing a sustainable business.[22–24]

A report on social firms in the UK noted that 83% of social firms operated in the service sector.[24] In Italy, with over 5000 social firms, 58% were in the service sector; 29% were in the manufacture of handicrafts; and the remainder were in areas described as building (4%), commercial (6%) and agricultural (3%) activities.[25]

In 2003, it was noted that there had not been any systematic evaluation of social firms.[26] To date, this seems not to have been remedied. This is a great pity because the evidence from industry groups suggests that this is a means by which people with mental illness could find work in an environment that is accommodating to the needs of their illness. There also seems to be longevity of employment, with less than 7% of staff leaving in a 1-year period.[24]

The downside to social firms is that, as with any business, a social firm requires a substantial amount of time and energy just to establish, let alone run successfully. Further, any individual social firm may not fit the vocational needs of an individual. Therefore, successful use of social firms involves not the establishment of one or two businesses, but the development of an employment sector. Italy has experienced substantial growth in this sector through the Italian government's mandate and support of its development as a means to create employment for those marginalised by their illnesses, disabilities or circumstances.[25] However, without research to examine the economic and health benefits of social firms, there is little leverage to encourage other governments, or those who might be described as social venture capitalists, to invest in the development of the social firm sector.

In comparison to both industrial therapy and social firms, there has been more research describing and examining two other interventions, the Clubhouse model and supported employment. Clubhouse programs typically involve prevocational training and transitional employment. Supported employment on the other hand, emphasises direct job placement and ongoing support and is best defined in the Individual Placement and Support (IPS) model of Becker and Drake.[27]

The Clubhouse model

The Clubhouse model was started by ex-psychiatric patients at Fountain House in New York in 1948.[28] At the Clubhouse, members contribute to the club by participating in voluntary work necessary to the running of the club (the work-ordered day).[20] The members are thus contributing to the club and developing skills necessary to succeed in employment, such as punctuality, confidence and responsibility. After this experience, members have access to a set period of employment in a local company. This transitional employment, which is central to the Clubhouse model,[29] involves an arrangement through which the company offers a number of positions that the job club guarantees to fill. The job club may then use 12 people working part-time to fill four full-time positions, so that no individual is required to work full-time. In order to be certified by the International Center for Clubhouse Development (ICCD), Clubhouses must have access to a wide range of different employment settings. Finally, at the end of this process, obtaining competitive employment is a potential goal for members.[30] While this has been the traditional Clubhouse model of employment (and Clubhouses are still misrepresented as offering only transitional employment),[31] more recently Clubhouses have viewed the work-ordered day and transitional employment as the first two steps of a hierarchy of vocational interventions which continues onto supported employment and then independent employment.[31] A worldwide survey of ICCD-certified Clubhouses in 2000 found that transitional employment provided 36.6% of job placements, supported employment 26.6% and independent employment 36.8%.[31,32]

Clubhouse studies

Research on the effectiveness of the Clubhouse model in achieving desired outcomes is one of the acknowledged neglected areas in its development over most of the last 50 years.[20,31] This led to a number of criticisms of Clubhouses. The lack of randomised controlled trials of transitional employment has possibly also affected the way that transitional employment has been viewed in widely cited systematic reviews of employment interventions for people with serious mental illness.

Three studies have examined either ICCD Clubhouse outcomes or compared them to other programs.[31,33,34] Only one study to date has actually compared ICCD-certified Clubhouses to another approach called Program of Assertive Community Treatment (PACT).[34] The outcome of competitive employment included transitional employment, even though it has not been viewed as competitive employment by all researchers of vocational interventions due to the 'set-aside' nature of transitional employment jobs.

Macias found that PACT and ICCD had similar outcomes on a number of measures, including the number of participants who started competitive work, the number of participants interested in work at baseline who started competitive work, job satisfaction and the amount of time from enrolment until commencing work. The ICCD Clubhouse performed better than PACT on measures of days worked, money earned, quality of jobs, hourly rate of pay and job tenure. PACT performed better than the ICCD Clubhouse on participant retention.[34]

Although the benefits of Clubhouses extend far beyond their role in employment rehabilitation, they, like social firms, are not easy to establish. Clubhouse budgets in America averaged just over US$400,000 in 1996.[28] Apart from cost, one of the other factors that mitigate against Clubhouses being established by and for young people with first-episode psychosis is that Clubhouses are the result of communities forming around a common issue. Typically, young people with first-episode psychosis are still coming to terms with their psychotic experiences and have not developed an identity based around their illness, nor have they necessarily developed the networks or skills required to establish an undertaking like a Clubhouse. To establish a Clubhouse for young people with first-episode psychosis would likely involve such significant input from non-consumers that those with first-episode psychosis might feel little ownership of the project, which would contravene the philosophy central to the Clubhouse model.

Individual placement and support

Supported employment is an approach to vocational intervention that is differentiated from pre-vocational training models by its focus on rapid job search and placement and by continued support following the acquisition of a competitive position.[35] Supported employment is most specifically defined in the IPS model, which has been developed for people with severe mental illness for just over a decade.

The IPS model has seven defining features:[27,29]

1. It is focused on competitive employment in integrated work settings, rather than sheltered or transitional employment;
2. The service is open to any person with mental illness who chooses to look for work, so that acceptance into the program is not determined by measures of work-readiness or illness variables;
3. Job searching commences directly on entry into the program;
4. The IPS program is integrated with the mental health treatment team, rather than constituting a separate vocational rehabilitation service;
5. Potential jobs are chosen based on consumer preference;
6. The support provided in the program continues after employment is obtained, rather than terminating at a set point, as needed by the individual; and
7. The IPS services are provided in the community, rather than at the mental health or rehabilitation facility.

In contrast to both social firms and Clubhouses, which developed largely from collectives of people experiencing mental illnesses, the supported employment model has been adapted by researchers and clinicians from its previous use in populations with intellectual disability. Consequently, it is the most studied of the various vocational interventions and the one most supported by systematic research.

The evidence for IPS in young people with first-episode psychosis

Much previous work in populations of people with chronic schizophrenia had established supported employment as the intervention with the most evidence of producing successful employment outcomes.[36] Of the various methods of supported employment, IPS was the most defined, most researched and most successful.[37] IPS has made a successful transition to early intervention, first with an open trial and then in a series of randomised controlled trials and further naturalistic studies.[38–43] In all of these studies, the importance of the addition of educational outcomes has been emphasised.

An example of one of the randomised controlled trials is described.[39] Forty-one young people with first-episode psychosis were randomised to either IPS or a control group consisting of referral to government-funded employment agencies. In the IPS group 13 out of 20 found employment compared to two out of 21 in the control group. In each group four people entered or completed an educational course. In sum, 17 out of the 20 people in the IPS group and six out of the 21 in the control group had a positive vocational outcome. Additionally, those in the IPS group earned more (median $2432 vs $0), worked more hours per week (38 vs 22.5) and worked more weeks (median 5 vs 0) than the control group. This study was conducted in Melbourne, Australia. The other randomised controlled trial of this intervention in first-episode psychosis was conducted in Los Angeles through UCLA. Where the Melbourne study had a positive vocational outcome rate of 85%, the Los Angeles study had 83% positive outcome in the IPS group. This indicates the robust nature of the intervention in different labour markets and economic systems.

A review of vocational intervention in early psychosis found that across all reviewed studies, a mean of 69% of young people with first-episode psychosis returned to work or study using IPS compared to 35% in a variety of control conditions.[2]

Importance of education

There is a clear relationship in the general population between the level of education and training achieved and both income level and employment status. People with higher levels of education earn more money and are more likely to be employed than people with lower levels of education.[44] In terms of employment, this holds true for people with psychotic illness too.[6] Because the onset of illness is often in late adolescence and early adulthood, secondary and post-secondary education and training are often disrupted. In our study conducted in Melbourne, Australia, only 25% of participants had finished high school or its equivalent,[39] compared to 84% of their same-age peers in the general population.[5] The obvious consequence of this is that in early psychosis, vocational interventions need to target educational outcomes as much as employment ones.[4] Where this has been done, there is a clear flow through of people finishing their educational course and transitioning to employment.[45] This is suggestive that with some support, people with early psychosis can reconnect with their original vocational trajectory.

The future

Opportunities

The concept of recovery has many definitions, but consistently it is stated that symptomatic recovery alone is not sufficient. Recovery needs to also take into account a return to functioning in a range of roles. As stated earlier, employment is not only an end in this, but a potential part of the process to achieving further goals, such as social and economic participation. Making vocational recovery a central part of the business of early intervention services significantly enhances the recovery goals of these services.

A role central to the vocational intervention is that of the employment consultant. However, as Browne and Waghorn point out,[42] there are no requisite qualifications for this position. There is also no defined career path. Therefore, an opportunity that presents itself here is to develop those two areas. Qualifications could include not only formal training and accreditation in the IPS model, but also in mental health literacy. Most often employment consultants come from outside of the traditional mental health workforce, instead coming from the employment services. In itself this is a great opportunity as it allows for the diversification of people providing services in mental health settings.

Challenges

In order to translate the research evidence into clinical practice there is a need for a convincing economic argument that providing high-fidelity IPS services saves money for funders. Given that costs associated with unemployment in schizophrenia make up over half of the total costs of illness,[12] this should not be a hard argument to make. However, to date there has been little economic analysis of IPS in chronic schizophrenia and none of IPS in early psychosis. This is a challenge to those designing studies because it is less likely that change will occur without such data.

In 1986, Richard Warner wrote that people with schizophrenia were the last to be employed in economic good times and the first to become unemployed in economic hard times.[46] It is a constant challenge to address the perceptions created by stigma about the capacity or willingness of people with psychotic illness to work. This challenge, as illustrated in the Meaningful Lives consensus guidelines (2010),[15] is one for all stakeholders to take up – consumers, carers, clinicians, researchers and other fellow travellers. At the same time, it should be remembered that the goal may not be to get all people with psychotic illness who want to work into work, but that the gap between the general unemployment rate and the unemployment rate of people with psychotic illness should be closed.

Another challenge is the difficulty in achieving collocation of employment and mental health services. In many countries the employment and mental health services are separately administered, located and funded. Additionally, they may have very different levels of knowledge about the services provided by each other. While in an ideal world, employment consultants would be directly employed in mental health agencies, it is more likely that IPS will be implemented in practice through interagency collaboration. This will take good will on both sides of the negotiation and a willingness to mutually educate and share resources. Further, most government-funded employment services are paid for employment rather than educational outcomes. This is a key area that needs to be addressed in collaboration around vocational interventions for young people with psychosis.

Conclusion

The unemployment rate in first-episode psychosis services averages about 50% and increases rapidly to 75–95% for those who develop schizophrenia.[1] Early intervention has an evidence-based method to address this problem and reduce the disability and social and economic exclusion associated with the illness. Importantly, given the phase of life in which early intervention services are provided, vocational intervention in this stage of illness takes a recovery-focused approach which places equal emphasis on education and the development of career capacity as it does on immediate employment outcomes. The initial evidence is in. The challenge now is to fill the evidence gaps and translate the research into policy and practice.

References

1 Killackey EJ, Jackson HJ, Gleeson J, Hickie IB, McGorry PD. Exciting career opportunity beckons! Early intervention and vocational rehabilitation in first-episode psychosis: employing cautious optimism. *Australian and New Zealand Journal of Psychiatry* 2006;40(11–12):951–62.
2 Rinaldi M, Killackey E, Smith J, Shepherd G, Singh SP, Craig T. First episode psychosis and employment: a review. *International Review of Psychiatry* 2010;22(2):148–62.
3 Marwaha S, Johnson S. Schizophrenia and employment – a review. *Social Psychiatry and Psychiatric Epidemiology* 2004;39(5):337–49.
4 Carmona VR, Gómez-Benito J, Rojo-Rodes JE. Employment support needs of people with schizophrenia: a scoping study. *Journal of Occupational Rehabilitation* 2019;29(1):1–10.
5 Department of Education and Training. *Department of Education and Training: annual report*. Melbourne: Department of Education and Training; 2006.
6 Waghorn G, Chant D, Whiteford H. The strength of self-reported course of illness in predicting vocational recovery for persons with schizophrenia. *Journal of Vocational Rehabilitation* 2003;18(1):33–41.
7 Saavedra J, López M, Gonzáles S, Cubero R. Does employment promote recovery? Meanings from work experience in people diagnosed with serious mental illness. *Culture, Medicine and Psychiatry* 2016;40(3):507–32.
8 Charzyńska K, Kucharska K, Mortimer A. Does employment promote the process of recovery from schizophrenia? A review of the existing evidence. *International Journal of Occupational Medicine and Environmental Health* 2015;28(3):407–18.
9 Secker J, Grove B, Seebohm P. Challenging barriers to employment, training and education for mental health service users: the service user's perspective. *Journal of Mental Health* 2001;10(4):395–404.
10 Ramsay CE, Broussard B, Goulding SM, Cristofaro S, Hall D, Kaslow NJ, et al. Life and treatment goals of individuals hospitalized for first-episode nonaffective psychosis. *Psychiatry Research* 2011;189(3):344–8.
11 SANE Australia. *Schizophrenia costs: an analysis of the burden of schizophrenia and related suicide in Australia*. Victoria: SANE Australia; 2002.
12 Wu EQ, Birnbaum HG, Shi L, Ball DE, Kessler RC, Moulis M, et al. The economic burden of schizophrenia in the United States in 2002. *Journal of Clinical Psychiatry* 2005;66(9):1122–9.
13 Löthgren M. Economic evidence in psychotic disorders: a review. *European Journal of Health Economics* 2004;5(1):S67–74.
14 Carr V, Neil A, Halpin S, Holmes S, on behalf of the low prevalence disorders study group. *Costs of psychosis in urban Australia: a bulletin of the low prevalence disorders study*. Canberra: Commonwealth Department of Health and Ageing; 2002.
15 International First Episode Vocational Recovery (iFEVR) group. Meaningful lives: supporting young people with psychosis in education, training and employment: an international consensus statement. *Early Intervention in Psychiatry* 2010;4(4):323–6.

16 Baron RC, Salzer MS. Accounting for unemployment among people with mental illness. *Behavioral Sciences and the Law* 2002;20(6):585–99.
17 Leff J. Can we manage without the mental hospital? *Australian and New Zealand Journal of Psychiatry* 2001;35(4):421–7.
18 Ungerleider JT, Shadowen PJ. The diagnostic and therapeutic value of work. *Hospital and Community Psychiatry* 1966;17(12):373–5.
19 O'Flynn D. Approaching employment: mental health, work projects and the care programme approach. *Psychiatric Bulletin* 2001;25(5):169–71.
20 Anonymous. The wellspring of the clubhouse model for social and vocational adjustment of persons with serious mental illness. *Psychiatric Services* 1999;50(11):1473–6.
21 Morrin M, Simmonds D, Somerville W. Social enterprise: mainstreamed from the margins? *Local Economy* 2004;19(1):69–84.
22 Social Firms England. *Types of social firms*. Retrieved from: www.socialfirmsengland.co.uk/types-of-social-firms/
23 Social Firms England. *Enterprise, employment and empowerment*. Retrieved from: www.socialfirmsengland.co.uk/enterprise-employment-empowerment/
24 Baker K. *Mapping the social firm sector 2005*. Surrey: Social Firms UK; 2005.
25 Ducci G, Stentella C, Vulterini P. The social enterprise in Europe: the state of the art. *International Journal of Mental Health* 2002;31(3):76–91.
26 Boardman J, Grove B, Perkins R, Shepherd G. Work and employment for people with psychiatric disabilities. *British Journal of Psychiatry* 2003;182:467–8.
27 Becker DR, Drake RE. *A working life for people with severe mental illness*. New York: Oxford University Press; 2003.
28 Macias C, Jackson R, Schroeder C, Wang Q. What is a clubhouse? Report on the ICCD 1996 survey of USA clubhouses. *Community Mental Health Journal* 1999;35(2):181–90.
29 Bond GR. Supported employment: evidence for an evidence-based practice. *Psychiatric Rehabilitation Journal* 2004;27(4):345–59.
30 Johnsen M, McKay C, Henry AD, Manning TD. What does competitive employment mean? A secondary analysis of employment approaches in the Massachusetts employment intervention demonstration project. In Fisher WH (Ed) *Research on employment for persons with severe mental illness*. Bingley: Emerald Group Publishing Limited; 2004. p 43–62.
31 McKay C, Johnsen M, Stein R. Employment outcomes in Massachusetts clubhouses. *Psychiatric Rehabilitation Journal* 2005;29(1):25–33.
32 Johnsen M, McKay C, Corcoran J, Lidz C. *Characteristics of Clubhouses across the world: findings from the International Survey of Clubhouses 2000*. Worcester, MA: University of Massachusetts Medical School; 2002.
33 Henry AD, Barreira P, Banks S, Brown JM, McKay C. A retrospective study of clubhouse-based transitional employment. *Psychiatric Rehabilitation Journal* 2001;24(4):344–54.
34 Macias C. *Final report Massachusetts Employment Intervention Demonstration Project 'An Experimental Comparison of PACT and Clubhouse'*. New York: Fountain House; 2001.
35 Cook JA, Leff HS, Blyler CR, Gold PB, Goldberg RW, Mueser KT, et al. Results of a multisite randomized trial of supported employment interventions for individuals with severe mental illness. *Archives of General Psychiatry* 2005;62(5):505–12.
36 Crowther RE, Marshall M, Bond GR, Huxley P. Helping people with severe mental illness to obtain work: systematic review. *British Medical Journal* 2001;322(7280):204–8.
37 Bond GR, Drake RE, Becker DR. An update on randomized controlled trials of evidence-based supported employment. *Psychiatric Rehabilitation Journal* 2008;31(4):280–90.

38 Rinaldi M, McNeil K, Firn M, Koletsi M, Perkins R, Singh SP. What are the benefits of evidence-based supported employment for patients with first-episode psychosis? *Psychiatric Bulletin* 2004;28(8):281–4.
39 Killackey E, Jackson HJ, McGorry PD. Vocational intervention in first-episode psychosis: individual placement and support v. treatment as usual. *British Journal of Psychiatry* 2008;193(2):114–20.
40 Major BS, Hinton MF, Flint A, Chalmers-Brown A, McLoughlin K, Johnson S. Evidence of the effectiveness of a specialist vocational intervention following first episode psychosis: a naturalistic prospective cohort study. *Social Psychiatry and Psychiatric Epidemiology* 2010;45(1):1–8.
41 Nuechterlein KH, Subotnik KL, Turner LR, Ventura J, Becker DR, Drake RE. Individual placement and support for individuals with recent-onset schizophrenia: integrating supported education and supported employment. *Psychiatric Rehabilitation Journal* 2008;31(4):340–9.
42 Browne DJ, Waghorn G. Employment services as an early intervention for young people with mental illness. *Early Intervention in Psychiatry* 2010;4(4):327–35.
43 Porteous N, Waghorn G. Implementing evidence-based employment services in New Zealand for young adults with psychosis: progress during the first five years. *British Journal of Occupational Therapy* 2007;70(12):521–6.
44 U.S. Bureau of Labor Statistics. *More education: lower unemployment, higher earnings*. Retrieved from: www.bls.gov/emp/education-pays-handout.pdf
45 Rinaldi M, Perkins R, McNeil K, Hickman N, Singh SP. The individual placement and support approach to vocational rehabilitation for young people with first episode psychosis in the UK. *Journal of Mental Health* 2010;19(6):483–91.
46 Warner R. Hard times and schizophrenia. *Psychology Today* 1986;20(6):50–2.

14 Youth suicide

Prevalence, predictors and prevention

Jo Robinson, Georgina Cox, Sarah Hetrick and Sadhbh Byrne

Introduction

Suicide is one of the leading causes of premature mortality among young people. Suicide-related behaviour, such as suicide attempt and self-harm, is more common and is one of the key indicators of future suicide. This chapter will begin by examining the rates of, and risk factors for, the full spectrum of suicide-related behaviour, including suicidal ideation, before moving on to consider a range of preventative approaches.

Definitions of suicide and suicide-related behaviour

Suicide is the deliberate act of killing oneself. The classification of a death as a suicide is complex. However, in Western countries like Australia, the death must be attributed to non-natural causes, and it must be established by coronial inquiry that the death resulted from a deliberate act of the deceased, with the intention of ending his or her own life.[1,2]

A suicide attempt is a non-fatal, self-inflicted, potentially injurious behaviour with explicit or inferred intent to die,[3] whether or not actual injury occurs.

Suicidal ideation is defined as thoughts of engaging in behaviour intended to end one's life[4] and may encompass voices, images, beliefs or cognitions.

For the purposes of this chapter, the term self-harm refers to a range of behaviours (including self-poisoning and self-injury) through which an individual directly causes harm to her or himself, irrespective of the type of motive or the degree of suicidal intent.[5] The conceptualisation of self-harming behaviours is contested,[6,7] with some researchers employing the term 'non-suicidal self-injury' when referring to the deliberate, self-inflicted destruction of body tissue *without suicidal intent* and for purposes not socially sanctioned, which explicitly excludes behaviours engaged in with any level of suicidal intention.[8] However, the intentions underlying an act of self-harm can be complex and can vary, with young people reporting that an episode of self-harm can serve multiple functions.[9] As such, we have used the more inclusive term 'self-harm' here.

Rates of suicide and suicide-related behaviour

Suicide

In 2016, approximately 793,000 people died from suicide worldwide,[10,11] representing one death every 40 seconds.[12] Of this total 52,750 were young people aged

15 to 19 years old, of which 27,060 were female (51.3% of suicides in this age group) and 25,690 were male.[13]

Among those aged 15 to 29 years old, suicide is the second-leading cause of death globally[13] and the leading cause of death in high-income countries and lower- to middle-income countries of the Southeast Asia region.[14] Suicide and accidental death from self-harm is the third-leading cause of mortality worldwide for younger adolescents (aged 10 to 19 years old) and the second-leading cause of death for older adolescent girls.[15]

Suicide ideation, self-harm and suicide attempts

Suicide ideation and attempts and self-harm are more common than suicide deaths.[16] A systematic review of population-based studies with adolescents demonstrated that 29.9% of participants reported thinking about suicide at some point.[17] For each suicide death globally in 2016, there were more than 20 suicide attempts.[12] A study using 2011–2013 data from the Multicentre Study of Self-Harm in England found that 171 adolescents aged 12–17 years died by suicide, while 1320 adolescents presented to the study hospitals following non-fatal self-harm.[18]

True rates of self-harm are difficult to estimate, and figures based on hospital presentations are likely to under-represent the extent of the problem.[19] A meta-analysis of community-based studies of self-harm among 12- to 18-year-olds found an overall lifetime prevalence of 16.9%.[20] This approximate figure is corroborated irrespective of definition used (i.e., 'non-suicidal self-injury' or 'deliberate self-harm')[21] and falls at the upper limit of previous estimates, which suggested that lifetime prevalence was between 12% and 17%.[22–25] Twelve-month estimates vary significantly depending on how self-harm is measured (i.e., whether a multiple-item or single-item measure was employed); studies variously suggest that between 5% and 28% of adolescents in Western countries have engaged in self-harm over the previous 12 months.[21,26]

Globally, rates of self-harm are higher among 15- to 19-year-old females than among same-age males, and this discrepancy has been consistently reported across the period 1990–2016.[11] For example, in a community study of 15- and 16-year-olds across seven countries, 8.9% of females and 2.6% of males reported self-harm in the past year, with females over three times as likely to report self-harm episodes in the last year or over their lifetime, and more than twice as likely as males to report episodes in the last month.[27] However, the gap between rates of male and female self-harm in young people has been closing over time.[11]

Whilst the mortality associated with suicide is a key concern in itself,[28] suicide attempt, ideation and self-harm in young people are also associated with a range of other negative outcomes, such as premature mortality from other causes,[29] low self-esteem, externalising issues, interpersonal difficulties, financial hardship, unemployment, substance use and emotional dysregulation.[30–33] A birth cohort study demonstrated that people who attempt suicide at a young age are at a significantly elevated risk for a range of adverse outcomes in later adulthood, including persistent mental and physical health problems, violence and poor functioning.[34]

Risk factors

Suicide-related behaviour is determined by a complex interplay of risk factors, which can be classified as distal and proximal risk factors.[35–38] Distal risk factors occur early in life and subsequently predispose an individual to vulnerable behaviours that could lead to suicide-related behaviours; these include psychiatric morbidity, past suicidal or self-harming behaviour, gender, social factors, familial factors and sexual orientation.

Distal risk factors

Psychiatric morbidity

A recent systematic review and meta-analysis found that the presence of mental disorder was associated with ten times greater risk of death by suicide among young people aged 12 to 26 years old.[39] These results align with those found in other systematic reviews of adult data.[40,41] Suicidal youth are six times more likely to have a psychiatric disorder compared with non-suicidal youth,[42] and psychiatric issues present at as early as eight years old can be predictive of future suicide-related behaviours.[43]

Common psychiatric disorders associated with suicide-related behaviour in young people include mood disorders, borderline personality disorder, any personality disorder, conduct disorders, substance abuse, co-morbid depression and generalised anxiety disorder, and first episode psychosis.[42,44–46] Depressive disorders show the strongest link with suicidality in adolescents;[39] between 60% and 80% have a depressive diagnosis either at the time of dying by suicide or when making a suicide attempt.[3] Repetition of self-harm is also frequently reported among young people who have been diagnosed with borderline personality disorder.[46] However, it is difficult to parse the distinct contribution of specific mental disorders to suicide risk, as comorbidity of disorders tends to be the rule, rather than the exception.

While depression is estimated to increase the likelihood of suicide by 20 fold in adolescent females, a previous suicide attempt is more predictive of subsequent suicide-related behaviour in young males, increasing risk by up to 30 times.[47] Substance misuse disorders, personality disorders and childhood disorders are also more strongly associated with male compared to female suicide-related behaviour.[40,47] Furthermore, one study found that a childhood diagnosis of attention-deficit/hyperactivity disorder (ADHD) is predictive of future suicide-related behaviour in young males, but not females.[48]

Past suicide-related behaviour

Prior suicidal ideation, suicidal intent and self-harming behaviour are also significant indicators of future suicidality in the general population, as well as in clinical samples.[28,49–53] Suicidal ideation, plans and attempts can begin as young as ten years of age and show the highest hazards at age 15.[54] However, while 60% of transitions from suicidal ideation to plan and attempt occur within one year of initial ideation onset,[55] risk remains elevated for as many as 37 years.[49]

Gender

Gender has been associated with differing rates of suicide-related behaviours. Girls and young women are at greater risk of suicide attempt, ideation and self-harm than are boys and young men.[17,25,38,56,57] Rates of suicide are higher among boys;[58,59] however, there have been sharp increases in suicide rates among girls.[60] For example, in Australia, there has been a 76.2% increase in suicides among females under 24 years over the past ten years, compared to a 34.3% increase in suicides among males under 24 years in the same time period.[61]

Young people who are transgender or gender diverse experience suicidal ideation and engage in suicide-related behaviours at a higher rate than their cisgender peers.[62–64] The Trans Pathways study in Australia involved the participation of transgender or gender diverse young people aged 14 to 25 years; 79.7% of participants had engaged in self-harm, 82.4% had experienced suicidal thoughts and 48.1% had attempted suicide.[65] Social transition to align one's gender identity with one's biological sex is associated with improved mental health among transgender young people.[66] Feeling supported to go by one's chosen name at home, in school, at work and among friends is associated with reduced suicidal ideation and behaviour.[67]

Sexual orientation

Gay, lesbian and bisexual young people experience suicide-related behaviour, most notably ideation and attempt, between two and six times more frequently than heterosexual youth,[68–73] and lifetime suicide attempt rates have been estimated as high as 42% within this population.[74] Furthermore, suicidal ideation and repetitive self-harm is associated with young people either unsure or worried about their sexual orientation.[69,75]

Social factors

Broader social factors are also known to impact upon young people's wellbeing[76–79] and to be associated with suicide-related behaviour. Worldwide, young Indigenous people have higher rates of suicide and suicide-related behaviour, as well as poorer mental health outcomes, than their non-Indigenous peers.[80,81] For example, in Australia, the suicide rate for Aboriginal and Torres Strait Islander Australians aged 15 to 24 years old is 40.5 per 100,000 – more than three times the rate of suicide among non-Indigenous young Australians.[82] This higher rate may be associated with the loss-related trauma (including loss of culture, identity and power) and discrimination experienced by Indigenous young people living in post-colonial societies.[83–88] Young people who experience racial and other forms of discrimination may also experience higher rates of suicide-related behaviour.[89–91] These challenges are often exacerbated for young people who identify with multiple minority groups.[92]

Family factors

Suicide-related behaviour has been observed to cluster in families. Evidence for the familial transmission of suicide-related behaviour (most notably suicide death and attempt) has come from studies assessing genetic linkage via twin studies, parental psychopathology and family history of suicide-related behaviour (for a comprehensive review, see Brent, 2010).[93]

Parental history of suicide attempt conveys approximately five-fold increased odds of suicide attempt in offspring, even when controlling for previous suicide attempt in offspring and the familial transmission of mood disorder.[94] Maternal suicide is a risk factor for suicide attempts leading to hospitalisation in adolescents, and this relationship remains significant after controlling for psychiatric disorders.[95,96] Suicide attempt and suicide death in young people is associated with suicide-related behaviour in first and second degree relatives, including siblings.[97–100]

Childhood adversity

Childhood adversity, including physical and/or sexual abuse, witnessing violent events and poverty, is associated with later suicide-related behaviours.[46,99,101–107] Childhood exposure to parental adversities (i.e., maternal and paternal substance abuse, psychiatric disorders, criminality and hospitalisations due to interpersonal violence or self-harm) has been associated with significantly increased risk of self-harm in adolescents.[108] Various pathways and mechanisms between childhood maltreatment and later suicide-related behaviour have been explored.[109,110] History of sexual abuse is a predictor of first time self-harm in adolescents.[75] Adolescents and young adults who are victims of violent life events, rather than just witnesses, are also more likely to attempt suicide.[111]

Psychological factors

Multiple facets of impulsivity are associated with suicide-related behaviour in young people.[112] It has also been postulated that impulsivity is the mediating factor between childhood abuse and suicide,[113] with impulsive behaviour proposed to be a consequence of trauma-related maladaptive emotion regulation processes and neurobiological changes.[114,115] Psychological autopsy studies have found higher levels of impulsivity and lifetime history of aggressive behaviour to be associated with death by suicide at a younger age.[116] In adolescents who die by suicide, both impulsivity and lifetime aggression are higher than in community controls.[117] Higher levels of impulsivity has been found to predict frequency of self-harm over time in young adults, controlling for other risk factors for self-harm,[118] and young adults who attempt suicide have higher levels of impulsivity than those who experience suicidal ideation (but have not made an attempt).[119]

Increased aggression and poor impulse control have been observed among adolescents who have made multiple suicide attempts and who report suicidal ideation.[120,121] Higher trait levels of anger and anger expressed outwardly is associated with an increased likelihood of suicide attempt in young adult males.[122]

Hopelessness

Hopelessness has long been linked to an increased risk of suicide-related behaviour,[123,124] including among young people,[125] even when controlled for the presence of psychiatric disorder, principally depression.[126,127] Not only is hopelessness one of the key factors mediating the relationship between depression and suicidal ideation, but it also increases risk among already suicidal patients.[128] A meta-analysis indicated that the presence of hopelessness increases the overall risk of eventual suicide by at least three-fold.[129] It appears that lack of positive expectations, rather than presence of negative expectations, accounted for the relationship between hopelessness and future depression and suicide-related behaviour among adolescents.[130] A recent study with 12- to 17-year-old young people undergoing acute medication treatment for depression found that a one-scale unit increase in baseline hopelessness total score was related to a 6.3% increase in the predicted or expected suicide ideation over the 6-week period of treatment.[131] However, this relationship differed for male and female adolescents; a one-scale unit increase in hopelessness was related to a 8.3% increase in predicted suicidal ideation for girls, while the same unit increase in hopelessness was related to a 2.3% increase in predicted suicidal ideation in boys.[131] This suggests that there may be particular clinical utility in identifying hopelessness among adolescent girls at an early stage in their treatment.

Hopelessness has also been postulated as a mediating factor between problem-solving ability and suicidal ideation.[132,133] Deficits in interpersonal and social problem-solving ability have been linked with both suicide attempts and suicidal ideation.[132,134] This has been reported when poor problem-solving is conceptualised as the inability to generate adequate solutions to one's problems,[135] when there is a focus on negative outcomes to suggested solutions,[135,136] when there is evidence of avoidance of presenting problems[137] and when people express low expectations with regard to their ability to solve their problems.[138]

Proximal risk factors

Proximal risk factors temporally precipitate an event and are often referred to as the 'tipping point' which lead an individual into suicide-related behaviour. These can include negative or adverse life events such as relationship difficulties; interpersonal losses or conflict with parents, peers or significant others; bullying; substance abuse; availability of means; media reporting of suicide; and social milieu such as self-harm or suicide in those close to the young person.

Adverse life events

A number of studies have demonstrated a link between stressful life events and suicide-related behaviour in adolescents,[97] for example, the loss of a parent, being assaulted, a romantic break up and/or being arrested.[139,140] Suicidal young people have reported experiencing more negative life events when compared with non-suicidal peers.[141] Preliminary findings from the Canadian Paediatric Surveillance Program (which monitors self-harm and suicide attempt admissions to the ICU among children under the age of 18 years) suggest that the most common events precipitating serious self-harm or suicide attempts were family conflict (51%), conflict with peer(s) (23%) and loss of a romantic relationship (23%).[142] A greater number of recent stressful life events, and particularly a romantic break-up, appears to distinguish adolescents with suicidal ideation from those who have attempted suicide, when accounting for covariates and comorbid psychiatric disorders.[143] A systematic review suggests that people under the age of 35 years may respond more impulsively to relationship conflict and that this may characterise the association between such conflict and suicidality.[144] It is important to note that the emergence of suicide-related behaviour may impact upon difficulties in relationships.

Bullying

Both victims and perpetrators of bullying show high levels of suicidal ideation and increased numbers of suicide attempts, compared with those not involved in bullying behaviour.[145] This association remains at 10-month follow-up and when controlled for psychiatric and sociodemographic risk factors.[146] Furthermore, bullying behaviour at eight years of age is predictive of future suicidality amongst girls, but not boys, when followed up at age 25.[147]

Cyberbullying, and its relationship to suicide risk, has also become a significant concern. One meta-analysis has found a stronger association between cyberbullying and suicide ideation than that between traditional bullying and suicide ideation.[148] However, this association is complicated by the fact that research suggests that cyberbullying creates few new victims, with one large-scale study in the UK finding that 85–90% of cyber-victimisation occurs alongside traditional victimisation.[149,150] In adolescents, both victims and offenders of cyberbullying report more suicidal thoughts and behaviours compared with peers who had not been involved in cyberbullying.[151,152]

Substance misuse

Drug and alcohol use (including binge drinking) by adolescents has been associated with an increased risk of suicide attempt and ideation.[153–155] However, evidence with regard to age is mixed, perhaps due to the complexity associated with distinguishing between episodic or isolated substance use problems and substance use issues meeting diagnostic criteria for substance use disorders. This is further compounded by methodological issues relating to dependence upon adolescents' self-report of substance use.[156]

Heavy episodic drinking was found to be more strongly associated with suicide attempt for adolescents under the age of 13 years than those over the age of 13.[157] Conversely, suicide risk in those over the age of 16 years is more strongly linked to substance use disorder, compared with those under 16 years.[58]

Moreover, reviews of autopsy reports consistently indicate that one-third of those who die by suicide had consumed alcohol, and one-quarter were intoxicated by alcohol at the time of their death.

Exposure to suicide-related behaviour in others

The term 'suicide cluster' describes a situation in which more suicides than expected occur in terms of time, place, or both.[158] Several mechanisms have been proposed to explain suicide clusters.[158] Young people are at elevated risk for suicide clusters compared to adults.[159–163] Cross-sectional and longitudinal analyses have revealed significant associations between exposure to a peer's suicide-related behaviour and suicide ideation and attempts among adolescents.[164–169] For example, a recent study found that adolescents exposed to self-harm in peers are eight times more likely to also report self-harm.[170] Adolescents who had attempted suicide are more likely to have been exposed to self-harm in others than are adolescents who had experienced suicidal ideation but had not attempted suicide.[171]

Gender differences have been documented with regards to modelling suicide-related behaviour; one study found that self-harm by peers was a significant risk factor for adolescent girls but not boys.[172] Girls are more likely to make a suicide attempt if they are aware of a peer that has attempted suicide, while boys are more likely to make a suicide attempt if they are aware of someone who has died by suicide.[173]

Young people appear to be particularly susceptible to contagion effects through media reporting of real-life suicide.[174–176] Depictions of suicide in popular media have also been linked to increased suicide-related behaviour among young people.[177–179] However, dispute continues regarding the link (or lack thereof) between young people's online behaviour and subsequent mental health issues and suicide risk.[180–185] Importantly, young people report that the internet can also be extremely helpful in terms of providing support and information about seeking help.[180,186–190]

For a review on suicide clusters, see Robinson et al. (2016),[191] and for a recent review on clustering of suicides among young people specifically, see Hawton et al. (2020).[158]

Help-seeking

Young people are often reluctant to seek help for mental health issues, suicidal ideation and self-harm.[192,193] Just 55% of young people who attempt suicide seek help within 30 days of their attempt.[194] When help is sought, it is most often from friends and family members in the first instance.[22,195]

A number of factors reduce the likelihood of help-seeking, including stigma, poor mental health literacy and/or emotional competence, the young person believing that they can and should be able to solve the problem themselves, a prior negative experience of help-seeking and experiencing suicidal thoughts and/or depression.[192]

Thus, suicide and suicide-related behaviour in young people is complex and multi-factorial, meaning no one single approach will be effective. The evidence for a range of preventative approaches is presented next.

Suicide prevention approaches

As described earlier, the pathways to suicide are complex and multi-factorial, hence prevention strategies need to adopt a range of approaches and operate across a range of settings.[196] For the most part, preventative approaches adopt a framework whereby interventions are classified as either universal, selective, or indicated on the basis of how their target groups are defined.[197] Universal approaches to youth suicide prevention target all young people, regardless of their current level of suicide ideation, with the aim of reducing risk factors or boosting protective factors across an entire population. Selective approaches seek to identify at-risk youth (e.g., those who possess one or more of the risk factors described previously), and indicated approaches target individuals already displaying suicide-related behaviour (e.g., have made a suicide attempt or expressed suicidal ideation).

One of the key challenges in suicide prevention is that, although suicide is a serious public health problem claiming a significant number of lives a year, statistically, suicide is considered a rare event. As such, although universal interventions which target entire populations are appealing, extremely large sample sizes are required if we are to adequately test their efficacy, thus decreasing their feasibility and cost-effectiveness. Selective or indicated interventions may be better placed to show an effect, given the defined (at-risk) populations targeted. However, the downside is that such interventions reach smaller numbers of people. Hence, there is a need for interventions to span the broad spectrum of approaches.

In addition to adopting a range of preventative approaches, suicide prevention activities also need to operate in a range of settings. Schools are an obvious and accepted environment for implementing suicide prevention initiatives for youth,[198–200] but others include juvenile justice settings, general practice, emergency departments, specialist mental health settings and general community settings.

We direct readers to our recent systematic review and meta-analysis of 99 individual studies of interventions designed to reduce suicide-related behaviours among young people, which found that interventions delivered in clinical, educational and community settings appear to reduce self-harm and/or suicidal ideation.[196] In addition, we will now describe a selection of prevention approaches that appear to have utility in addressing youth suicide and suicide-related behaviour.

Universal interventions

Reducing access to means of suicide

Good evidence exists regarding the effectiveness of reducing access to means of suicide.[201–210] For example, evidence from the UK shows that reducing the pack sizes of analgesics has reduced suicide rates by this method.[211] However, few studies have examined the impact of means restriction on youth suicide rates specifically. Those that have focus on firearm restriction and demonstrate a reduction in firearm suicides, but no effect on overall youth suicide rates.[196]

Awareness and education programs

Another popular universal approach is awareness and education programs, aimed either at the general population or in specific settings. Schools are a common location for delivering these programs to young people. The focus of such programs is generally to enhance awareness regarding suicide among students, to reduce suicide stigma, to educate students to recognise possible signs of suicide-related behaviour and to provide students with information about available school and community resources.[212] A review of six curriculum-based suicide prevention programs reported overall positive findings in terms of improved knowledge, attitudes and help-seeking, and reduced suicidal ideation.[213] Only one suicide-specific education and awareness program has been tested in Australian secondary schools, and it shows promising results.[214] Historically, concerns have existed regarding the potentially negative effects of such programs,[215] such as the lack of support services available to meet growing demand, should these programs effectively increase help-seeking behaviour. Additionally, the long-term effectiveness of universal education programs is unclear; research that incorporates follow-up testing is required.

Other universal programs employ techniques such as cognitive behavioural therapy and apply these techniques to whole school populations with a view towards reducing depressive symptoms in those who are displaying them and preventing the onset of illness in those who are not (for a review see Neil and Christensen [2007]).[216]

Selective interventions

As noted earlier, selective interventions target subgroups of the population who are not necessarily showing signs of suicide-related behaviour but possess risk factors (e.g., symptoms of mental illness) which may place them at greater risk in the future. Selective interventions with evidence of efficacy, and which can be readily employed with young people, include gatekeeper training and screening programs.

Gatekeeper training

The rationale behind 'gatekeeper training' is to better equip professionals to identify people at risk and enable them to provide front-line support whilst positioning them to refer the individual on for a thorough assessment and treatment. When it comes to reducing suicide among young people, school staff are an obvious target for such training programs. A systematic review of school-based gatekeeper training programs reported increases in gatekeepers' knowledge and skills in suicide prevention, but the impact of such training on behavioural change is less clear.[217]

Promisingly, however, individual studies have reported referral of youth to services by trained gatekeepers.[218]

Screening programs

Screening programs focus upon the early identification of people who may be at risk but who have not sought help or been identified by professionals as needing support. The key difference between screening and gatekeeper training is that screening is implemented via an instrument or tool and therefore can be more readily scaled-up to reach larger numbers of people. Screening programs may focus on identifying people already showing suicide risk, although they may also seek to identify people at risk of other difficulties which would place them at elevated risk of suicide, such as depression or anxiety. Research shows that screening successfully facilitates the identification of at-risk students, including those who have not previously sought help, and is not associated with iatrogenic effects.[219,220] Screening can be implemented across settings including schools, general health settings and juvenile justice settings, and can also be implemented using paper or computerised assessment tools.[199,201,221,222]

In the past, it had been argued that both staff and students consider school-wide screening programs to be less acceptable than curriculum-based programs and staff training programs.[223,224] However, more recent research indicates that students, parents and school staff found a screening program to be acceptable and appropriate for delivery in a school setting.[199] Research demonstrates that adolescents often do not reveal their suicidal thoughts or behaviours to others,[225–227] and they are more likely to report information that could be potentially stigmatising in a self-administered instrument (including online and app-based self-monitoring)[228,229] than they are during a face-to-face evaluation.[230,231] As such, screening for suicidal ideation has been demonstrated to be an effective way of identifying young people as at risk when risk was previously unknown[232] and can be an important catalyst in ensuring that these young people receive early prevention and intervention services.

Yet, the subsequent engagement of identified individuals with treatment remains unclear. Whilst there is some evidence to suggest that screening can increase the likelihood of accessing treatment,[233] more research is required into health outcomes for young people following screening. Additionally, future studies may examine cost-effectiveness, the predictive validity and reliability of particular screening instruments and the appropriateness of screening instruments across different cultures and settings.

Indicated interventions

For the most part, indicated interventions, which target those people who have come to the attention of professionals as a result of having already displayed signs of suicide risk, fall into the category of treatment interventions, such as pharmacological or psychosocial therapies.

Pharmacological interventions

One of the difficulties in this field is the relative paucity of large, well-conducted trials in young people,[234–236] a particular concern being the exclusion of young people with severe and complex disorders who also report suicidality. Guidelines, while varying, consistently recommend close monitoring of symptoms and side effects and typically recommend judicious use of medication.[237–240]

In the treatment of schizophrenia, clozapine has been found to reduce suicide risk,[241] however this has not been specifically tested in an adolescent sample. Similarly, mood stabilisers, such as lithium, have been shown to have anti-suicidal effects in patients with mood disorders.[242] We direct readers to Zalpuri and Singh (2019) for a thorough review of current knowledge of pharmacological treatment options for suicidal adolescents.[243] For a review of pharmacological interventions for self-harm in adults, see Hawton et al. (2016).[244]

Psychosocial interventions

Psychosocial interventions for suicide risk fall into two main categories: those which aim to reduce risk by attempting to enhance access to and engagement with specialist services, most frequently mental health or emergency services, and those which aim to reduce risk via the provision of group or individual psychological therapy, either delivered face-to-face or via the internet.

Psychosocial interventions delivered to indicated populations have been associated with significant reductions in suicidal ideation among young people in systematic reviews.[196,245] In particular, Mentalisation Based Treatment (MBT; adapted for adolescents), Dialectical Behavioural Therapy (DBT; again, adapted for adolescents), and cognitive behavioural therapy appear to be potentially effective interventions to reduce suicide-related behaviour, with MBT and DBT showing the most promise for targeting self-harm specifically.[246–250]

However, there remains simply too little evidence from good-quality, sufficiently powered trials to enable us to say with any certainty what types of interventions do and do not work with this population;[247,251] replication of DBT and MBT trials among adolescent samples is particularly required.

e-Health interventions

The effects of internet-based or 'e-Health' treatment interventions among young people have been explored in various studies and show promise (see Chapter 9). Use of the internet is common among young people, and delivering therapy in this way potentially affords greater anonymity and may be viewed as less stigmatising and more accessible.[252,253] The growing capacity of online platforms has seen the development of an abundance of internet-based interventions for mental health problems, including depression and anxiety, of which many have been shown to reduce symptoms.[254]

Internet-based cognitive behavioural therapy has been shown to be an effective form of treatment for depression and anxiety among adults.[255–263] It has also been shown to have the potential both to prevent and reduce symptoms of depression and anxiety in adolescents.[264–267] Internet-based and other digital interventions directly targeting suicide-related behaviours also show signs of efficacy among young people.[268–272] For example, the Reframe IT intervention, which was developed with the specific aim of preventing suicide, has been tested among young people; was found to be safe, feasible to deliver and acceptable to participants; and also appeared to lead to decreases in suicidal ideation.[190,273–275] Online screening to assess suicidal thoughts and behaviours has been deemed acceptable among young people.[276] However, few randomised controlled trials have been conducted on online and smartphone apps for the self-management of suicidal ideation and self-harm, thus impeding our ability to draw conclusions regarding effectiveness.[277]

In addition to online interventions, recent research suggests that social media holds potential for the treatment of suicidal ideation among at-risk youth and can also be successfully utilised to support young people bereaved by suicide.[189] One online social networking intervention for suicidal young people is currently being trialled.[278] However, there remains a paucity of controlled trials that target suicide outcomes specifically, are designed for young people and do not exclude those at highest risk.

Future directions

Overall, despite suicide prevention being a national priority in many countries, the evidence regarding the effectiveness of interventions for suicidal youth is limited. There is a distinct lack of well-conducted, sufficiently powered studies for us to draw any robust conclusions. Other gaps include the lack of suicide prevention studies for young people in university and other tertiary education settings, in workplace settings and in primary care.[196] All too often, young people at risk of suicide are specifically excluded from research, partly due to ethical concerns, but also as a result of fear of talking about suicide with young people. Further, in many cases, studies testing the effects of depression interventions do not include suicide-related outcomes. Therefore, their effect on suicide risk remains unknown.

However, that said, there are some interventions that do appear to show promise, and these include reducing access to means of suicide, gatekeeper training programs, screening programs and psychological therapies delivered face-to-face and online.[196]

References

1 Jowett S, Carpenter B, Tait G. Determining a suicide under Australian law. *University of New South Wales Law Journal* 2018;41(2):355–79.

2 Jowett S, Carpenter B, Tait G. Determining a suicide under Australian law: a comparative study of coronial practice. *University of New South Wales Law Journal* 2019;42(2):534–56.

3 Cash SJ, Bridge JA. Epidemiology of youth suicide and suicidal behavior. *Current Opinion in Pediatrics* 2009;21(5):613.
4 Nock MK, Borges G, Bromet EJ, Cha CB, Kessler RC, Lee S. Suicide and suicidal behavior. *Epidemiologic Reviews* 2008;30(1):133–54.
5 Robinson J, McCutcheon L, Browne V, Witt K. *Looking the other way: young people and self-harm.* Melbourne: Orygen, The National Centre of Excellence in Youth Mental Health; 2016.
6 Silverman MM, Berman AL, Sanddal ND, O'Carroll PW, Joiner Jr TE. Rebuilding the Tower of Babel: a revised nomenclature for the study of suicide and suicidal behaviors part 2: suicide-related ideations, communications, and behaviors. *Suicide and Life-Threatening Behavior* 2007;37(3):264–77.
7 Silverman MM, Berman AL, Sanddal ND, O'Carroll PW, Joiner Jr TE. Rebuilding the Tower of Babel: a revised nomenclature for the study of suicide and suicidal behaviors part 1: background, rationale, and methodology. *Suicide and Life-Threatening Behavior* 2007;37(3):248–63.
8 Nock MK. Self-injury. *Annual Review of Clinical Psychology* 2010;6:339–63.
9 Rasmussen S, Hawton K, Philpott-Morgan S, O'Connor RC. Why do adolescents self-harm? *Crisis* 2016;37(3):176–83.
10 World Health Organization. *Suicide rates (per 100 000 population).* Geneva: World Health Organization; 2018. Retrieved from: www.who.int/gho/mental_health/suicide_rates/en/
11 Naghavi M. Global, regional, and national burden of suicide mortality 1990 to 2016: systematic analysis for the Global Burden of Disease Study 2016. *BMJ* 2019;364:l94.
12 World Health Organization. *Suicide prevention.* Geneva: World Health Organization. Retrieved from: www.who.int/health-topics/suicide
13 World Health Organization. *Suicide data 2016.* Geneva: World Health Organization. Retrieved from: www.who.int/mental_health/prevention/suicide/suicideprevent/en/
14 World Health Organization. *Preventing suicide: a global imperative.* Geneva: World Health Organization; 2014.
15 World Health Organization. *More than 1.2 million adolescents die every year, nearly all preventable* [press release]. Geneva: World Health Organization; 16 May 2017.
16 Grunbaum JA, Kann L, Kinchen S, Ross J, Hawkins J, Lowry R, et al. Youth risk behavior surveillance – United States, 2003. *Morbidity and Mortality Weekly Report: Surveillance Summaries* 2004;53(2):1–96.
17 Evans E, Hawton K, Rodham K, Deeks J. The prevalence of suicidal phenomena in adolescents: a systematic review of population-based studies. *Suicide and Life-Threatening Behavior* 2005;35(3):239–50.
18 Geulayov G, Casey D, McDonald KC, Foster P, Pritchard K, Wells C, et al. Incidence of suicide, hospital-presenting non-fatal self-harm, and community-occurring non-fatal self-harm in adolescents in England (the iceberg model of self-harm): a retrospective study. *Lancet Psychiatry* 2018;5(2):167–74.
19 Arensman E, Corcoran P, McMahon E. The iceberg model of self-harm: new evidence and insights. *Lancet Psychiatry* 2018;5(2):100–1.
20 Gillies D, Christou MA, Dixon AC, Featherston OJ, Rapti I, Garcia-Anguita A, et al. Prevalence and characteristics of self-harm in adolescents: meta-analyses of community-based studies 1990–2015. *Journal of the American Academy of Child and Adolescent Psychiatry* 2018;57(10):733–41.
21 Muehlenkamp JJ, Claes L, Havertape L, Plener PL. International prevalence of adolescent non-suicidal self-injury and deliberate self-harm. *Child and Adolescent Psychiatry and Mental Health* 2012;6(1):10.

22 De Leo D, Heller TS. Who are the kids who self-harm? An Australian self-report school survey. *Medical Journal of Australia* 2004;181(3):140–4.
23 Hawton K, Rodham K, Evans E, Weatherall R. Deliberate self harm in adolescents: self report survey in schools in England. *BMJ* 2002;325(7374):1207–11.
24 Nixon MK, Cloutier P, Jansson SM. Nonsuicidal self-harm in youth: a population-based survey. *CMAJ* 2008;178(3):306–12.
25 Patton GC, Harris R, Carlin JB, Hibbert M, Coffey C, Schwartz M, et al. Adolescent suicidal behaviours: a population-based study of risk. *Psychological Medicine* 1997;27(3):715–24.
26 Skegg K. Self-harm. *Lancet* 2005;366(9495):1471–83.
27 Madge N, Hewitt A, Hawton K, de Wilde EJ, Corcoran P, Fekete S, et al. Deliberate self-harm within an international community sample of young people: comparative findings from the Child & Adolescent Self-harm in Europe (CASE) Study. *Journal of Child Psychology and Psychiatry* 2008;49(6):667–77.
28 Castellví P, Lucas-Romero E, Miranda-Mendizábal A, Parés-Badell O, Almenara J, Alonso I, et al. Longitudinal association between self-injurious thoughts and behaviors and suicidal behavior in adolescents and young adults: a systematic review with meta-analysis. *Journal of Affective Disorders* 2017;215:37–48.
29 Hawton K, Fagg J. Suicide, and other causes of death, following attempted suicide. *British Journal of Psychiatry* 1988;152(3):359–66.
30 Adrian M, Zeman J, Erdley C, Lisa L, Sim L. Emotional dysregulation and interpersonal difficulties as risk factors for nonsuicidal self-injury in adolescent girls. *Journal of Abnormal Child Psychology* 2011;39(3):389–400.
31 Boudewyn AC, Liem JH. Psychological, interpersonal, and behavioral correlates of chronic self-destructiveness: an exploratory study. *Psychological Reports* 1995;77(3):1283–97.
32 Lundh L-G, Karim J, Quilisch E. Deliberate self-harm in 15-year-old adolescents: a pilot study with a modified version of the Deliberate Self-Harm Inventory. *Scandinavian Journal of Psychology* 2007;48(1):33–41.
33 Borschmann R, Becker D, Coffey C, Spry E, Moreno-Betancur M, Moran P, et al. 20-year outcomes in adolescents who self-harm: a population-based cohort study. *Lancet Child & Adolescent Health* 2017;1(3):195–202.
34 Goldman-Mellor SJ, Caspi A, Harrington H, Hogan S, Nada-Raja S, Poulton R, et al. Suicide attempt in young people: a signal for long-term health care and social needs. *JAMA Psychiatry* 2014;71(2):119–27.
35 Mościcki EK. Identification of suicide risk factors using epidemiologic studies. *Psychiatric Clinics of North America* 1997;20(3):499–517.
36 Hankin BL, Abela JR. Nonsuicidal self-injury in adolescence: prospective rates and risk factors in a 2 ½ year longitudinal study. *Psychiatry Research* 2011;186(1):65–70.
37 Carballo J, Llorente C, Kehrmann L, Flamarique I, Zuddas A, Purper-Ouakil D, et al. Psychosocial risk factors for suicidality in children and adolescents. *European Child & Adolescent Psychiatry* 2019; in press.
38 Fliege H, Lee J-R, Grimm A, Klapp BF. Risk factors and correlates of deliberate self-harm behavior: a systematic review. *Journal of Psychosomatic Research* 2009;66(6):477–93.
39 Gili M, Castellví P, Vives M, de la Torre-Luque A, Almenara J, Blasco MJ, et al. Mental disorders as risk factors for suicidal behavior in young people: a meta-analysis and systematic review of longitudinal studies. *Journal of Affective Disorders* 2019;245:152–62.
40 Arsenault-Lapierre G, Kim C, Turecki G. Psychiatric diagnoses in 3275 suicides: a meta-analysis. *BMC Psychiatry* 2004;4:37.
41 Conner KR, Bridge JA, Davidson DJ, Pilcher C, Brent DA. Metaanalysis of mood and substance use disorders in proximal risk for suicide deaths. *Suicide and Life-Threatening Behavior* 2019;49(1):278–92.

42 Foley DL, Goldston DB, Costello EJ, Angold A. Proximal psychiatric risk factors for suicidality in youth: the Great Smoky Mountains Study. *Archives of General Psychiatry* 2006;63(9):1017–24.
43 Sourander A, Klomek AB, Niemelä S, Haavisto A, Gyllenberg D, Helenius H, et al. Childhood predictors of completed and severe suicide attempts: findings from the Finnish 1981 Birth Cohort Study. *Archives of General Psychiatry* 2009;66(4):398–406.
44 Bella ME, Fernández RA, Willington JM. Depression and the conduct disorder are the most frequent pathologies in child and adolescent suicide attempt. *Archivos Argentinos de Pediatria* 2010;108(2):124–9.
45 Falcone T, Mishra L, Carlton E, Lee C, Butler RS, Janigro D, et al. Suicidal behavior in adolescents with first-episode psychosis. *Clinical Schizophrenia & Related Psychoses* 2010;4(1):34–40.
46 Witt K, Milner A, Spittal MJ, Hetrick S, Robinson J, Pirkis J, et al. Population attributable risk of factors associated with the repetition of self-harm behaviour in young people presenting to clinical services: a systematic review and meta-analysis. *European Child & Adolescent Psychiatry* 2019;28(1):5–18.
47 Shaffer D, Gould MS, Fisher P, Trautman P, Moreau D, Kleinman M, et al. Psychiatric diagnosis in child and adolescent suicide. *Archives of General Psychiatry* 1996;53(4):339–48.
48 Chronis-Tuscano A, Molina BS, Pelham WE, Applegate B, Dahlke A, Overmyer M, et al. Very early predictors of adolescent depression and suicide attempts in children with attention-deficit/hyperactivity disorder. *Archives of General Psychiatry* 2010;67(10):1044–51.
49 Suominen K, Isometsä E, Suokas J, Haukka J, Achte K, Lönnqvist J. Completed suicide after a suicide attempt: a 37-year follow-up study. *American Journal of Psychiatry* 2004;161(3):562–3.
50 Hawton K, Zahl D, Weatherall R. Suicide following deliberate self-harm: long-term follow-up of patients who presented to a general hospital. *British Journal of Psychiatry* 2003;182(6):537–42.
51 Suominen K, Isometsä E, Ostamo A, Lönnqvist J. Level of suicidal intent predicts overall mortality and suicide after attempted suicide: a 12-year follow-up study. *BMC Psychiatry* 2004;4(1):11.
52 Robinson J, Cotton S, Conus P, Schimmelmann BG, McGorry P, Lambert M. Prevalence and predictors of suicide attempt in an incidence cohort of 661 young people with first-episode psychosis. *Australian and New Zealand Journal of Psychiatry* 2009;43(2):149–57.
53 Robinson J, Harris MG, Harrigan SM, Henry LP, Farrelly S, Prosser A, et al. Suicide attempt in first-episode psychosis: a 7.4 year follow-up study. *Schizophrenia Research* 2010;116(1):1–8.
54 Borges G, Benjet C, Medina-Mora ME, Orozco R, Nock M. Suicide ideation, plan, and attempt in the Mexican adolescent mental health survey. *Journal of the American Academy of Child and Adolescent Psychiatry* 2008;47(1):41–52.
55 Nock MK, Borges G, Bromet EJ, Alonso J, Angermeyer M, Beautrais A, et al. Cross-national prevalence and risk factors for suicidal ideation, plans and attempts. *British Journal of Psychiatry* 2008;192(2):98–105.
56 An H, Ahn JH, Bhang SY. The association of psychosocial and familial factors with adolescent suicidal ideation: a population-based study. *Psychiatry Research* 2010;177(3):318–22.
57 Mitrou F, Gaudie J, Lawrence D, Silburn SR, Stanley FJ, Zubrick SR. Antecedents of hospital admission for deliberate self-harm from a 14-year follow-up study using data-linkage. *BMC Psychiatry* 2010;10(1):82.

58 Brent DA, Baugher M, Bridge J, Chen T, Chiappetta L. Age-and sex-related risk factors for adolescent suicide. *Journal of the American Academy of Child and Adolescent Psychiatry* 1999;38(12):1497–505.
59 Lee S, Dwyer J, Paul E, Clarke D, Treleaven S, Roseby R. Differences by age and sex in adolescent suicide. *Australian and New Zealand Journal of Public Health* 2019;43(3):248–53.
60 Ruch DA, Sheftall AH, Schlagbaum P, Rausch J, Campo JV, Bridge JA. Trends in suicide among youth aged 10 to 19 years in the United States, 1975 to 2016. *JAMA Network Open* 2019;2(5):e193886.
61 Australian Bureau of Statistics. *3303.0 – causes of death, Australia, 2017*. Canberra: Australian Bureau of Statistics; 2018.
62 Grossman AH, Park JY, Russell ST. Transgender youth and suicidal behaviors: applying the interpersonal psychological theory of suicide. *Journal of Gay & Lesbian Mental Health* 2016;20(4):329–49.
63 Rimes KA, Goodship N, Ussher G, Baker D, West E. Non-binary and binary transgender youth: comparison of mental health, self-harm, suicidality, substance use and victimization experiences. *International Journal of Transgenderism* 2019;20(2–3):230–40.
64 Taliaferro LA, McMorris BJ, Rider GN, Eisenberg ME. Risk and protective factors for self-harm in a population-based sample of transgender youth. *Archives of Suicide Research* 2019;23(2):203–21.
65 Strauss P, Cook A, Winter S, Watson V, Wright Toussaint D, Lin A. Associations between negative life experiences and the mental health of trans and gender diverse young people in Australia: findings from Trans Pathways. *Psychological Medicine* 2020;50(5):808–17.
66 Steensma TD, McGuire JK, Kreukels BP, Beekman AJ, Cohen-Kettenis PT. Factors associated with desistence and persistence of childhood gender dysphoria: a quantitative follow-up study. *Journal of the American Academy of Child and Adolescent Psychiatry* 2013;52(6):582–90.
67 Russell ST, Pollitt AM, Li G, Grossman AH. Chosen name use is linked to reduced depressive symptoms, suicidal ideation, and suicidal behavior among transgender youth. *Journal of Adolescent Health* 2018;63(4):503–5.
68 McDaniel JS, Purcell D, D'Augelli AR. The relationship between sexual orientation and risk for suicide: research findings and future directions for research and prevention. *Suicide and Life-Threatening Behavior* 2001;31(1):84–105.
69 Zhao Y, Montoro R, Igartua K, Thombs BD. Suicidal ideation and attempt among adolescents reporting "unsure" sexual identity or heterosexual identity plus same-sex attraction or behavior: forgotten groups? *Journal of the American Academy of Child and Adolescent Psychiatry* 2010;49(2):104–13.
70 Marshal MP, Dietz LJ, Friedman MS, Stall R, Smith HA, McGinley J, et al. Suicidality and depression disparities between sexual minority and heterosexual youth: a meta-analytic review. *Journal of Adolescent Health* 2011;49(2):115–23.
71 Oginni OA, Robinson EJ, Jones A, Rahman Q, Rimes KA. Mediators of increased self-harm and suicidal ideation in sexual minority youth: a longitudinal study. *Psychological Medicine* 2019;49(15):2524–32.
72 Plöderl M, Tremblay P. Mental health of sexual minorities. A systematic review. *International Review of Psychiatry* 2015;27(5):367–85.
73 Miranda-Mendizábal A, Castellví P, Parés-Badell O, Almenara J, Alonso I, Blasco M, et al. Sexual orientation and suicidal behaviour in adolescents and young adults: systematic review and meta-analysis. *British Journal of Psychiatry* 2017;211(2):77–87.
74 Hershberger SL, D'Augelli AR. The impact of victimization on the mental health and suicidality of lesbian, gay, and bisexual youths. *Developmental Psychology* 1995;31(1): 65–74.

75 O'Connor RC, Rasmussen S, Hawton K. Predicting deliberate self-harm in adolescents: a six month prospective study. *Suicide and Life-Threatening Behavior* 2009;39(4):364–75.
76 Viner RM, Ozer EM, Denny S, Marmot M, Resnick M, Fatusi A, et al. Adolescence and the social determinants of health. *Lancet* 2012;379(9826):1641–52.
77 Currie C, Zanotti C, Morgan A, Currie D, de Looze M, Roberts C, et al. *Social determinants of health and well-being among young people. Health Behaviour in School-aged Children (HBSC) study: international report from the 2009/2010 survey*. Copenhagen: WHO Regional Office for Europe; 2012.
78 Reiss F. Socioeconomic inequalities and mental health problems in children and adolescents: a systematic review. *Social Science & Medicine* 2013;90:24–31.
79 Harding S, Read UM, Molaodi OR, Cassidy A, Maynard MJ, Lenguerrand E, et al. The Determinants of young Adult Social well-being and Health (DASH) study: diversity, psychosocial determinants and health. *Social Psychiatry and Psychiatric Epidemiology* 2015;50(8):1173–88.
80 Leenaars AA. Suicide among indigenous peoples: introduction and call to action. *Archives of Suicide Research* 2006;10(2):103–15.
81 Eckhoff C, Sørvold MT, Kvernmo S. Adolescent self-harm and suicidal behavior and young adult outcomes in indigenous and non-indigenous people. *European Child & Adolescent Psychiatry* 2019; in press.
82 Australian Bureau of Statistics. *3303.0 – causes of death, Australia, 2018*. Canberra: Australian Bureau of Statistics; 2019.
83 Lawson-Te Aho K, Liu JH. Indigenous suicide and colonization: the legacy of violence and the necessity of self-determination. *International Journal of Conflict and Violence* 2010;4(1):124–33.
84 Heart MY, Chase J, Elkins J, Altschul DB. Historical trauma among indigenous peoples of the Americas: concepts, research, and clinical considerations. *Journal of Psychoactive Drugs* 2011;43(4):282–90.
85 Hunter E, Milroy H. Aboriginal and Torres Strait Islander suicide in context. *Archives of Suicide Research* 2006;10(2):141–57.
86 Tucker RP, Wingate LR, O'Keefe VM, Hollingsworth DW, Cole AB. An examination of historical loss thinking frequency and rumination on suicide ideation in American Indian young adults. *Suicide and Life-Threatening Behavior* 2016;46(2):213–22.
87 Bals M, Turi AL, Skre I, Kvernmo S. Internalization symptoms, perceived discrimination, and ethnic identity in indigenous Sami and non-Sami youth in Arctic Norway. *Ethnicity & Health* 2010;15(2):165–79.
88 Harder HG, Rash J, Holyk T, Jovel E, Harder K. Indigenous youth suicide: a systematic review of the literature. *Pimatisiwin: a Journal of Aboriginal and Indigenous Community Health* 2012;10(1):125–42.
89 Cheref S, Lane R, Polanco-Roman L, Gadol E, Miranda R. Suicidal ideation among racial/ethnic minorities: moderating effects of rumination and depressive symptoms. *Cultural Diversity and Ethnic Minority Psychology* 2015;21(1):31–40.
90 Castle K, Conner K, Kaukeinen K, Tu X. Perceived racism, discrimination, and acculturation in suicidal ideation and suicide attempts among black young adults. *Suicide and Life-Threatening Behavior* 2011;41(3):342–51.
91 Gomez J, Miranda R, Polanco L. Acculturative stress, perceived discrimination, and vulnerability to suicide attempts among emerging adults. *Journal of Youth and Adolescence* 2011;40(11):1465–76.
92 Thoma BC, Huebner DM. Health consequences of racist and antigay discrimination for multiple minority adolescents. *Cultural Diversity and Ethnic Minority Psychology* 2013;19(4):404–13.

93 Brent D. What family studies teach us about suicidal behavior: implications for research, treatment, and prevention. *European Psychiatry* 2010;25(5):260–3.
94 Brent DA, Melhem NM, Oquendo M, Burke A, Birmaher B, Stanley B, et al. Familial pathways to early-onset suicide attempt: a 5.6-year prospective study. *JAMA Psychiatry* 2015;72(2):160–8.
95 Kuramoto SJ, Stuart EA, Runeson B, Lichtenstein P, Långström N, Wilcox HC. Maternal or paternal suicide and offspring's psychiatric and suicide-attempt hospitalization risk. *Pediatrics* 2010;126(5):e1026–32.
96 Brent DA, Bridge J, Johnson BA, Connolly J. Suicidal behavior runs in families: a controlled family study of adolescent suicide victims. *Archives of General Psychiatry* 1996;53(12):1145–52.
97 Gould MS, Fisher P, Parides M, Flory M, Shaffer D. Psychosocial risk factors of child and adolescent completed suicide. *Archives of General Psychiatry* 1996;53(12):1155–62.
98 Mittendorfer-Rutz E, Rasmussen F, Wasserman D. Familial clustering of suicidal behaviour and psychopathology in young suicide attempters. *Social Psychiatry and Psychiatric Epidemiology* 2008;43(1):28–36.
99 Brent DA, Perper JA, Moritz G, Liotus L, Schweers J, Balach L, et al. Familial risk factors for adolescent suicide: a case-control study. *Acta Psychiatrica Scandinavica* 1994;89(1):52–8.
100 Agerbo E, Nordentoft M, Mortensen PB. Familial, psychiatric, and socioeconomic risk factors for suicide in young people: nested case-control study. *BMJ* 2002;325(7355):74.
101 Fergusson DM, Boden JM, Horwood LJ. Exposure to childhood sexual and physical abuse and adjustment in early adulthood. *Child Abuse & Neglect* 2008;32(6):607–19.
102 Johnson JG, Cohen P, Gould MS, Kasen S, Brown J, Brook JS. Childhood adversities, interpersonal difficulties, and risk for suicide attempts during late adolescence and early adulthood. *Archives of General Psychiatry* 2002;59(8):741–9.
103 Fergusson DM, Horwood LJ, Lynskey MT. Childhood sexual abuse and psychiatric disorder in young adulthood: II. Psychiatric outcomes of childhood sexual abuse. *Journal of the American Academy of Child and Adolescent Psychiatry* 1996;35(10):1365–74.
104 Serafini G, Canepa G, Adavastro G, Nebbia J, Belvederi Murri M, Erbuto D, et al. The relationship between childhood maltreatment and non-suicidal self-injury: a systematic review. *Frontiers in Psychiatry* 2017;8:149.
105 Wang YR, Sun JW, Lin PZ, Zhang HH, Mu GX, Cao FL. Suicidality among young adults: unique and cumulative roles of 14 different adverse childhood experiences. *Child Abuse & Neglect* 2019;98:104183.
106 Bernburg JG, Thorlindsson T, Sigfusdottir ID. The spreading of suicidal behavior: the contextual effect of community household poverty on adolescent suicidal behavior and the mediating role of suicide suggestion. *Social Science & Medicine* 2009;68(2):380–9.
107 Chen CY, Yeh HH, Huang N, Lin YC. Socioeconomic and clinical characteristics associated with repeat suicide attempts among young people. *Journal of Adolescent Health* 2014;54(5):550–7.
108 Pitkänen J, Remes H, Aaltonen M, Martikainen P. Experience of maternal and paternal adversities in childhood as determinants of self-harm in adolescence and young adulthood. *Journal of Epidemiology & Community Health* 2019;73(11):1040–6.
109 Kaess M. Differential pathways from childhood maltreatment to self-harm and suicidal ideation. *European Child & Adolescent Psychiatry* 2019;28(10):1281–2.
110 Duprey EB, Oshri A, Liu S. Developmental pathways from child maltreatment to adolescent suicide-related behaviors: the internalizing and externalizing comorbidity hypothesis. *Development and Psychopathology* 2019; in press.

111 Nrugham L, Holen A, Sund AM. Associations between attempted suicide, violent life events, depressive symptoms, and resilience in adolescents and young adults. *Journal of Nervous and Mental Disease* 2010;198(2):131–6.
112 McHugh CM, Chun Lee RS, Hermens DF, Corderoy A, Large M, Hickie IB. Impulsivity in the self-harm and suicidal behavior of young people: a systematic review and meta-analysis. *Journal of Psychiatric Research* 2019;116:51–60.
113 Braquehais MD, Oquendo MA, Baca-García E, Sher L. Is impulsivity a link between childhood abuse and suicide? *Comprehensive Psychiatry* 2010;51(2):121–9.
114 Teicher MH, Samson JA. Annual research review: enduring neurobiological effects of childhood abuse and neglect. *Journal of Child Psychology and Psychiatry* 2016;57(3):241–66.
115 Cross D, Fani N, Powers A, Bradley B. Neurobiological development in the context of childhood trauma. *Clinical Psychology: Science and Practice* 2017;24(2):111–24.
116 McGirr A, Renaud J, Bureau A, Seguin M, Lesage A, Turecki G. Impulsive-aggressive behaviours and completed suicide across the life cycle: a predisposition for younger age of suicide. *Psychological Medicine* 2008;38(3):407–17.
117 Brent DA, Johnson BA, Perper J, Connolly J, Bridge J, Bartle S, et al. Personality disorder, personality traits, impulsive violence, and completed suicide in adolescents. *Journal of the American Academy of Child and Adolescent Psychiatry* 1994;33(8):1080–6.
118 Hamza CA, Willoughby T. Impulsivity and nonsuicidal self-injury: a longitudinal examination among emerging adults. *Journal of Adolescence* 2019;75:37–46.
119 Dhingra K, Boduszek D, O'Connor RC. Differentiating suicide attempters from suicide ideators using the Integrated Motivational – Volitional model of suicidal behaviour. *Journal of Affective Disorders* 2015;186:211–8.
120 Stein D, Apter A, Ratzoni G, Har-Even D, Avidan G. Association between multiple suicide attempts and negative affects in adolescents. *Journal of the American Academy of Child and Adolescent Psychiatry* 1998;37(5):488–94.
121 Pfeffer CR, Hurt SW, Peskin JR, Siefker CA. Suicidal children grow up: ego functions associated with suicide attempts. *Journal of the American Academy of Child and Adolescent Psychiatry* 1995;34(10):1318–25.
122 Daniel SS, Goldston DB, Erkanli A, Franklin JC, Mayfield AM. Trait anger, anger expression, and suicide attempts among adolescents and young adults: a prospective study. *Journal of Clinical Child and Adolescent Psychology* 2009;38(5):661–71.
123 Beck AT, Kovacs M, Weissman A. Hopelessness and suicidal behavior: an overview. *JAMA* 1975;234(11):1146–9.
124 Kovacs M, Beck AT, Weissman A. Hopelessness: an indicator of suicidal risk. *Suicide and Life-Threatening Behavior* 1975;5(2):98–103.
125 Hetrick SE, Parker AG, Robinson J, Hall N, Vance A. Predicting suicidal risk in a cohort of depressed children and adolescents. *Crisis* 2012;33(1):13–20.
126 Kwok SY, Shek DT. Hopelessness, parent-adolescent communication, and suicidal ideation among Chinese adolescents in Hong Kong. *Suicide and Life-Threatening Behavior* 2010;40(3):224–33.
127 Kazdin AE, French NH, Unis AS, Esveldt-Dawson K, Sherick RB. Hopelessness, depression, and suicidal intent among psychiatrically disturbed inpatient children. *Journal of Consulting and Clinical Psychology* 1983;51(4):504–10.
128 Dahlsgaard KK, Beck AT, Brown GK. Inadequate response to therapy as a predictor of suicide. *Suicide and Life-Threatening Behavior* 1998;28(2):197–204.
129 McMillan D, Gilbody S, Beresford E, Neilly L. Can we predict suicide and non-fatal self-harm with the Beck Hopelessness Scale? A meta-analysis. *Psychological Medicine* 2007;37(6):769–78.

130 Horwitz AG, Berona J, Czyz EK, Yeguez CE, King CA. Positive and negative expectations of hopelessness as longitudinal predictors of depression, suicidal ideation, and suicidal behavior in high-risk adolescents. *Suicide and Life-Threatening Behavior* 2017;47(2):168–76.
131 Wolfe KL, Nakonezny PA, Owen VJ, Rial KV, Moorehead AP, Kennard BD, et al. Hopelessness as a predictor of suicide ideation in depressed male and female adolescent youth. *Suicide and Life-Threatening Behavior* 2019;49(1):253–63.
132 Wilson KG, Stelzer J, Bergman JN, Kral MJ, Inayatullah M, Elliott CA. Problem solving, stress, and coping in adolescent suicide attempts. *Suicide and Life-Threatening Behavior* 1995;25(2):241–52.
133 Hetrick S, Yuen HP, Cox G, Bendall S, Yung A, Pirkis J, et al. Does cognitive behavioural therapy have a role in improving problem solving and coping in adolescents with suicidal ideation? *The Cognitive Behaviour Therapist* 2014;7:e13.
134 McAuliffe C, Corcoran P, Keeley HS, Perry IJ. Risk of suicide ideation associated with problem-solving ability and attitudes toward suicidal behavior in university students. *Crisis* 2003;24(4):160–7.
135 Schotte DE, Clum GA. Problem-solving skills in suicidal psychiatric patients. *Journal of Consulting and Clinical Psychology* 1987;55(1):49–54.
136 Jeglic EL, Sharp IR, Chapman JE, Brown GK, Beck AT. History of family suicide behaviors and negative problem solving in multiple suicide attempters. *Archives of Suicide Research* 2005;9(2):135–46.
137 Orbach I, Bar-Joseph H, Dror N. Styles of problem solving in suicidal individuals. *Suicide and Life-Threatening Behavior* 1990;20(1):56–64.
138 Rudd MD, Rajab MH, Dahm PF. Problem-solving appraisal in suicide ideators and attempters. *American Journal of Orthopsychiatry* 1994;64(1):136–49.
139 Fordwood SR, Asarnow JR, Huizar DP, Reise SP. Suicide attempts among depressed adolescents in primary care. *Journal of Clinical Child and Adolescent Psychology* 2007;36(3):392–404.
140 Agerbo E, Nordentoft M, Mortensen P. Suicide among young people – familial, psychiatric and socioeconomic risk factors. A nested case-control study. *Ugeskrift for Laeger* 2002;164(49):5786–90.
141 Paykel ES, Prusoff BA, Myers JK. Suicide attempts and recent life events: a controlled comparison. *Archives of General Psychiatry* 1975;32(3):327–33.
142 Korczak DJ, Skinner R, Dopko R. Serious self-harm requiring intensive care unit admission: understanding near-fatal suicide attempts. *Paediatrics & Child Health* 2019;24(1):58–9.
143 Paul E. Proximally-occurring life events and the first transition from suicidal ideation to suicide attempt in adolescents. *Journal of Affective Disorders* 2018;241:499–504.
144 Kazan D, Calear AL, Batterham PJ. The impact of intimate partner relationships on suicidal thoughts and behaviours: a systematic review. *Journal of Affective Disorders* 2016;190:585–98.
145 Klomek AB, Sourander A, Gould M. The association of suicide and bullying in childhood to young adulthood: a review of cross-sectional and longitudinal research findings. *Canadian Journal of Psychiatry* 2010;55(5):282–8.
146 Kim YS, Leventhal BL, Koh Y-J, Boyce WT. Bullying increased suicide risk: prospective study of Korean adolescents. *Archives of Suicide Research* 2009;13(1):15–30.
147 Klomek AB, Sourander A, Niemelä S, Kumpulainen K, Piha J, Tamminen T, et al. Childhood bullying behaviors as a risk for suicide attempts and completed suicides: a population-based birth cohort study. *Journal of the American Academy of Child and Adolescent Psychiatry* 2009;48(3):254–61.

148 Van Geel M, Vedder P, Tanilon J. Relationship between peer victimization, cyberbullying, and suicide in children and adolescents: a meta-analysis. *JAMA Pediatrics* 2014;168(5):435–42.
149 Przybylski AK, Bowes L. Cyberbullying and adolescent well-being in England: a population-based cross-sectional study. *Lancet Child & Adolescent Health* 2017;1(1):19–26.
150 Wolke D. Cyberbullying: how big a deal is it? *Lancet Child & Adolescent Health* 2017;1(1):2–3.
151 Hinduja S, Patchin JW. Bullying, cyberbullying, and suicide. *Archives of Suicide Research* 2010;14(3):206–21.
152 John A, Glendenning AC, Marchant A, Montgomery P, Stewart A, Wood S, et al. Self-harm, suicidal behaviours, and cyberbullying in children and young people: systematic review. *Journal of Medical Internet Research* 2018;20(4):e129.
153 Clarke MC, Coughlan H, Harley M, Connor D, Power E, Lynch F, et al. The impact of adolescent cannabis use, mood disorder and lack of education on attempted suicide in young adulthood. *World Psychiatry* 2014;13(3):322–3.
154 Schilling EA, Aseltine Jr RH, Glanovsky JL, James A, Jacobs D. Adolescent alcohol use, suicidal ideation, and suicide attempts. *Journal of Adolescent Health* 2009;44(4):335–41.
155 Schaffer M, Jeglic EL, Stanley B. The relationship between suicidal behavior, ideation, and binge drinking among college students. *Archives of Suicide Research* 2008;12(2):124–32.
156 Meyers K, Hagan TA, Zanis D, Webb A, Frantz J, Ring-Kurtz S, et al. Critical issues in adolescent substance use assessment. *Drug and Alcohol Dependence* 1999;55(3):235–46.
157 Aseltine Jr RH, Schilling EA, James A, Glanovsky JL, Jacobs D. Age variability in the association between heavy episodic drinking and adolescent suicide attempts: findings from a large-scale, school-based screening program. *Journal of the American Academy of Child and Adolescent Psychiatry* 2009;48(3):262–70.
158 Hawton K, Hill N, Gould M, John A, Lascelles K, Robinson J. Clustering of suicides in children and adolescents. *Lancet Child & Adolescent Health* 2020;4(1):58–67.
159 Gould MS, Wallenstein S, Kleinman MH, O'Carroll P, Mercy J. Suicide clusters: an examination of age-specific effects. *American Journal of Public Health* 1990;80(2):211–2.
160 Robinson J, San Too L, Pirkis J, Spittal MJ. Spatial suicide clusters in Australia between 2010 and 2012: a comparison of cluster and non-cluster among young people and adults. *BMC Psychiatry* 2016;16:417.
161 Too LS, Pirkis J, Milner A, Spittal MJ. Clusters of suicides and suicide attempts: detection, proximity and correlates. *Epidemiology and Psychiatric Sciences* 2017;26(5):491–500.
162 Cox GR, Robinson J, Williamson M, Lockley A, Cheung YT, Pirkis J. Suicide clusters in young people. *Crisis* 2012;33(4):208–14.
163 Haw C, Hawton K, Niedzwiedz C, Platt S. Suicide clusters: a review of risk factors and mechanisms. *Suicide and Life-Threatening Behavior* 2013;43(1):97–108.
164 Insel BJ, Gould MS. Impact of modeling on adolescent suicidal behavior. *Psychiatric Clinics of North America* 2008;31(2):293–316.
165 Feigelman W, Gorman BS. Assessing the effects of peer suicide on youth suicide. *Suicide and Life-Threatening Behavior* 2008;38(2):181–94.
166 Ho TP, Leung PW, Hung SF, Lee CC, Tang CP. The mental health of the peers of suicide completers and attempters. *Journal of Child Psychology and Psychiatry* 2000;41(3):301–8.
167 Randall JR, Nickel NC, Colman I. Contagion from peer suicidal behavior in a representative sample of American adolescents. *Journal of Affective Disorders* 2015;186:219–25.
168 Abrutyn S, Mueller AS. Are suicidal behaviors contagious in adolescence? Using longitudinal data to examine suicide suggestion. *American Sociological Review* 2014;79(2):211–27.

169 Swanson SA, Colman I. Association between exposure to suicide and suicidality outcomes in youth. *CMAJ* 2013;185(10):870–7.
170 McMahon EM, Corcoran P, Keeley H, Perry IJ, Arensman E. Adolescents exposed to suicidal behavior of others: prevalence of self-harm and associated psychological, lifestyle, and life event factors. *Suicide and Life-Threatening Behavior* 2013;43(6):634–45.
171 Mars B, Heron J, Klonsky ED, Moran P, O'Connor RC, Tilling K, et al. What distinguishes adolescents with suicidal thoughts from those who have attempted suicide? A population-based birth cohort study. *Journal of Child Psychology and Psychiatry* 2019;60(1):91–9.
172 O'Connor RC, Rasmussen S, Hawton K. Predicting depression, anxiety and self-harm in adolescents: the role of perfectionism and acute life stress. *Behaviour Research and Therapy* 2010;48(1):52–9.
173 Cutler DM, Glaeser EL, Norberg KE. Explaining the rise in youth suicide. In Gruber J (Ed) *Risky behavior among youths: an economic analysis*. Chicago: University of Chicago Press; 2001. p 219–70.
174 Romer D, Jamieson PE, Jamieson KH. Are news reports of suicide contagious? A stringent test in six US cities. *Journal of Communication* 2006;56(2):253–70.
175 Gould M, Jamieson P, Romer D. Media contagion and suicide among the young. *American Behavioral Scientist* 2003;46(9):1269–84.
176 Phillips DP, Carstensen LL. Clustering of teenage suicides after television news stories about suicide. *New England Journal of Medicine* 1986;315(11):685–9.
177 Niederkrotenthaler T, Stack S, Till B, Sinyor M, Pirkis J, Garcia D, et al. Association of increased youth suicides in the United States with the release of 13 Reasons Why. *JAMA Psychiatry* 2019;76(9):933–40.
178 Sinyor M, Williams M, Tran US, Schaffer A, Kurdyak P, Pirkis J, et al. Suicides in young people in Ontario following the release of "13 Reasons Why". *Canadian Journal of Psychiatry* 2019;64(11):798–804.
179 Cooper MT Jr, Bard D, Wallace R, Gillaspy S, Deleon S. Suicide attempt admissions from a single children's hospital before and after the introduction of Netflix series 13 Reasons Why. *Journal of Adolescent Health* 2018;63(6):688–93.
180 Bell J. Harmful or helpful? The role of the internet in self-harming and suicidal behaviour in young people. *Mental Health Review Journal* 2014;19(1):61–71.
181 Recupero PR, Harms SE, Noble JM. Googling suicide: surfing for suicide information on the internet. *Journal of Clinical Psychiatry* 2008;69(6):878–88.
182 Marchant A, Hawton K, Stewart A, Montgomery P, Singaravelu V, Lloyd K, et al. A systematic review of the relationship between internet use, self-harm and suicidal behaviour in young people: the good, the bad and the unknown. *PLoS One* 2017;12(8):e0181722.
183 Jensen M, George MJ, Russell MR, Odgers CL. Young adolescents' digital technology use and mental health symptoms: little evidence of longitudinal or daily linkages. *Clinical Psychological Science* 2019;7(6):1416–33.
184 Przybylski AK, Weinstein N. A large-scale test of the Goldilocks Hypothesis: quantifying the relations between digital-screen use and the mental well-being of adolescents. *Psychological Science* 2017;28(2):204–15.
185 Twenge JM, Joiner TE, Rogers ML, Martin GN. Increases in depressive symptoms, suicide-related outcomes, and suicide rates among US adolescents after 2010 and links to increased new media screen time. *Clinical Psychological Science* 2018;6(1):3–17.
186 Robinson J, Hill NT, Thorn P, Battersby R, Teh Z, Reavley NJ, et al. The #chatsafe project. Developing guidelines to help young people communicate safely about suicide on social media: a Delphi study. *PLoS One* 2018;13(11):e0206584.

187 Rice S, Robinson J, Bendall S, Hetrick S, Cox G, Bailey E, et al. Online and social media suicide prevention interventions for young people: a focus on implementation and moderation. *Journal of the Canadian Academy of Child and Adolescent Psychiatry* 2016;25(2):80–6.
188 Robinson J, Bailey E, Hetrick S, Paix S, O'Donnell M, Cox G, et al. Developing social media-based suicide prevention messages in partnership with young people: exploratory study. *JMIR Mental Health* 2017;4(4):e40.
189 Robinson J, Cox G, Bailey E, Hetrick S, Rodrigues M, Fisher S, et al. Social media and suicide prevention: a systematic review. *Early Intervention in Psychiatry* 2016;10(2):103–21.
190 Robinson J, Hetrick S, Cox G, Bendall S, Yuen HP, Yung A, et al. Can an internet-based intervention reduce suicidal ideation, depression and hopelessness among secondary school students: results from a pilot study. *Early Intervention in Psychiatry* 2016;10(1):28–35.
191 Robinson J, Pirkis J, O'Connor RC. Suicide clusters. In O'Connor RC, Pirkis J (Eds) *The international handbook of suicide prevention*. Chichester: John Wiley & Sons Ltd; 2016. p 758–74.
192 Rickwood DJ, Deane FP, Wilson CJ. When and how do young people seek professional help for mental health problems? *Medical Journal of Australia* 2007;187(S7):S35–9.
193 Michelmore L, Hindley P. Help-seeking for suicidal thoughts and self-harm in young people: a systematic review. *Suicide and Life-Threatening Behavior* 2012;42(5):507–24.
194 Swahn MH, Potter LB. Factors associated with the medical severity of suicide attempts in youths and young adults. *Suicide and Life-Threatening Behavior* 2001;32(1):21–9.
195 Evans E, Hawton K, Rodham K. In what ways are adolescents who engage in self-harm or experience thoughts of self-harm different in terms of help-seeking, communication and coping strategies? *Journal of Adolescence* 2005;28(4):573–87.
196 Robinson J, Bailey E, Witt K, Stefanac N, Milner A, Currier D, et al. What works in youth suicide prevention? A systematic review and meta-analysis. *EClinicalMedicine* 2018;4–5:52–91.
197 Silverman MM, Maris RW. The prevention of suicidal behaviors: an overview. *Suicide and Life-Threatening Behavior* 1995;25(1):10–21.
198 Brophy M, Holmstrom R. *Truth hurts: report of the national inquiry into self-harm among young people*. London: Mental Health Foundation; 2006.
199 Robinson J, Yuen HP, Martin C, Hughes A, Baksheev GN, Dodd S, et al. Does screening high school students for psychological distress, deliberate self-harm, or suicidal ideation cause distress – and is it acceptable? An Australian-based study. *Crisis* 2011;32(5):254–63.
200 Robinson J, Calear AL, Bailey E. Suicide prevention in educational settings: a review. *Australasian Psychiatry* 2018;26(2):132–40.
201 Mann JJ, Apter A, Bertolote J, Beautrais A, Currier D, Haas A, et al. Suicide prevention strategies: a systematic review. *JAMA* 2005;294(16):2064–74.
202 Gunnell D, Frankel S. Prevention of suicide: aspirations and evidence. *BMJ* 1994;308(6938):1227–33.
203 Gunnell D, Middleton N, Frankel S. Method availability and the prevention of suicide – a re-analysis of secular trends in England and Wales 1950–1975. *Social Psychiatry and Psychiatric Epidemiology* 2000;35(10):437–43.
204 Beautrais A, Fergusson D, Coggan C, Collings C, Doughty C, Ellis P, et al. Effective strategies for suicide prevention in New Zealand: a review of the evidence. *New Zealand Medical Journal* 2007;120(1251):U2459.
205 Ohberg A, Lonnqvist J, Sarna S, Vuori E, Penttila A. Trends and availability of suicide methods in Finland: proposals for restrictive measures. *British Journal of Psychiatry* 1995;166(1):35–43.

206 Beautrais A. Suicide by jumping: a review of research and prevention strategies. *Crisis* 2007;28(1):58–63.
207 Beautrais AL, Fergusson D, Horwood L. Firearms legislation and reductions in firearm-related suicide deaths in New Zealand. *Australian and New Zealand Journal of Psychiatry* 2006;40(3):253–9.
208 Knipe DW, Chang SS, Dawson A, Eddleston M, Konradsen F, Metcalfe C, et al. Suicide prevention through means restriction: impact of the 2008–2011 pesticide restrictions on suicide in Sri Lanka. *PLoS One* 2017;12(3):e0172893.
209 Barber CW, Miller MJ. Reducing a suicidal person's access to lethal means of suicide: a research agenda. *American Journal of Preventive Medicine* 2014;47(3):S264–72.
210 Yip PS, Caine E, Yousuf S, Chang SS, Wu KC, Chen YY. Means restriction for suicide prevention. *Lancet* 2012;379(9834):2393–9.
211 Hawton K, Simkin S, Deeks J, Cooper J, Johnston A, Waters K, et al. UK legislation on analgesic packs: before and after study of long term effect on poisonings. *BMJ* 2004;329(7474):1076.
212 Shaffer D, Garland A, Gould M, Fisher P, Trautman P. Preventing teenage suicide: a critical review. *Journal of the American Academy of Child and Adolescent Psychiatry* 1988;27(6):675–87.
213 Cusimano MD, Sameem M. The effectiveness of middle and high school-based suicide prevention programmes for adolescents: a systematic review. *Injury Prevention* 2011;17(1):43–9.
214 Bailey E, Spittal MJ, Pirkis J, Gould M, Robinson J. Universal suicide prevention in young people: an evaluation of the safeTALK program in Australian high schools. *Crisis* 2017;38(5):300–8.
215 Shaffer D, Gould M. Suicide prevention in schools. In Hawton K, van Heeringen K (Eds) *The international handbook of suicide and attempted suicide*. Chichester: John Wiley & Sons Ltd; 2000. p 645–60.
216 Neil AL, Christensen H. Australian school-based prevention and early intervention programs for anxiety and depression: a systematic review. *Medical Journal of Australia* 2007;186(6):305–8.
217 Mo PKH, Ko TT, Xin MQ. School-based gatekeeper training programmes in enhancing gatekeepers' cognitions and behaviours for adolescent suicide prevention: a systematic review. *Child and Adolescent Psychiatry and Mental Health* 2018;12:29.
218 Rodi MS, Garraza LG, Walrath C, Stephens RL, Condron DS, Hicks BB, et al. Referral patterns for youths identified at risk for suicide by trained gatekeepers. *Crisis* 2012;33(2):113–9.
219 Peña JB, Caine ED. Screening as an approach for adolescent suicide prevention. *Suicide and Life-Threatening Behavior* 2006;36(6):614–37.
220 Gould MS, Marrocco FA, Kleinman M, Thomas JG, Mostkoff K, Cote J, et al. Evaluating iatrogenic risk of youth suicide screening programs: a randomized controlled trial. *JAMA* 2005;293(13):1635–43.
221 Nemeroff R, Levitt JM, Faul L, Wonpat-Borja A, Bufferd S, Setterberg S, et al. Establishing ongoing, early identification programs for mental health problems in our schools: a feasibility study. *Journal of the American Academy of Child and Adolescent Psychiatry* 2008;47(3):328–38.
222 Shaffer D, Scott M, Wilcox H, Maslow C, Hicks R, Lucas CP, et al. The Columbia Suicide Screen: validity and reliability of a screen for youth suicide and depression. *Journal of the American Academy of Child and Adolescent Psychiatry* 2004;43(1):71–9.
223 Eckert TL, Miller DN, Riley-Tillman TC, DuPaul GJ. Adolescent suicide prevention: gender differences in students' perceptions of the acceptability and intrusiveness of school-based screening programs. *Journal of School Psychology* 2006;44(4):271–85.

224 Miller DN, Eckert TL, DuPaul GJ, White GP. Adolescent suicide prevention: acceptability of school-based programs among secondary school principals. *Suicide and Life-Threatening Behavior* 1999;29(1):72–85.
225 Cantwell DP, Lewinsohn PM, Rohde P, Seeley JR. Correspondence between adolescent report and parent report of psychiatric diagnostic data. *Journal of the American Academy of Child and Adolescent Psychiatry* 1997;36(5):610–9.
226 Velez CN, Cohen P. Suicidal behavior and ideation in a community sample of children: maternal and youth reports. *Journal of the American Academy of Child and Adolescent Psychiatry* 1988;27(3):349–56.
227 Young TL, Zimmerman R. Clueless: parental knowledge of risk behaviors of middle school students. *Archives of Pediatrics & Adolescent Medicine* 1998;152(11):1137–9.
228 Hetrick SE, Robinson J, Burge E, Blandon R, Mobilio B, Rice SM, et al. Youth codesign of a mobile phone app to facilitate self-monitoring and management of mood symptoms in young people with major depression, suicidal ideation, and self-harm. *JMIR Mental Health* 2018;5(1):e9.
229 Hetrick SE, Goodall J, Yuen HP, Davey CG, Parker AG, Robinson J, et al. Comprehensive online self-monitoring to support clinicians manage risk of suicide in youth depression. *Crisis* 2017;38(3):147–57.
230 Van Griensven F, Naorat S, Kilmarx PH, Jeeyapant S, Manopaiboon C, Chaikummao S, et al. Palmtop-assisted self-interviewing for the collection of sensitive behavioral data: randomized trial with drug use urine testing. *American Journal of Epidemiology* 2005;163(3):271–8.
231 Newman JC, Des Jarlais DC, Turner CF, Gribble J, Cooley P, Paone D. The differential effects of face-to-face and computer interview modes. *American Journal of Public Health* 2002;92(2):294–7.
232 Scott MA, Wilcox HC, Schonfeld IS, Davies M, Hicks RC, Turner JB, et al. School-based screening to identify at-risk students not already known to school professionals: the Columbia Suicide Screen. *American Journal of Public Health* 2009;99(2):334–9.
233 Gould MS, Marrocco FA, Hoagwood K, Kleinman M, Amakawa L, Altschuler E. Service use by at-risk youths after school-based suicide screening. *Journal of the American Academy of Child and Adolescent Psychiatry* 2009;48(12):1193–201.
234 Hetrick SE, McKenzie JE, Merry SN. The use of SSRIs in children and adolescents. *Current Opinion in Psychiatry* 2010;23(1):53–7.
235 Jensen PS. After TADS, can we measure up, catch up, and ante up? *Journal of the American Academy of Child and Adolescent Psychiatry* 2006;45(12):1456–60.
236 Hickie IB, McGorry PD. Guidelines for youth depression: time to incorporate new perspectives. *Medical Journal of Australia* 2010;193(3):133–4.
237 Birmaher B, Brent D, AACAP Work Group on Quality Issues. Practice parameter for the assessment and treatment of children and adolescents with depressive disorders. *Journal of the American Academy of Child and Adolescent Psychiatry* 2007;46(11):1503–26.
238 Cheung AH, Zuckerbrot RA, Jensen PS, Laraque D, Stein REK, GLAD-PC Steering Group. Guidelines for Adolescent Depression in Primary Care (GLAD-PC): part II. Treatment and ongoing management. *Pediatrics* 2018;141(3):e20174082.
239 National Institute for Health and Care Excellence. *Depression in children and young people: identification and management.* London: National Institute for Health and Care Excellence; 2019.
240 Zuckerbrot RA, Cheung A, Jensen PS, Stein REK, Laraque D, GLAD-PC Steering Group. Guidelines for Adolescent Depression in Primary Care (GLAD-PC): part I. Practice preparation, identification, assessment, and initial management. *Pediatrics* 2018;141(3):e20174081.

241 Meltzer HY, Alphs L, Green AI, Altamura AC, Anand R, Bertoldi A, et al. Clozapine treatment for suicidality in schizophrenia: International Suicide Prevention Trial (InterSePT). *Archives of General Psychiatry* 2003;60(1):82–91.

242 Cipriani A, Hawton K, Stockton S, Geddes JR. Lithium in the prevention of suicide in mood disorders: updated systematic review and meta-analysis. *BMJ* 2013;346:f3646.

243 Zalpuri I, Singh MK. Pharmacological approaches for treating suicidality in adolescents. In Berk M (Ed) *Evidence-based treatment approaches for suicidal adolescents: translating science into practice.* Washington, DC: American Psychiatric Association Publishing; 2019. p 293–332.

244 Hawton K, Witt KG, Taylor Salisbury TL, Arensman E, Gunnell D, Hazell P, et al. Pharmacological interventions for self-harm in adults. *BJPsych Advances* 2016;22(1):2.

245 Calear AL, Christensen H, Freeman A, Fenton K, Grant JB, Van Spijker B, et al. A systematic review of psychosocial suicide prevention interventions for youth. *European Child & Adolescent Psychiatry* 2016;25(5):467–82.

246 Hawton K, Witt KG, Taylor Salisbury TL, Arensman E, Gunnell D, Townsend E, et al. Interventions for self-harm in children and adolescents. *Cochrane Database of Systematic Reviews* 2015;12:CD012013.

247 Robinson J, Hetrick SE, Martin C. Preventing suicide in young people: systematic review. *Australian and New Zealand Journal of Psychiatry* 2011;45(1):3–26.

248 Cox G, Hetrick S. Psychosocial interventions for self-harm, suicidal ideation and suicide attempt in children and young people: What? How? Who? and Where? *Evidence-Based Mental Health* 2017;20(2):35–40.

249 Carter G, Page A, Large M, Hetrick S, Milner AJ, Bendit N, et al. Royal Australian and New Zealand College of Psychiatrists clinical practice guideline for the management of deliberate self-harm. *Australian and New Zealand Journal of Psychiatry* 2016;50(10):939–1000.

250 Rossouw TI, Fonagy P. Mentalization-based treatment for self-harm in adolescents: a randomized controlled trial. *Journal of the American Academy of Child and Adolescent Psychiatry* 2012;51(12):1304–13.

251 Burns J, Dudley M, Hazell P, Patton G. Clinical management of deliberate self-harm in young people: the need for evidence-based approaches to reduce repetition. *Australian and New Zealand Journal of Psychiatry* 2005;39(3):121–8.

252 Cuijpers P, Van Straten A, Andersson G. Internet-administered cognitive behavior therapy for health problems: a systematic review. *Journal of Behavioral Medicine* 2008;31(2):169–77.

253 Berger M, Wagner TH, Baker LC. Internet use and stigmatized illness. *Social Science & Medicine* 2005;61(8):1821–7.

254 Saddichha S, Al-Desouki M, Lamia A, Linden IA, Krausz M. Online interventions for depression and anxiety – a systematic review. *Health Psychology and Behavioral Medicine* 2014;2(1):841–81.

255 Gerhards S, De Graaf L, Jacobs L, Severens J, Huibers M, Arntz A, et al. Economic evaluation of online computerised cognitive – behavioural therapy without support for depression in primary care: randomised trial. *British Journal of Psychiatry* 2010;196(4):310–8.

256 Kessler D, Lewis G, Kaur S, Wiles N, King M, Weich S, et al. Therapist-delivered internet psychotherapy for depression in primary care: a randomised controlled trial. *Lancet* 2009;374(9690):628–34.

257 Spek V, Cuijpers P, Nyklíček I, Riper H, Keyzer J, Pop V. Internet-based cognitive behaviour therapy for symptoms of depression and anxiety: a meta-analysis. *Psychological Medicine* 2007;37(3):319–28.

258 Titov N. Status of computerized cognitive behavioural therapy for adults. *Australian and New Zealand Journal of Psychiatry* 2007;41(2):95–114.

259 Kaltenthaler E, Parry G, Beverley C. Computerized cognitive behaviour therapy: a systematic review. *Behavioural and Cognitive Psychotherapy* 2004;32(1):31–55.
260 Griffiths KM, Farrer L, Christensen H. The efficacy of internet interventions for depression and anxiety disorders: a review of randomised controlled trials. *Medical Journal of Australia* 2010;192(S11):S4–11.
261 Proudfoot J, Ryden C, Everitt B, Shapiro DA, Goldberg D, Mann A, et al. Clinical efficacy of computerised cognitive-behavioural therapy for anxiety and depression in primary care: randomised controlled trial. *British Journal of Psychiatry* 2004;185(1):46–54.
262 Richards D, Richardson T. Computer-based psychological treatments for depression: a systematic review and meta-analysis. *Clinical Psychology Review* 2012;32(4):329–42.
263 Mohr DC, Weingardt KR, Reddy M, Schueller SM. Three problems with current digital mental health research . . . and three things we can do about them. *Psychiatric Services* 2017;68(5):427–9.
264 Richardson T, Stallard P, Velleman S. Computerised cognitive behavioural therapy for the prevention and treatment of depression and anxiety in children and adolescents: a systematic review. *Clinical Child and Family Psychology Review* 2010;13(3):275–90.
265 Calear AL, Christensen H. Review of internet-based prevention and treatment programs for anxiety and depression in children and adolescents. *Medical Journal of Australia* 2010;192(S11):S12–4.
266 O'Kearney R, Kang K, Christensen H, Griffiths K, Gibson M. A CBT internet program for depression in adolescents (MoodGYM): effects on depressive symptoms, attributional style, self-esteem and beliefs about depression. In Einstein DA (Ed) *Innovations and advances in cognitive behaviour therapy*. Bowen Hills, Queensland: Australian Academic Press; 2007. p 197–203.
267 Neil A, Christensen H, Griffiths K. Evaluation of MoodGYM with an adolescent population. *Acta Neuropsychiatrica* 2006;18(6):263.
268 Silverstone PH, Bercov M, Suen VY, Allen A, Cribben I, Goodrick J, et al. Long-term results from the Empowering a Multimodal Pathway Toward Healthy Youth Program, a multimodal school-based approach, show marked reductions in suicidality, depression, and anxiety in 6,227 students in grades 6–12 (aged 11–18). *Frontiers in Psychiatry* 2017;8:81.
269 Perry Y, Werner-Seidler A, Calear AL, Christensen H. Web-based and mobile suicide prevention interventions for young people: a systematic review. *Journal of the Canadian Academy of Child and Adolescent Psychiatry* 2016;25(2):73–9.
270 Tighe J, Shand F, Ridani R, Mackinnon A, De La Mata N, Christensen H. Ibobbly mobile health intervention for suicide prevention in Australian indigenous youth: a pilot randomised controlled trial. *BMJ Open* 2017;7(1):e013518.
271 McManama O'Brien KH, LeCloux M, Ross A, Gironda C, Wharff EA. A pilot study of the acceptability and usability of a smartphone application intervention for suicidal adolescents and their parents. *Archives of Suicide Research* 2017;21(2):254–64.
272 Stallard P, Porter J, Grist R. A smartphone app (BlueIce) for young people who self-harm: open phase 1 pre-post trial. *JMIR mHealth and uHealth* 2018;6(1):e32.
273 Hetrick SE, Yuen HP, Bailey E, Cox GR, Templer K, Rice SM, et al. Internet-based cognitive behavioural therapy for young people with suicide-related behaviour (Reframe-IT): a randomised controlled trial. *Evidence-Based Mental Health* 2017;20(3):76–82.
274 Robinson J, Hetrick S, Cox G, Bendall S, Yung A, Pirkis J. The safety and acceptability of delivering an online intervention to secondary students at risk of suicide: findings from a pilot study. *Early Intervention in Psychiatry* 2015;9(6):498–506.

275 Robinson J, Hetrick S, Cox G, Bendall S, Yung A, Yuen HP, et al. The development of a randomised controlled trial testing the effects of an online intervention among school students at risk of suicide. *BMC Psychiatry* 2014;14(1):155.
276 Christensen H, Batterham P, O'Dea B. E-health interventions for suicide prevention. *International Journal of Environmental Research and Public Health* 2014;11(8):8193–212.
277 Witt K, Spittal MJ, Carter G, Pirkis J, Hetrick S, Currier D, et al. Effectiveness of online and mobile telephone applications ('apps') for the self-management of suicidal ideation and self-harm: a systematic review and meta-analysis. *BMC Psychiatry* 2017;17(1):297.
278 Bailey E, Rice S, Robinson J, Nedeljkovic M, Alvarez-Jimenez M. Theoretical and empirical foundations of a novel online social networking intervention for youth suicide prevention: a conceptual review. *Journal of Affective Disorders* 2018;238:499–505.

15 Family interventions

Catharine McNab

Introduction

Families often play a key role in supporting young people with emergent mental illness. At any age, the development of mental illness will have clear impact on both patients and their families, but this is likely to be especially true when the patient is a young person. For example, the vast majority of young people live with family and are to some extent financially and emotionally reliant on them. It is also often families who will initially seek help for their relative, and only after members feel they have done everything they can to manage the young person's difficulties. Additionally, family involvement in supporting people with mental illness, regardless of phase, may have increased in the last four decades as a consequence of changes in service delivery. With a higher emphasis globally on outpatient treatment, families may be increasingly used by clinical services as de facto members of the treating team, for example, as key monitors of early warning signs of relapse and key bearers of responsibility in accessing services at these times.

The way that families support young people during this period may have some effect on the young person's recovery. The 'expressed emotion' literature, although limited in its application to outcome in early onset disorder and difficult to draw conclusions from, suggests that particular types of family interactions may be stressful for patients and thereby worsen the course of illness. A separate literature focusing on 'emotion socialisation', or families' responses to particular emotions in young people, also suggests that these responses may influence the course of depressive and anxious illnesses in adolescents.

However, a focus on families as potentially problematic factors in patient recovery, or as informal members of the treating team, must be partnered with recognition of the challenges of parenting young people generally and those with emergent mental illness in particular. Family experiences such as bewilderment, grief, loss, guilt, and stigma are all appropriate targets for clinical services in their own right.

This chapter reviews relationships between family experiences and patient outcomes, the experiences of families of young people with early-onset mental illness; the evidence-base for family interventions targeted at these families, and implications for what interventions should include. Its focus is primarily on first-episode psychosis (FEP), with a smaller emphasis on depression and anxiety, as the vast majority of the limited research on family experiences of mental illness in young people has been in these fields.

Families and the cause and course of mental illness

Historical factors

The roles and challenges of families caring for people with mental illness have been the subject of clinical and research interest for decades. However, this has been largely restricted in terms of diagnosis (with schizophrenia being the primary mental illness of interest) and of outcome (with the focus being overwhelmingly one of examining family factors as a way of preventing onset and relapse of psychiatric disorder in patients, rather than family experiences in their own right).

Early research suggested that families could cause mental illness generally and specifically psychotic disorders. These theories focused particularly on the role of mothers, who caused schizophrenia by having a 'perverted maternal instinct' or being 'schizophrenogenic', or using confusing communication styles that placed patients in a 'double bind' and led to psychotic symptoms.[1] These theories were largely based on anecdotal or methodologically problematic evidence.

Expressed emotion

The clinical and research focus has since shifted from family factors contributing to onset to those contributing to relapse. The construct of expressed emotion (EE) has dominated this field. Brown and colleagues coined this term after observing that the prognosis for patients with psychosis appeared related to their living situation after discharge.[2] According to these authors, patients returning from admission to live with parents or partners relapsed more quickly than those who returned to live with siblings or in shared accommodation. These findings seemed particularly strong when parents or spouses demonstrated a number of behaviours in a semi-structured interview: criticism (comment on behaviours or characteristics of the patient that were regarded as annoying or which caused resentment), hostility (generalised criticism or rejection), and emotional over-involvement (over-intrusive or self-sacrificing behaviour, exaggerated responses, or over-identification with the patient).[3] Two positive subscales were also included – warmth and positive comments – and were hypothesised to be protective.

The 'negative' subscales of EE have demonstrated considerable predictive validity. EE is highly predictive of psychotic relapse, with rates in families with high EE ranging between 50% and 65%, while those for families with low EE range from 23% to 35%.[4] EE appears even more strongly predictive of relapse in other chronic disorders, despite the initial reservations of Brown and colleagues regarding the construct's generalisability beyond psychosis.[2] Disorders in which EE predicts worsening symptomatology and/or relapse include depression, bipolar disorder, eating disorders, substance use, comorbid substance use and psychotic disorder, and post-traumatic stress disorder. EE also appears to play a role in the prognosis of physical health disorders.[5] The relationship between the negative subscales of EE and relapse also emerges across many cultures, although with some reference to culturally normative levels of EE.[6] The major moderating factor in the link between EE and relapse is the amount of time spent with the carer: EE is more strongly related to relapse when carers have more contact with patients. The positive subscales have shown limited predictive validity.

Informal caregivers are not the only carers to demonstrate behaviours consistent with high EE. Formal caregivers, such as case managers and inpatient unit staff, also score on EE measures, although rates of high EE are generally lower in this group than amongst informal caregivers, perhaps because of under-report or a lower level of emotional investment in patients.[7] High EE in formal caregivers is also associated with poorer patient outcome.

The role of EE in patient outcome can be more broadly positioned within the diathesis-stress literature,[8,9] in which family interactions serve as a stressor which, interacting with an organic diathesis, lead to patient illness. EE research has led to the development of family interventions with a key focus on changing communication patterns in order to reduce EE and therefore risk of relapse in patients.

EE in early onset disorders

Most studies report rates of high EE in early-onset psychiatric disorders that are similar to those in chronic samples, although the range is very broad, with rates of high EE ranging from 20% to 71%. Most of these early-onset samples consist of patients with early-onset (although not necessarily first episode) psychosis and their families; this may include young people presenting with mania with psychotic features. Although there is no reason theoretically why EE should not predict relapse in first episode disorder (i.e., predict the first relapse),[10] this link is less consistently detected in the FEP group. Although some studies have detected a relationship between EE and outcome in the first episode group, other studies have suggested that this relationship is more complicated in FEP. For example, some have suggested that EE's impact on outcome is limited in FEP once controlling for other factors, like duration of untreated symptoms, is delayed, or that EE is not predictive at all in this group.

A number of factors may account for the less problematic nature of high EE in the FEP group, although none have been examined empirically. It may be that families may be better able to censor interpersonal interactions with the patient early in the course of illness but feel more able to speak freely with others – this would then mean that high EE assessed at interview did not relate to interactions with patients, with the assessment of EE in this instance becoming less valid. Alternatively, EE interactions may be less stressful for adolescents in their first episode than they are for older people, as criticism and emotional over-involvement may be regarded, both by parents and young people, as normative – and therefore perceived as less stressful – than expectations of relationships between older adults and their families. Other reasons why the link may be less consistently detected in the FEP group are outlined in McNab and Linszen.[11]

There is a related but distinct literature that has emerged over the past two decades linking EE cross-sectionally and longitudinally with non-psychotic psychopathology in children and adolescents with mental illness. This literature is relevant, given that this population is likely early in the course of mental illness, although this is generally not specified in the literature. This literature on the whole suggests a consistent cross-sectional relationship between symptom levels and EE, with a particular focus on maternal criticism, but a less consistent longitudinal relationship between EE and outcome. Cross-sectional studies show a link between maternal high EE and child diagnosis of ADHD, conduct disorder, or substance abuse; adolescent anorexia; depression; and child diagnosis of obsessive-compulsive disorder and/or disruptive behaviour disorder. This reasonably consistent cross-sectional literature has led some to suggest that high EE, particularly criticism, is a risk factor for child and adolescent psychopathology more broadly, of both internalising and externalising forms. The role of emotional over-involvement (EOI) seems more questionable; only two studies have detected a cross-sectional relationship between childhood EOI and poorer outcome in the form of increased rates of anxiety disorders. Problematically, however, there is very limited longitudinal research examining the predictive validity of EE in the more general childhood/adolescence mental illness domain, and that which exists is inconsistent and complex, with some researchers finding this is influenced by comorbidity as well as the age, sex, and social functioning of the patient.

Therefore, while EE's (and particularly criticism's) cross-sectional link with higher levels of psychopathology and/or different disorders has been established in childhood and adolescent mental illness, the degree to which EE predicts outcome is less settled. This clearly has implications for an understanding of the development of EE and the degree to which it is a valid target for intervention in these groups, given any 'causative', or even influential, role of EE in first episode/early-onset patient presentation is unclear.

Adverse family relationships and adolescent depression and anxiety

A different literature has focused on 'adverse family relationships' in adolescent depression and has found that these, particularly absence of support and elevated criticism, conflict, and anger in the family (including when assessing both mothers and fathers), appear cross-sectionally related to adolescent depressive symptoms.[12] For example, this literature demonstrates that depressed adolescents may be more 'reactive' to aversive interactions with parents, in that such aversive interactions provoke dysphoria to a greater extent in those with depression. Family relationships seem more reliably associated with adolescent depressive symptomatology than peer relationships.[13]

A more specific literature has focused on the longitudinal relationship between adolescent mental illness, most notably depression, and parenting behaviours (emotion modelling, specific parenting practices, and the family emotional climate) that appear to shape the development of children's understanding, experience, expression, and regulation of emotion (also known as 'parental socialisation of emotion').[14] This literature demonstrates complex relationships between parental behaviour and mental health outcomes for children and adolescents. Parent management of emotions may both contribute to and maintain depression in young people. Anxiety in children and adolescents is cross-sectionally and longitudinally associated with parental controlling behaviours.[15] Both anxiety and depression are predicted by parental aggression in otherwise benign circumstances.[16] The relationship between parent and adolescent behaviour is reciprocal, though; particular adolescent behaviour may evoke reactions in parents that lead to later psychiatric problems. Negative responses to negative adolescent behaviour (e.g., parental aggressive or dysphoric responses to adolescent aggression) predict later depressive onset, perhaps because these parental behaviours represent ineffective attempts to manage adolescent aggression.[17] Parents may also respond to positive emotions in adolescents in ways that increase the chances of adolescent depression: dysphoric responses to adolescents' positive emotions predict depression onset.[18] It is not just the presence of a negative emotional environment but also of a less positive emotional environment that may contribute to poor psychiatric outcomes in adolescents, although this may be specific to depression.[19] Complicating this research further, the emotion socialisation behaviours of mothers may have a different impact on adolescents than that of fathers and, as noted earlier, may have different impacts on boys compared to girls.[20] Limited research has examined the intrapersonal processes that may precipitate or maintain psychiatric problems in adolescents in the face of particular parenting behaviours, but as an example, a recent paper suggests parental conflict may be longitudinally associated with adolescent depression because adolescents engage in experiential avoidance in order to reduce the impact of this conflict.[21] Similarly, adolescents may ruminate more in the face of a less positive family environment, which then increases the risk of depression onset, particularly in girls.[22] Different parenting behaviours may also be associated with physiological stress reactivity and brain structure.[23,24] There has to date been limited exploration of the extent to which these observed behaviours may be related to the more traditional EE construct, and there are no published studies using the data from the adverse family relationships literature to establish whether, and, if so, what kinds of interventions reduce parental behaviours that are linked to poorer patient outcome.

It is also important to note that high EE / criticism / conflict / low levels of support may in fact be an understandable reaction to parenting a young person with mental illness. EOI and intermittent criticism may both be reasonable responses to the parenting of adolescents generally or to the grief and loss that may accompany the experience of learning that a son or daughter has developed difficulties that may mean he or she goes on to develop a serious or chronic illness. This may be the reason that EE and parental distress are so strongly related in the literature. EE may in part be formed as a function of particular thoughts or attributions that many of us share – that psychiatric illness is controllable and that criticism or emotional over-involvement may help patients control their symptoms.[25,26] However, reasonable or understandable responses may still be problematic.

Summary

Different literatures suggest that interactions between adolescents and their families may contribute to the onset and maintenance of mental illness, although the evidence seems stronger in depressive than psychotic disorders. This may, however, be due to differences in the constructs explored across these different diagnostic groups (adverse family relationships / parental socialisation of emotion vs. expressed emotion) rather than a reflection of different roles for family interactions generally across these two groups. Further research is required to establish whether adolescents' interactions with their families are also related to prognosis in other psychiatric disorders.

Experiences of families

Although most research has focused on the impact of families on patient psychopathology, it is remiss to focus only on this as it disregards the importance of the wellbeing of caregivers in its own right. Family experience is also likely to influence patient prognosis beyond the construct of EE or quality of family relationships more broadly. For example, higher family burden may be related to lower levels of contact with patients, which then may be linked with later detection of relapse and higher levels of service use. It is therefore important to examine family's experiences independent of EE, as this provides important pointers to family's needs and some indications for effective intervention.

While results are inconsistent, it appears that levels of distress in caregivers of people with recent-onset psychosis are at least comparable to those in carers of people with more chronic difficulties. Indeed, some research has suggested that distress is highest at onset of FEP, falling over time.[27,28] Qualitative results suggest that some experience disorder onset as particularly stressful. Symptomatology may be experienced as emerging suddenly and without warning, with the patient seeming significantly different from their 'former self', with associated abrupt changes in family roles. Families often describe these difficulties as magnified by inexperience in coping with symptoms and in navigating mental health systems.

There is a dearth of literature relating to experiences of families of young people with early-onset non-psychotic illness. The experience may be qualitatively different, given that onset may be more likely to be insidious in non-psychotic disorders. There is some suggestion that youth depression may be related to maternal distress,[29] consistent with interpersonal theories of depression that depressed adults negatively impact those with whom they interact closely. However, considerable extra research is required to establish more clearly what it is like to parent a young person with a non-psychotic mental illness.

Needs of carers

Recent qualitative and, to a lesser extent, quantitative research has explored perceived needs of families of people with FEP. Families have described factors they most highly value as the opportunity to engage with others in similar situations, by learning that they are not alone in their experiences or responses to them.[30] They have also reported wanting more involvement in treatment, support from the treating team, advice on managing symptoms, help with understanding and moving through the service system, and the opportunity for contact with other families. Families have described wanting a formal diagnosis, something that may be elusive early in the course of illness due to diagnostic ambiguity.

Family interventions: the research base

The EE literature has led to a strong research base demonstrating the effectiveness of interventions for those with chronic schizophrenia,[31] although others challenge this, given the diversity of interventions and outcome measures.[32] This chapter focuses on those interventions developed for and/or studied specifically in young people and their families.

It is difficult to compare family interventions provided during early stages of illness. Firstly, the dominant focus has been on psychotic disorders, rather than youth mental illness more broadly. Secondly, interventions differ significantly in their components (though most will include a sampling of the elements listed next, their relative weight, for example, is rarely described) and in their format, including the length of intervention and delivery format (in the presence or absence of the young person; in group or individual formats). Few studies explore the effectiveness of stand-alone family interventions, normally nesting these within a broader intensive approach to patient care. Much of the focus in this research is on patient outcome exclusively, rather than assessing impact of interventions on family wellbeing. Finally, research methodologies differ substantially, including in follow-up periods.

The data that does exist suggests intervention for families of young people with FEP can be effective in improving negative and positive symptoms and relatives' perception of patients' social role performance, and more recent data suggests that family intervention can reduce levels of attenuated positive symptoms in young people at risk of developing psychosis.[33] It is also effective for reducing admission rates, total time in inpatient care, and symptoms in bipolar affective disorder such as aggression, mania, psychotic symptoms, depressive features, sleep disturbance, and global functioning, as well as 'behaviour problems' and externalising and internalising behaviour.[11] Family interventions may provide a significant additive effect when combined with individual interventions in terms of patient outcome. However, the advantages of family intervention in FEP on patient outcome are not consistently detected, and as many null findings as significant findings seem to exist.[34] Family interventions appear less effective than in more chronic samples in reducing patient relapse rates, particularly interventions that are shorter (i.e., 2–10 hours in length).[35] Even when interventions are effective, there is some evidence that treatment effects do not persist beyond the period in which the intervention is delivered. Further, they appear less effective in reducing the behaviours represented by the EE construct. Reasons for this lesser impact might include that families could have less intrinsic motivation to change behaviour after a first episode in the hope that this will be the only episode and that a focus purely on behaviour change within the family may preclude space being given to important issues such as grief and loss.

The equivocal nature of EE findings in FEP suggest that traditional ways of targeting EE may not be effective in this group and that the goal of reducing EE may itself be questionable. Interventions may be useful in this period instead by targeting loss and psychological comorbidity in families and by providing resources to enable families to stay involved with patients. This not only facilitates early intervention in case of relapse, but also potentially reduces factors that might contribute to the development or maintenance of high EE.

The data regarding impact of family interventions on families themselves appears more consistent. Family interventions enhance family outcomes, such as improving knowledge and understanding of mental illness generally and psychotic illness in particular; increasing confidence and a subjective sense of coping in the caring role; and reducing family burden, negative appraisal of the impact of caregiving, and feelings of isolation and guilt.[30] Shorter interventions may also have considerable effects on family outcome despite having more limited effects on patient outcome.[36] However, as treatment effects may not persist long beyond the intervention period,[37] family interventions may need to more explicitly recruit other caring networks, such as carer support groups, to maintain gains of intervention.

Systemic problems in implementation

A primary difficulty is that support programs are not universally available and, when they are, uptake rates can be poor.[38] The focus on resolving crises in the patient may at times prevent services from adequately focusing on supporting families, or from families focusing on themselves. There may be limited workforce training or development in implementation of family interventions. Further, families may be reluctant to engage in these interventions if they have an understandable 'sealing over' response to FEP in the hope that this will be the only episode. Patients may also be reluctant to support or encourage family involvement in care. Assertive engagement of carers, and significant financial and organisational investment in the delivery of interventions, are required before routine implementation of interventions is possible.

Implications for interventions

The aforementioned literature – on the role of families in supporting young people with mental illness and the needs that these families identify in these circumstances – suggests a number of components that can be usefully incorporated into attempts to engage families in caring for patients and themselves.

Systems negotiation and information on rights and responsibilities

Families often describe seeking help when they feel they can no longer handle the young person's difficulties,[39] particularly when insidious symptom onset means that difficulties are more likely to be interpreted (by patients, families, and other support structures) as normal adolescence. The later emergence of more significant difficulties can then lead to family guilt for delayed help-seeking.[40] Even when help is sought, services are not always responsive.[41] An often-overlooked intervention that would ease family experiences of distress and burden is therefore that of provision of early intervention services, promotion of early help-seeking, and provision of information to families about service structures and how to access and negotiate these, including providing information on service recipient rights and responsibilities.

Psychoeducation

The clearest evidence coming from the family intervention literature is that interventions are useful in enhancing knowledge and understanding of mental illness generally and psychotic illness in particular. It is likely to be useful to clarify what particular families feel they specifically need in terms of information and to engage clinicians for whom this work is routine to discuss these issues with patients (e.g., drug and alcohol specialists to discuss substance use and psychiatric comorbidity). Families in particular need information about the likelihood of recovery, realistically partnered with information about relapse. Although there is limited evidence to this effect, it is possible that such knowledge prevents the entrenchment of beliefs relating to illness, particularly the degree to which symptoms are under the patient's voluntary control, the degree to which families blame young people for their problems, or that particular family behaviours (such as criticism or overprotection) might help patients. These beliefs have also been related to EE, parental control, aggression, and low levels of facilitative behaviour[42–44] and therefore may drive family behaviours that increase patient stress.

Coping strategies, communication skills, and problem-solving

Anecdotally, a key unmet need of families of young people is information and coping strategies, especially for situations in which the patient is symptomatic. Families may, for example, be concerned that they need to develop entirely new ways of coping with stress (including, perhaps, eliminating stress at home) for fear of exacerbating patients' symptoms. On the other hand, 'walking on eggshells' might inhibit clear and open communication and lead to resentment and anger. It is likely that at least some of the coping strategies that families are using are effective and useful, and bolstering strengths and validation are important components of family intervention. Enlisting the assistance of family peer support workers in delivering interventions may have particular benefits. Family peer support workers are in an invaluable position of having 'lived experience' that can enable modelling of effective coping and facilitate a greater felt sense in families of feeling understood. The experience of coping with feelings of shame, guilt, and loss may particularly resonate between carers. Although research on the role of trained family peer support workers in delivering interventions has been primarily limited to the chronic mental illness field, qualitative data in FEP suggests that supportive psychoeducational interventions run by graduate carers of previous groups, together with clinicians, have demonstrated positive results, including lowering levels of isolation and guilt, and increasing confidence, understanding of psychosis, and a subjective sense of coping in the caring role.[45]

The rationale for including communication skills and problem-solving elements in family interventions is largely EE based, given that EE may be seen to be a prime example of problematic communication. Such interventions, which are normally behavioural in focus, may enhance families' capacity to discuss and problem-solve issues that emerge within the home that relate to symptoms and stress, thereby reducing the likelihood of communicating in ways that manifest high EE. However, as noted earlier, a focus on this domain within interventions to the exclusion of others may be inappropriate for families of young people with emergent mental illness, given (a) there is limited evidence linking problematic communication with outcome in early onset mental illness, and (b) this may be perceived by families as neglecting other key needs such as support in the particularly distressing time that this may represent.

Timing of intervention

Interventions should not only be sensitive in their delivery, but also sensitively timed. There is limited data on phase-based appropriateness of interventions, but it stands to reason that some interventions may be more appropriate at particular stages than others. For example, interventions including a focus on relapse prevention are likely to be more appropriately delivered outside the acute phase of illness, when clear, concise psychoeducation is likely to be most beneficial to families. There may also be individual differences in support-seeking, related to the family members' general coping style. Some may feel isolated unless offered support early, while others may need some time to withdraw and reflect, using informal support networks, before engaging in service-based support. Assertive attempts to assess this by service workers are likely to enhance appropriate service delivery.

Conclusions

It is unclear whether and what type of family interventions benefit young people with mental illness. However, these interventions may benefit families and might thereby benefit patients who progress to longer courses of illness. Fostering a spirit of partnership in care also requires services to support families and attempt to meet their needs, even in the absence of empirical data suggesting this then benefits patients. It may also be useful to identify predictors of prolonged distress and difficulties coping for families, in order to develop 'stepped-care' models that accurately identify 'high-risk' families who could then be offered more comprehensive family services and/or family therapy. However, considerable engagement and investment is likely to be required before family interventions can be routinely delivered in clinical practice.

References

1 Bateson G, Jackson DD, Haley J, Weakland J. Toward a theory of schizophrenia. *Behavioral Science* 1956;1(4):251–64.
2 Brown GW, Carstairs GM, Topping G. Post-hospital adjustment of chronic mental patients. *Lancet* 1958;2(7048):685–8.
3 Leff JP, Vaughn C. *Expressed emotion in families: its significance for mental illness.* New York: Guilford Press; 1985.
4 Hooley JM, Hiller JB. Expressed emotion and the pathogenesis of relapse in schizophrenia. In Lenzenweger MF, Dworkin RH (Eds) *Origins and development of schizophrenia: advances in experimental psychopathology.* Washington, DC: American Psychological Association; 1998. p 447–68.
5 Wearden AJ, Tarrier N, Barrowclough C, Zastowny TR, Rahill AA. A review of expressed emotion research in health care. *Clinical Psychology Review* 2000;20(5):633–66.
6 Karno M, Jenkins JH. Cross-cultural issues in the course and treatment of schizophrenia. *Psychiatric Clinics of North America* 1993;16(2):339–50.
7 Barrowclough C, Haddock G, Lowens I, Connor A, Pidliswyj J, Tracey N. Staff expressed emotion and causal attributions for client problems on a low security unit: an exploratory study. *Schizophrenia Bulletin* 2001;27(3):517–26.
8 Meehl PE. Schizotaxia, schizotypy, and schizophrenia. *American Psychologist* 1962;17: 827–38.
9 Lenzenweger MF. Schizotaxia, schizotypy, and schizophrenia: Paul E. Meehl's blueprint for the experimental psychopathology and genetics of schizophrenia. *Journal of Abnormal Psychology* 2006;115(2):195–200.
10 Kavanagh DJ. Recent developments in expressed emotion and schizophrenia. *British Journal of Psychiatry* 1992;160:601–20.
11 McNab C, Linszen D. Family intervention in early psychosis. In McGorry PD, Jackson HJ (Eds) *The recognition and management of early psychosis: a preventive approach.* 2nd ed. Cambridge: Cambridge University Press; 2009. p 305–29.
12 Sheeber L, Hops H, Davis B. Family processes in adolescent depression. *Clinical Child and Family Psychology Review* 2001;4(1):19–35.
13 Auerbach RP, Bigda-Peyton JS, Eberhart NK, Webb CA, Ho MH. Conceptualizing the prospective relationship between social support, stress, and depressive symptoms among adolescents. *Journal of Abnormal Child Psychology* 2011;39(4):475–87.
14 Denham SA, Bassett HH, Wyatt T. The socialization of emotional competence. In Grusec JE, Hastings PD (Eds) *Handbook of socialization: theory and research.* 2nd ed. New York: Guilford Press; 2014. p 590–613.

15 Bayer JK, Sanson AV, Hemphill SA. Parent influences on early childhood internalizing difficulties. *Journal of Applied Developmental Psychology* 2006;27(6):542–59.

16 Schwartz OS, Dudgeon P, Sheeber LB, Yap MB, Simmons JG, Allen NB. Parental behaviors during family interactions predict changes in depression and anxiety symptoms during adolescence. *Journal of Abnormal Child Psychology* 2012;40(1):59–71.

17 Schwartz OS, Dudgeon P, Sheeber LB, Yap MB, Simmons JG, Allen NB. Observed maternal responses to adolescent behavior predict the onset of major depression. *Behaviour Research and Therapy* 2011;49(5):331–8.

18 Schwartz OS, Byrne ML, Simmons JG, Whittle S, Dudgeon P, Yap MB, et al. Parenting during early adolescence and adolescent-onset major depression: a 6-year prospective longitudinal study. *Clinical Psychological Science* 2014;2(3):272–86.

19 Luebbe AM, Bell DJ. Positive and negative family emotional climate differential predict youth anxiety and depression via distinct affective pathways. *Journal of Abnormal Child Psychology* 2014;42(6):897–911.

20 Shortt JW, Katz LF, Allen N, Leve C, Davis B, Sheeber L. Emotion socialization in the context of risk and psychopathology: mother and father socialization of anger and sadness in adolescents with depressive disorder. *Social Development* 2016;25(1):27–46.

21 Biglan A, Gau JM, Backen Jones L, Hinds E, Rusby JC, Cody C, et al. The role of experiential avoidance in the relationship between family conflict and depression among early adolescents. *Journal of Contextual Behavioral Science* 2015;4(1):30–6.

22 Gaté MA, Watkins ER, Simmons JG, Byrne ML, Schwartz OS, Whittle S, et al. Maternal parenting behaviors and adolescent depression: the mediating role of rumination. *Journal of Clinical Child and Adolescent Psychology* 2013;42(3):348–57.

23 Kulhman KR, Olson SL, Lopez-Duran NL. Predicting developmental changes in internalizing symptoms: examining the interplay between parenting and neuroendocrine stress reactivity. *Developmental Psychology* 2014;56(5):908–23.

24 Whittle S, Simmons JG, Dennis M, Vijayakumar N, Schwartz O, Yap MB, et al. Positive parenting predicts the development of adolescent brain structure: a longitudinal study. *Developmental Cognitive Neuroscience* 2014;8:7–17.

25 Barrowclough C, Hooley JM. Attributions and expressed emotion: a review. *Clinical Psychology Review* 2003;23(6):849–80.

26 McNab C, Haslam N, Burnett P. Expressed emotion, attributions, utility beliefs, and distress in parents of young people with first episode psychosis. *Psychiatry Research* 2007;151(1–2):97–106.

27 Martens L, Addington J. The psychological well-being of family members of individuals with schizophrenia. *Social Psychiatry and Psychiatric Epidemiology* 2001;36(3):128–33.

28 Koutra K, Vgontzas AN, Lionis C, Triliva S. Family functioning in first-episode psychosis: a systematic review of the literature. *Social Psychiatry and Psychiatric Epidemiology* 2014;49(7):1023–36.

29 Sheeber L, Sorensen E. Maternal affect during mother-adolescent interactions: the role of adolescent depression. Paper presented at the annual Kansas Conference in Clinical Child Psychology, Lawrence, KS; 1998.

30 Lowenstein JA, Butler DW, Ashcroft K. The efficacy of a cognitively orientated carers group in an early intervention in psychosis service – a pilot study. *Journal of Psychiatric and Mental Health Nursing* 2010;17(7):628–35.

31 Pilling S, Bebbington P, Kuipers E, Garety P, Geddes J, Orbach G, et al. Psychological treatments in schizophrenia: I. Meta-analysis of family intervention and cognitive behaviour therapy. *Psychological Medicine* 2002;32(5):763–82.

32 Pharoah F, Mari J, Rathbone J, Wong W. Family intervention for schizophrenia. *Cochrane Database of Systematic Reviews* 2010;12:CD000088.
33 Miklowitz DJ, O'Brien MP, Schlosser DA, Addington J, Candan KA, Marshall C, et al. Family-focused treatment for adolescents and young adults at high risk for psychosis: results of a randomized trial. *Journal of the American Academy of Child and Adolescent Psychiatry* 2014;53(8):848–58.
34 Alvarez-Jiménez M, Parker AG, Hetrick SE, McGorry PD, Gleeson JF. Preventing the second episode: a systematic review and meta-analysis of psychosocial and pharmacological trials in first-episode psychosis. *Schizophrenia Bulletin* 2011;37(3):619–30.
35 Glynn SM, Cohen AN, Niv N. New challenges in family interventions for schizophrenia. *Expert Review of Neurotherapeutics* 2007;7(1):33–43.
36 Birchwood M, Smith J, Cochrane R. Specific and non-specific effects of educational intervention for families living with schizophrenia: a comparison of three methods. *British Journal of Psychiatry* 1992;160:806–14.
37 Hogarty GE, Anderson CM, Reiss DJ, Kornblith SJ, Greenwald DP, Ulrich RF, et al. Family psychoeducation, social skills training, and maintenance chemotherapy in the aftercare treatment of schizophrenia. II. Two-year effects of a controlled study on relapse and adjustment. *Archives of General Psychiatry* 1991;48(4):340–7.
38 Leavey G, Gulamhussein S, Papadopoulos C, Johnson-Sabine E, Blizard B, King M. A randomized controlled trial of a brief intervention for families of patients with a first episode of psychosis. *Psychological Medicine* 2004;34(3):423–31.
39 Gerson R, Davidson L, Booty A, McGlashan T, Malespina D, Pincus HA, et al. Families' experience with seeking treatment for recent-onset psychosis. *Psychiatric Services* 2009;60(6):812–6.
40 Chen EY, Dunn EL, Miao MY, Yeung WS, Wong CK, Chan WF, et al. The impact of family experience on the duration of untreated psychosis (DUP) in Hong Kong. *Social Psychiatry and Psychiatric Epidemiology* 2005;40(5):350–6.
41 McCann TV, Lubman DI, Clark E. First-time primary caregivers' experience accessing first-episode psychosis services. *Early Intervention in Psychiatry* 2011;5(2):156–62.
42 Sheeber LB, Johnston C, Chen M, Leve C, Hops H, Davis B. Mothers' and fathers' attributions for adolescent behavior: an examination in families of depressed, subdiagnostic, and non-depressed youth. *Journal of Family Psychology* 2009;23(6):871–81.
43 Domínguez-Martínez T, Medina-Pradas C, Kwapil TR, Barrantes-Vidal N. Relatives' illness attributions mediate the association of expressed emotion with early psychosis symptoms and functioning. *Psychiatry Research* 2014;218(1–2):48–53.
44 Vasoncelos E Sa D, Wearden A, Barrowclough C. Expressed emotion, types of behavioural control and controllability attributions in relatives of people with recent-onset psychosis. *Social Psychiatry and Psychiatric Epidemiology* 2013;48(9):1377–88.
45 Riley G, Gregory N, Bellinger J, Davies N, Mabbott G, Sabourin R. Carer's education groups for relatives with a first episode of psychosis: an evaluation of an eight-week education group. *Early Intervention in Psychiatry* 2011;5(1):57–63.

16 Psychopharmacology in youth mental health

Andrew Thompson and Alison R. Yung

Introduction

Over the last decade there has been a marked increase in the prescribing of psychotropic substances in youth populations.[1–3] This has included a number of psychotropic classes such as antipsychotics, stimulants, antidepressants and mood stabilisers.[4–7] Whilst these higher rates of prescribing have been particularly highlighted in the US, high rates of prescribing have been reported in a number of other countries.[8,9] Although this increase to some extent mirrors the acceptance of the high rates of emerging mental illness in this population, it has not been without controversy.[9] For example, there has been extensive debate over the use of Selective Serotonin Reuptake Inhibitors (SSRIs) in an adolescent population, given the less convincing efficacy data and the concerns regarding particular side effects such as the potential for increased suicidal ideation.[10–15] Similarly, the increasing use of stimulant medication and mood stabilisers is to be acknowledged but will not be discussed further in this review. Suffice to say, the debate over whether psychotropic medications are used appropriately and safely in these populations will continue; medication prescription should not be a substitute for lack of good clinical services if there is not a good clinical indication. Despite these reservations, it seems that psychopharmacology for youth mental health is becoming a more accepted part of modern clinical practice.

It is however, beyond the scope of this chapter to review all the evidence regarding all established psychotropic treatments, given the extensive and growing literature in this area (for example, see reviews[16–20] and Cochrane collaboration reviews[13,21–23]). There is also a growing literature on the use of herbal medicines in young people with mental disorders[24] which will not be reviewed in detail. Instead, we aim to concentrate on the general principles of prescribing in this population and the developing area of preventative pharmacotherapy for emerging mental disorders, either to prevent or to delay the occurrence of major mental disorders in at-risk groups or the progression of psychopathology.

Psychotropic prescribing in youth: general issues

Before describing the overall principles of prescribing in a youth (15–25) population, it is worth discussing a few issues that relate to the specifics of this age group and to those experiencing the early episode of mental illness.

The traditional child psychiatry / adult psychiatry "divide"

When reviewing the literature on psychopharmacology in youth one is faced with the conventional age distinction between what constitutes child and adolescent psychiatry and adult psychiatry. Traditionally this has been set at the age of 18. This somewhat artificial divide created by the current systems of psychiatric service delivery is often adopted by regulatory bodies, such as the Food and Drug Administration (FDA) in the US and the Therapeutic Goods Administration (TGA) in Australia, who have also divided the legislative mechanisms for drug regulations at this age. Some regulatory boards have different recommendation for the use of some medications, such as fluoxetine in under 18s. Whilst it is difficult to imagine that the effect of a medication on someone at the age of 18 may be vastly different from someone at 20, only a few studies have specifically addressed a youth population that spans the traditional age cut-off of 18 years old. Thus data is often available for the under 18 group and data for 18–25 is extrapolated or extracted from trials that include the full adult age range of 18–65. This has a number of drawbacks, most notably the lack of data on this specific population and therefore combination of data from studies that may be methodologically quite different.

We would argue that for youth populations it is not sufficient to extrapolate efficacy or side effect data from adult studies. For example, the debate on the efficacy and side effects of SSRIs in the youth population is fuelled by the suggestion that both the efficacy of the compounds[12,25] and the side effects or risks[13] may be subtly different in youth populations to adult populations.

There are also reports of side effect profile differences for antipsychotics between adolescents and adults. For example, children and adolescents taking antipsychotic medications seem to be more vulnerable to prolactin abnormalities and extrapyramidal side effects (EPS), especially akathisia and withdrawal dyskinesia, as well as more difficulty with weight gain and metabolic abnormalities.[16] It has also been suggested that young people experience more behavioural and cognitive side effects in general, whereas adults experience more somatic problems,[26] but there is limited empirical data for this outside of the SSRI studies to support this generalisation. One of the reasons for these differences may be the effect of these compounds on the developing brain.[27,28] This is an area that needs further research.

The growth in specific services for the youth population will help to address some of these difficulties over the next few years, and we would encourage youth-specific treatment trials to improve this evidence base.

Pharmacokinetic and pharmacodynamic issues

It is necessary to highlight some of the pharmacological issues which are related to an individual's age. Pharmacokinetics describes the way an individual treats a drug and includes absorption, drug distribution, drug metabolism and drug excretion. Pharmacodynamics describes the way in which the brain (or intended organ) responds to a drug and includes drug receptor interactions, specificity and selectivity of drug action, and mechanisms of drug action. There appears to be distinct differences in youth populations compared to adult populations, especially for pharmacokinetic issues. For example, dependent on the age and stage of development of the young person, the smaller body size (higher peak plasma concentration due to differences in volume of drug distribution), larger liver parenchyma (higher first pass metabolism)[29] and relatively higher kidney parenchyma (higher levels of excretion)[26] can lead to particular differences in drug pharmacokinetics from adult populations. Such differences in youth population are often hard to quantify, there is a lack of trial evidence and, therefore, the drug dosage of many agents are extrapolated from adult study data. The consequences of these differences are the need for possible difference in dosing regimes, the likelihood of needing to use lower doses if peak plasma concentrations are higher and the potential for greater susceptibility to drug side effects if these plasma levels are elevated in young people. There has been little research for psychopharmacological agents, and most research has been directed towards the SSRIs. For example, there has been shown to be some similarities in accumulation profile and steady-state concentrations between adults and adolescents for fluoxetine.[30]

Principles for prescribing in youth populations

General issues in young people

From our experience in working with young people we have a few clinical insights into the approach that might be beneficial when prescribing psychotropic medications. Often for the young person, they have had relatively little previous contact with doctors and especially with psychiatrists. They are probably not used to taking any medications on a regular basis, let alone psychotropic medication. Adolescent lifestyles may not lend themselves to medication compliance, and sometimes the need to look after one's health is not prioritised to the same extent as social lives and other activities. Allied to this can be the problems inherent in those with major psychiatric illnesses. These include poor insight and chaotic lifestyles as well as symptoms such as cognitive disturbance that may impede compliance with medications. The aim is to help the young person understand why the clinician would *want* to prescribe medication and the reason they think medication will help them and their situation in particular. Often the use of specific psychoeducational materials can be helpful in stimulating a discussion with the young person. Helping the young person to maintain control by being involved in the choice of medication to use (for example, discussing possible side effects of antipsychotics with equal efficacy and letting the young person choose which one they would prefer) has been beneficial with a number of young people. Therefore, a therapeutic alliance and shared model/understanding of how medication may help their current situation in our view is essential. If there is no clinical urgency, this may be best done over a number of sessions. This practice is consistent with the Royal Australasian College of Physicians recommendations that children and adolescents should be involved in decision-making about their health.[31]

Often particular side effects such as weight gain or sexual disturbance are particularly important in young people, and our experience is that the young person is more likely to stop taking their medication if you have not warned them of these potential side effects at the outset rather than when they occur. Side effects such as weight gain may also be more of a problem in a youth population due to the young person not having been previously exposed to psychotropic medications.[32] There is a difficult balance between encouraging compliance with something the doctor thinks is beneficial and informing the young person of any anticipated side effects. Our experience also suggests that particularly reinforcing both the expected time delay in efficacy when initiating and the reasons for continued prescribing in the face of improvements, important in all populations, are particularly important in young people.

Consent and parental assent

Most young people from the age of 15 will be competent to consent to treatment, but some will not, and this should be assessed on an individual basis. A judgment about whether a young person understands the situation, is able to make decisions and apply these to their own health care needs to made. The ability of a young person under the age of 16 to consent to treatment is often called "Gillick competence" (following a ruling in the English House of Lords).[33] The maturity and intelligence of a young person need to be taken into account, along with the gravity of the decision.[33]

For young people who want parents and carers involved in their treatment, especially those under the age of 18, obtaining assent from the guardian and involving them in the decision to start medication is important. In cases where the young person does not want the parent/guardian involved in treatment, we would suggest that confidentiality and engagement are often paramount unless the current risks to the individual or others override them.

Principles for prescribing

Given this information, we propose a number of principles for prescribing medication in young people (see Box 16.1).

Box 16.1 Principles for prescribing medication in young people

1) Consider the appropriate use of evidence-based non-pharmacological interventions (such as Cognitive Behavioural Therapy [CBT], family interventions) before prescribing psychotropic medications.

2) Consider the use of putative neuroprotective agents with lower side effects, such as omega-3 fatty acids, in line with recent evidence on the staging of illness in young people if this is clinically appropriate and evidence based.
3) Use lower doses than in adult populations and if poor efficacy at low doses, increase the dose slowly (a "start low go slow" policy).
4) Pay particular attention to side effects, especially those with effects on sexual and physical development, weight gain, cognition, sedation and suicidal ideation in those prescribed antidepressant medications.
5) Pay attention to compliance and provide a clear rationale for prescribing to the young person. If possible, try to involve the young person in choice of medication and be open about possible side effects as well as benefits. Develop a therapeutic alliance. Obtaining parental assent or involving the family/carers in decisions about medication is important depending on the young person's wishes.
6) Use the medication for the shortest period of time to treat or prevent the recurrence of the illness. Continue to provide a rationale to the young person and/or carer for the continued use if prescribing for prevention of recurrence.
7) As with adult populations, try to avoid the use of regular benzodiazepines or stimulants if there are specific concerns regarding abuse or dependence.
8) Whilst we would generally discourage off-label prescribing, a proportion of prescribing in youth populations will be off label. The same procedures should be followed for off-label prescribing in adults.

Developments in psychopharmacological approaches for emerging psychiatric disorders in young people: preventative psychopharmacology

Prevention strategies

Prevention strategies can be distinguished in two overlapping categories: primary, secondary, tertiary and quaternary; or universal, selective and indicated. Primary prevention strategies describe strategies that intend to avoid the development of disease. Most population-based health promotion activities are primary preventive measures. Within primary prevention, the concept of universal prevention aimed at the general population is difficult in psychiatry when specific pathological processes have not been identified. Selective prevention is aimed at subgroups of populations at higher risk, for example, high-vulnerability and high-risk groups. This is somewhat similar to taking measures to prevent obesity in a patient who has a first-degree relative with diabetes.

Secondary prevention strategies attempt to diagnose and treat an existing disease in its early stages before it results in significant morbidity. Under the umbrella of secondary prevention is the idea of indicated prevention. This involves the use of a screening process and aims to identify individuals who exhibit early symptoms or signs of a disease. This has been an area of recent interest in psychiatric disorders with a particular focus on young people when the majority of major mental disorders first present.[34]

The staging model and secondary or indicated prevention

The approach of identifying and treating psychiatric disorders early in young people has been influenced by the findings and the growth of early intervention/detection paradigms that have been previously outlined in this book. Early intervention approaches were initially concentrated on psychotic disorders but have more recently been directed towards other major mental disorders that are highly incident in youth populations such as bipolar affective disorder and depression. More recently, thinking on this subject has been enhanced by the introduction of the concept of "clinical staging". This concept has been successfully applied in a number of areas of medicine, most notably in the treatment of cancer. The proposed staging model of psychiatric disorders by McGorry and colleagues posits that the majority of mental illness will progress through a number of distinct clinical stages, such as in cancer, where more diffuse, less severe pathology may present in an early stage of a disorder and in turn may respond to or necessitate more benign interventions at this early stage.[35] This has considerable implications for the use of psychopharmacological agents in these disorders and can potentially provide a framework for medication prescribing. It would follow that medications with more or more serious side effects would be reserved for the later stages of a disorder (an example being the use of clozapine in schizophrenia). It also has implications for indicated prevention approaches.

A number of potential examples of the staging approach are worth mentioning. First, for the illness schizophrenia, the first stage of an illness might be a diffuse "prodromal" stage, which consists of non-specific symptoms such as sleep disturbance as well as low-grade, psychotic-like experiences such as fleeting hallucinations or paranoid thoughts.[36] This has led to the development of clinical criteria based on such "prodromal" symptoms and other risk factors such as family history and lower functioning; those meeting these criteria have been termed "ultra high risk" (UHR) for psychosis or "clinical high risk" (CHR).[37–39] The potential to prevent or delay the development of a psychotic disorder in this group is an intriguing possibility and one that is the focus of much research activity.[40]

Second, bipolar disorder also may present with a different set of "prodromal" symptoms, which again may respond to a different treatment approach than an established bipolar disorder. A number of authors have proposed a similar "at-risk" state for bipolar disorder.[41,42] Whilst the immediate predictive validity for these criteria are lower than for psychotic disorders, there is still optimism in the field that such criteria may be clinically useful. The predictive validity for these criteria has been calculated in a review paper suggesting relatively high specificity but poor sensitivity.[41] However, instruments to detect those at risk still need refining.[43]

Third, it may also be possible to apply a staging model approach to depressive disorders with the aim of early detection and prevention of poor outcome, including recurrent depression in adulthood. Hetrick and colleagues have outlined an early potential risk stage or set of risk factors that might respond to more benign interventions.[44] The utility of the "prodrome" for diagnosis and early intervention in depressive disorders has also been proposed.[45,46] It has been somewhat complicated by poor discriminative value of early signs and symptoms. This is especially evident in the overlap between the prodromal stage of depressive disorders, bipolar disorders[47,48] and other psychotic disorders,[49] with diagnosis only becoming more apparent once the disorder has progressed. Furthermore, the categorical distinctiveness of disorders is also unclear, highlighted by recent work showing overlap between bipolar disorder with hypomanic symptoms and major depression. Authors continue to highlight the psychosocial and functional deficits associated with subsyndromal depression and the associated burden to society of these symptoms.[50] The predictive validity of these symptoms as a "prodrome" of a major depressive episode need further refining if pharmacological trials are to be recommended. Whilst identifying a high-risk group for depression may be less sensitive given the higher prevalence of depressive disorders in the community, it appears a promising public health approach.

These suggestions of early diffuse disorders that evolve into more specific illness types are substantiated by the results of imaging studies, especially for those at UHR for psychosis and those at risk for bipolar affective disorder. A staging model would predict that in such disorders a less severe form of the pathological deficit would be present in the early stages of the illness. Whilst there is no definitive pathological deficit universally described in schizophrenia and other psychotic disorders, imaging studies consistently report reduction in brain volume and specific grey and white matter changes in patients with schizophrenia, for example. It is therefore interesting that similar patterns may be present in those at risk for developing psychosis and progress as the illness proceeds. A review of the literature states that longitudinal magnetic resonance imaging findings in individuals at ultra high risk for developing a psychotic illness show that there are excessive neuroanatomical changes in those who convert to psychosis. These aberrant changes are observed most prominently in medial temporal and prefrontal cortical regions.[51] There is also some evidence to suggest that changes are specific to the type of psychotic disorder experienced, with anatomical changes being different in those who develop schizophrenia to an affective psychosis.[52] For other types of bipolar disorder, the picture may be somewhat different. Gross brain structure may be relatively preserved, and it is only with recurrences that there is a sequential, but marked loss of brain volume.[53]

All these proposed "at-risk" groups are not without considerable scientific and ethical questions. However, given the developments in identifying these possible indicated prevention targets in youth populations, it is timely to review the literature on pharmacological interventions for these targets.

New pharmacological treatments for emerging psychiatric disorders / "at-risk" states

There have been a number of approaches to the treatment of emerging psychiatric disorders or "at-risk" states. These have included both the use of medications known to be efficacious in the full-blown disorder and the use of new medications aimed at arresting or preventing the onset of the illness. In the youth population the focus on at-risk states has often been on the major psychiatric disorders of schizophrenia, bipolar disorder and major depression that have high incidence in this age group, and we will concentrate on these three disorders here.

1) Use of medications known to be efficacious in the full-threshold disorder

"At risk" for psychosis

There have been a number of small randomised controlled trials using antipsychotic medications in the UHR or CHR for psychosis group in a youth population. The first of these trials reported that the number of individuals developing a psychotic disorder was significantly lower after six months in those receiving a low dose of risperidone.[54] However, the effect was lost at 12-month follow-up.[55] Another similar trial suggested a trend difference in "transition" to a full-threshold psychotic disorder at 12 months in those treated with olanzapine.[56] However, the prevalence of side effects (especially weight gain) was much greater in those on active medication in both trials.[56] A third antipsychotic medication trial failed to find a difference between those receiving low dose risperidone, CBT and befriending,[57,58] with all groups having lower than expected rates of onset of frank psychotic illness. This, and the positive reports of psychological interventions in this group,[59,60] has led to caution regarding the use of antipsychotics in this "at-risk" population. Other considerations include the relatively high number of individuals in the recent trials who do not go on to develop a psychotic disorder even if not receiving antipsychotic medication (so-called false positives)[58,61] and the concern over the stigma of a relatively aggressive treatment for what still remains an "at-risk" state and not a full-blown disorder.[62] We suggest that the risks outweigh the benefits for using these medications in "at-risk" individuals.[63]

Ruhrmann and colleagues reported a non-placebo controlled randomised trial of the antipsychotic amisulpiride with or without a "needs-focused" intervention in a UHR group.[64] They reported that the amisulpiride plus needs-focused group (n = 56) produced superior effects on attenuated and full-blown psychotic symptoms; basic, depressive and negative symptoms; and global functioning. They reported that the main side effects were prolactin related. However, they concluded that the "effects require confirmation by a placebo-controlled study".[64]

Bipolar "at-risk" populations

There has been less research into traditional treatments in this population, primarily because the "prodromal" criteria are less well defined and at present do not have the short-term positive predictive value of the UHR criteria. This makes the argument for using traditional psychopharmacological agents in this group much weaker. However, one placebo-controlled trial has investigated the use of divalproaex sodium in a sample of young people deemed at risk of developing a bipolar illness. This was on the basis of a diagnosis of bipolar illness "not otherwise specified", or cyclothymia or a family history of bipolar disorder.[65] The population ($n = 56$) was young (mean age of ten), although it included patients up to the age of 17. The primary outcome was time to discontinuation for any reason. Neither time to discontinuation due to a mood event nor mood symptoms were significantly different in the divalproaex group, and the authors concluded that it did not produce "clinically meaningful improvements in the treatment of this potential 'at-risk' group". One possible explanation, as noted earlier, is that the "at-risk" criteria were not sensitive enough to identify a properly "at-risk" group.

Emerging depressive disorders or "at-risk" states

There are no trials to our knowledge of traditional antidepressant agents in those deemed at risk for depression. The approach of "at risk" for depression is less well developed than for the other two disorders as previously discussed. Allied to this is the questionable efficacy of antidepressants in mild depressive disorder and efficacy in a youth population.[66] Importantly, there are concerns about increases in suicidal ideation and behaviour related to use of SSRI antidepressants in young people.[10] These concerns make the rationale and ethics for such trials much less robust.

2) Use of novel agents

Neuroprotective agents and neutraceuticals

Current approaches to novel pharmacotherapy in this area are influenced by the idea of neuroprotection. Researchers have proposed that disruptions in the normal neuroprotective pathways are important in the development of psychotic and bipolar disorders and, therefore, these pathways may be important targets for pharmacological interventions.[67,68] The concept of neuroprotective interventions is established in neurological disorders.[69] The concept appears theoretically attractive to those who are displaying some signs of a disorder but not a full-blown syndrome/disorder. The idea is that neuroprotective strategies can possibly arrest or delay further pathological processes. One of the theories is that alteration in apoptosis occurs in these disorders and is responsible for altered synaptic pruning during critical developmental periods.[68,70]

Interestingly, a number of current psychopharmacological treatments such as atypical antipsychotic medication, mood stabilisers (lithium, anticonvulsants) and antidepressants all exhibit neuroprotective effects.[71–76]

Some of the novel agents proposed to be neuroprotective also come under the rubric of "neutraceuticals", a term combining the words "nutrition" and "pharmaceutical" and being a food or food product that provides health and medical benefits, including the prevention and treatment of disease. One with the most research interest is long-chain omega-3 polyunsaturated fatty acids or "fish oil". It should be noted that these trials of neutraceuticals are dissimilar to other psychopharmacological trials in that they rarely have pharmaceutical industry sponsorship; as such, compounds are rarely novel and often widely available for other uses.

"At risk" for psychosis or UHR

Given the impact and burden of psychotic disorders and the more accepted concept of a "prodrome" in these disorders, most of these trials have focused on the UHR group. Again, they have almost all been in youth populations aged 15–25 or 15–30.

Putative neuroprotective agents

A group from New York reported a possible beneficial effect of antidepressant medication on progression to a full-threshold psychotic disorder in a UHR group, arguing that antidepressants have neuroprotective properties.[77]

The study was a prospective naturalistic treatment study of 48 patients, 20 prescribed antidepressants and 28 prescribed second-generation antipsychotics. They reported a rate developing a psychotic disorder of 25% in the group treated primarily with antipsychotics whereas there were no "conversions" to a psychotic disorder in the primarily antidepressant-treated group. There were differences between the two groups at baseline, with the antipsychotic group having more disorganised thinking, and over the follow-up period they were more likely to be non-compliant with medications. Despite these methodological shortcomings, the study does indicate that this may be an important treatment approach in this population. However, as the rates of lifetime depressive disorders in UHR individuals can be as high as 60%,[78,79] the possibility of a randomised controlled trial to further investigate this treatment approach (which would mean randomising to placebo) is ethically difficult.[80]

Lithium is also thought to have neuroprotective properties and its efficacy in reducing risk of psychosis in the UHR population has been investigated, however the findings from this study have yet to be published. Preliminary results suggest that lithium has some neuroprotective effects but does not delay psychosis onset in itself. However, the trial was a small, single-site study.[68,81,82]

Whilst these therapies are established in the treatment of psychiatric disorder in general, they are not without well-documented and significant side effects, which in a population who are not "destined" to develop the full-threshold disorder raises a number of questions about the balance between risk and potential benefit. Attention has therefore turned to more benign pharmacological interventions.

Of these more benign interventions, supplementation or treatment with long-chain omega-3 polyunsaturated fatty acids (PUFAs) (fish oil) has received considerable research interest in psychotic disorders. Research into the beneficial effects of omega-3 PUFAs as an adjunctive treatment in individuals with established schizophrenia and first-episode psychosis has yielded some positive results.[83] In the UHR population, 12 weeks of omega-3 PUFAs reduced risk of development of psychotic disorder at 12-month follow-up,[84] and even at a later 7-year follow-up.[85] A significant reduction in positive and negative symptoms and improved functioning was also found in the omega-3–treated group compared to placebo. Adverse effects did not differ between the two groups. However, two subsequent replication studies failed to find a benefit of omega-3 PUFAs in transition rate or reduction in symptoms.[86,87]

There is some data to suggest those whose omega-3 levels increase with supplementation or have higher baseline levels may have more improvement in symptoms and functioning.[88] Other centres conducting similar studies are yet to report findings. There is recent interest in the use of the cannabinoid cannabidiol (CBD) as a possible preventative treatment in the UHR population,[89] although it is not clear what the proposed mechanism of action may be.

The recently published British Association of Psychopharmacology guidelines made no specific recommendations for medication use in young people "at risk" of psychosis.[90]

Bipolar "at risk" and emerging depressive disorders

A number of neutraceuticals have been investigated in depression and bipolar affective disorder. Despite there being no trials of indicated prevention in "at-risk" groups, it is worth briefly mentioning some of these compounds used either on their own or as adjunct in established disorders. The use of omega-3 PUFAs as an adjunct in the treatment of depression and bipolar depression has some evidence of efficacy.[83,91,92] The evidence for the efficacy of omega-3 PUFAs as a treatment alone is less robust. There has been one trial of the efficacy of omega-3 treatment alone in childhood depression (aged 6–12)[93] but nothing specifically to an older or youth population. Again, there is encouraging evidence to support the notion that supplementation may be beneficial. Epidemiological studies indicate an association between depression and low dietary intake of omega-3 fatty acids, and biochemical studies have shown reduced levels of omega-3 fatty acids in red blood cell membranes in depressed patients. Animal studies of fatty acid supplementation have also shown reduced "depression-like" behaviours in rats.[94]

Another neutraceutical of interest in depression is folate. This is based on the findings of low levels of plasma and red cell folate in people with depression, especially in those with poor response to treatment.[95,96] There is no convincing evidence of the use of folate in adults as yet,[97] although two trials using folate as an adjunct to treatment reported a reduction in depressive symptomatology[98] and schizophrenia.[99] Both of these trials were in patients above the age of 18 and in established disorders.

There have been no trials in those "at risk" for bipolar affective disorder, but in established bipolar affective disorder the addition of the neutraceutical ginseng (Acanthopanax senficosus) to lithium compared to fluoxetine was compared in an adolescent population (aged 12–17).[100] They did not find any difference in response rate, remission or depressive symptoms in this trial. There is evidence that N-acetylcysteine may be an effective adjunct in bipolar depression in adults,[101] but there are no trials in a youth population.

Conclusions

There is a growing acceptance of the use of psychopharmacological agents to treat mental illness in young people in conjunction with other treatments. However, there is also an understanding that young people are often not the same as adults in terms of response to these medications and their side effects. We have outlined some of the principles of prescribing medication in a youth population and encourage the development of an open and honest therapeutic alliance with the young person and/or their carer(s). The emergence of early intervention paradigms and the clinical staging model for major mental illness has encouraged investigation of more benign pharmacological treatments including neutraceuticals to treat the early symptoms of mental illness or illness progression in young people. Although the area of indicated prevention in psychopharmacology is in its infancy and subject to some ethical dilemmas, there are promising signs that some of these agents may have a preventative role, or potentially a neuroprotective role, in these disabling disorders and, therefore, potentially a wider public health benefit.

References

1 Zuvekas SH. Prescription drugs and the changing patterns of treatment for mental disorders, 1996–2001. *Health Affairs* 2005;24(1):195–205.
2 Zito JM, Safer DJ, DosReis S, Gardner JF, Magder L, Soeken K, et al. Psychotropic practice patterns for youth: a 10-year perspective. *Archives of Pediatrics & Adolescent Medicine* 2003;157(1):17–25.
3 Wong IC, Murray ML, Camilleri-Novak D, Stephens P. Increased prescribing trends of paediatric psychotropic medications. *Archives of Disease in Childhood* 2004;89(12):1131–2.
4 Olfson M, Blanco C, Liu L, Moreno C, Laje G. National trends in the outpatient treatment of children and adolescents with antipsychotic drugs. *Archives of General Psychiatry* 2006;63(6):679–85.
5 Wong IC, Asherson P, Bilbow A, Clifford S, Coghill D, DeSoysa R, et al. Cessation of attention deficit hyperactivity disorder drugs in the young (CADDY) – a pharmacoepidemiological and qualitative study. *Health Technology Assessment* 2009;13(50):1–120.
6 Olfson M, Marcus SC. National patterns in antidepressant medication treatment. *Archives of General Psychiatry* 2009;66(8):848–56.
7 Moreno C, Laje G, Blanco C, Jiang H, Schmidt AB, Olfson M. National trends in the outpatient diagnosis and treatment of bipolar disorder in youth. *Archives of General Psychiatry* 2007;64(9):1032–9.

8 Zito JM, Safer DJ, de Jong-van den Berg LT, Janhsen K, Fegert JM, Gardner JF, et al. A three-country comparison of psychotropic medication prevalence in youth. *Child and Adolescent Psychiatry and Mental Health* 2008;2(1):26.
9 Wong IC, Camilleri-Novak D, Stephens P. Rise in psychotropic drug prescribing in children in the UK: an urgent public health issue. *Drug Safety* 2003;26(15):1117–8.
10 Hammad TA, Laughren T, Racoosin J. Suicidality in pediatric patients treated with antidepressant drugs. *Archives of General Psychiatry* 2006;63(3):332–9.
11 Hebebrand J. Commentary on 'Forum: use of antidepressants in children and adolescents'. *Current Opinion in Psychiatry* 2010;23(1):62–3.
12 Hetrick SE, McKenzie JE, Merry SN. The use of SSRIs in children and adolescents. *Current Opinion in Psychiatry* 2010;23(1):53–7.
13 Hetrick S, Merry S, McKenzie J, Sindahl P, Proctor M. Selective serotonin reuptake inhibitors (SSRIs) for depressive disorders in children and adolescents. *Cochrane Database of Systematic Reviews* 2007;3:CD004851.
14 Goodyer IM, Wilkinson P, Dubicka B, Kelvin R. Forum: the use of selective serotonin reuptake inhibitors in depressed children and adolescents: commentary on the meta-analysis by Hetrick et al. *Current Opinion in Psychiatry* 2010;23(1):58–61.
15 Dubicka B, Hadley S, Roberts C. Suicidal behaviour in youths with depression treated with new-generation antidepressants: meta-analysis. *British Journal of Psychiatry* 2006;189:393–8.
16 Carlisle LL, McClellan J. Psychopharmacology of schizophrenia in children and adolescents. *Pediatric Clinics of North America* 2011;58(1):205–18.
17 Thomas T, Stansifer L, Findling RL. Psychopharmacology of pediatric bipolar disorders in children and adolescents. *Pediatric Clinics of North America* 2011;58(1):173–87.
18 Kodish I, Rockhill C, Ryan S, Varley C. Pharmacotherapy for anxiety disorders in children and adolescents. *Pediatric Clinics of North America* 2011;58(1):55–72.
19 Kaplan G, Ivanov I. Pharmacotherapy for substance abuse disorders in adolescence. *Pediatric Clinics of North America* 2011;58(1):243–58.
20 Smiga SM, Elliott GR. Psychopharmacology of depression in children and adolescents. *Pediatric Clinics of North America* 2011;58(1):155–71.
21 Hazell P, Mirzaie M. Tricyclic drugs for depression in children and adolescents. *Cochrane Database of Systematic Reviews* 2013;6:CD002317.
22 Ipser JC, Stein DJ, Hawkridge S, Hoppe L. Pharmacotherapy for anxiety disorders in children and adolescents. *Cochrane Database of Systematic Reviews* 2009;3:CD005170.
23 Kennedy E, Kumar A, Datta SS. Antipsychotic medication for childhood-onset schizophrenia. *Cochrane Database of Systematic Reviews* 2007;3:CD004027.
24 Feucht C, Patel DR. Herbal medicines in pediatric neuropsychiatry. *Pediatric Clinics of North America* 2011;58(1):33–54.
25 Bylund DB, Reed AL. Childhood and adolescent depression: why do children and adults respond differently to antidepressant drugs? *Neurochemistry International* 2007;51(5):246–53.
26 Feucht C, Patel DR. Principles of pharmacology. *Pediatric Clinics of North America* 2011;58(1):11–9.
27 Vitiello B. An international perspective on pediatric psychopharmacology. *International Review of Psychiatry* 2008;20(2):121–6.
28 Vitiello B, Jensen PS. Medication development and testing in children and adolescents. Current problems, future directions. *Archives of General Psychiatry* 1997;54(9):871–6.
29 Kearns GL, Abdel-Rahman SM, Alander SW, Blowey DL, Leeder JS, Kauffman RE. Developmental pharmacology – drug disposition, action, and therapy in infants and children. *New England Journal of Medicine* 2003;349(12):1157–67.

30 Wilens TE, Cohen L, Biederman J, Abrams A, Neft D, Faird N, et al. Fluoxetine pharmacokinetics in pediatric patients. *Journal of Clinical Psychopharmacology* 2002;22(6):568–75.
31 Hudson N, Spriggs M, Gillam L. Telling the truth to young children: ethical reasons for information disclosure in paediatrics. *Journal of Paediatrics and Child Health* 2019;55(1):13–7.
32 Alvarez-Jiménez M, González-Blanch C, Crespo-Facorro B, Hetrick S, Rodríguez-Sánchez JM, Pérez-Iglesias R, et al. Antipsychotic-induced weight gain in chronic and first-episode psychotic disorders: a systematic critical reappraisal. *CNS Drugs* 2008;22(7):547–62.
33 Griffith R. What is Gillick competence? *Human Vaccines and Immunotherapeutics* 2016;12(1):244–7.
34 Mrazek PJ, Haggerty RJ. *Reducing risks for mental disorders: frontiers for preventive intervention research*. Washington, DC: National Academies Press; 1994.
35 McGorry PD, Hickie IB, Yung AR, Pantelis C, Jackson HJ. Clinical staging of psychiatric disorders: a heuristic framework for choosing earlier, safer and more effective interventions. *Australian and New Zealand Journal of Psychiatry* 2006;40(8):616–22.
36 Yung AR, McGorry PD. The initial prodrome in psychosis: descriptive and qualitative aspects. *Australian and New Zealand Journal of Psychiatry* 1996;30(5):587–99.
37 Yung A, Phillips L, McGorry PD. *Treating schizophrenia in the prodromal phase*. London: Taylor & Francis; 2004.
38 Miller TJ, McGlashan TH, Rosen JL, Cadenhead K, Cannon T, Ventura J, et al. Prodromal assessment with the structured interview for prodromal syndromes and the scale of prodromal symptoms: predictive validity, interrater reliability, and training to reliability. *Schizophrenia Bulletin* 2003;29(4):703–15.
39 Yung AR, McGorry PD, McFarlane CA, Jackson HJ, Patton GC, Rakkar A. Monitoring and care of young people at incipient risk of psychosis. *Schizophrenia Bulletin* 1996;22(2):283–303.
40 Fusar-Poli P, Borgwardt S, Bechdolf A, Addington J, Riecher-Rössler A, Schultze-Lutter F, et al. The psychosis high-risk state: a comprehensive state-of-the-art review. *JAMA Psychiatry* 2013;70(1):107–20.
41 Howes OD, Lim S, Theologos G, Yung AR, Goodwin GM, McGuire P. A comprehensive review and model of putative prodromal features of bipolar affective disorder. *Psychological Medicine* 2011;41(8):1567–77.
42 Bechdolf A, Nelson B, Cotton SM, Chanen A, Thompson A, Kettle J, et al. A preliminary evaluation of the validity of at-risk criteria for bipolar disorders in help-seeking adolescents and young adults. *Journal of Affective Disorders* 2010;127(1–3):316–20.
43 Waugh MJ, Meyer TD, Young EA, Scott J. A review of self-rating instruments to identify young people at risk of bipolar spectrum disorders. *Journal of Affective Disorders* 2014;160:113–21.
44 Hetrick SE, Parker AG, Hickie IB, Purcell R, Yung AR, McGorry PD. Early identification and intervention in depressive disorders: towards a clinical staging model. *Psychotherapy and Psychosomatics* 2008;77(5):263–70.
45 Fava GA, Grandi S, Canestrari R, Molnar G. Prodromal symptoms in primary major depressive disorder. *Journal of Affective Disorders* 1990;19(2):149–52.
46 Fava GA, Tossani E. Prodromal stage of major depression. *Early Intervention in Psychiatry* 2007;1(1):9–18.
47 Biederman J, Mick E, Faraone SV, Spencer T, Wilens TE, Wozniak J. Pediatric mania: a developmental subtype of bipolar disorder? *Biological Psychiatry* 2000;48(6):458–66.

48 Hillegers MH, Reichart CG, Wals M, Verhulst FC, Ormel J, Nolen WA. Five-year prospective outcome of psychopathology in the adolescent offspring of bipolar parents. *Bipolar Disorders* 2005;7(4):344–50.
49 Häfner H, Maurer K, Trendler G, an der Heiden W, Schmidt M, Könnecke R. Schizophrenia and depression: challenging the paradigm of two separate diseases – a controlled study of schizophrenia, depression and healthy controls. *Schizophrenia Research* 2005;77(1):11–24.
50 Sadek N, Bona J. Subsyndromal symptomatic depression: a new concept. *Depression and Anxiety* 2000;12(1):30–9.
51 Wood SJ, Pantelis C, Velakoulis D, Yücel M, Fornito A, McGorry PD. Progressive changes in the development toward schizophrenia: studies in subjects at increased symptomatic risk. *Schizophrenia Bulletin* 2008;34(2):322–9.
52 Dazzan P, Soulsby B, Mechelli A, Wood SJ, Velakoulis D, Phillips LJ, et al. Volumetric abnormalities predating the onset of schizophrenia and affective psychoses: an MRI study in subjects at ultrahigh risk of psychosis. *Schizophrenia Bulletin* 2012;38(5):1083–91.
53 Berk M, Hallam K, Malhi GS, Henry L, Hasty M, Macneil C, et al. Evidence and implications for early intervention in bipolar disorder. *Journal of Mental Health* 2010;19(2):113–26.
54 McGorry PD, Yung AR, Phillips LJ, Yuen HP, Francey S, Cosgrave EM, et al. Randomized controlled trial of interventions designed to reduce the risk of progression to first-episode psychosis in a clinical sample with subthreshold symptoms. *Archives of General Psychiatry* 2002;59(10):921–8.
55 Phillips LJ, McGorry PD, Yuen HP, Ward J, Donovan K, Kelly D, et al. Medium term follow-up of a randomized controlled trial of interventions for young people at ultra high risk of psychosis. *Schizophrenia Research* 2007;96(1–3):25–33.
56 McGlashan TH, Zipursky RB, Perkins D, Addington J, Miller T, Woods SW, et al. Randomized, double-blind trial of olanzapine versus placebo in patients prodromally symptomatic for psychosis. *American Journal of Psychiatry* 2006;163(5):790–9.
57 McGorry PD, Nelson B, Phillips LJ, Yuen HP, Francey SM, Thampi A, et al. Randomized controlled trial of interventions for young people at ultra-high risk of psychosis: twelve-month outcome. *Journal of Clinical Psychiatry* 2013;74(4):349–56.
58 Yung AR, Phillips LJ, Nelson B, Francey SM, PanYuen H, Simmons MB, et al. Randomized controlled trial of interventions for young people at ultra high risk for psychosis: 6-month analysis. *Journal of Clinical Psychiatry* 2011;72(4):430–40.
59 Morrison AP, French P, Walford L, Lewis SW, Kilcommons A, Green J, et al. Cognitive therapy for the prevention of psychosis in people at ultra-high risk: randomised controlled trial. *British Journal of Psychiatry* 2004;185:291–7.
60 van der Gaag M, Smit F, Bechdolf A, French P, Linszen DH, Yung AR, et al. Preventing a first episode of psychosis: meta-analysis of randomized controlled prevention trials of 12 month and longer-term follow-ups. *Schizophrenia Research* 2013;149(1–3):56–62.
61 Yung AR, Yuen HP, Berger G, Francey S, Hung TC, Nelson B, et al. Declining transition rate in ultra high risk (prodromal) services: dilution or reduction of risk? *Schizophrenia Bulletin* 2007;33(3):673–81.
62 Corcoran C, Malaspina D, Hercher L. Prodromal interventions for schizophrenia vulnerability: the risks of being "at risk". *Schizophrenia Research* 2005;73(2–3):173–84.
63 Yung AR. Antipsychotic treatment of UHR ('prodromal') individuals. *Early Intervention in Psychiatry* 2010;4(3):197–9.

64 Ruhrmann S, Bechdolf A, Kühn KU, Wagner M, Schultze-Lutter F, Janssen B, et al. Acute effects of treatment for prodromal symptoms for people putatively in a late initial prodromal state of psychosis. *British Journal of Psychiatry* 2007;51:s88–95.
65 Findling RL, Frazier TW, Youngstrom EA, McNamara NK, Stansbrey RJ, Gracious BL, et al. Double-blind, placebo-controlled trial of divalproex monotherapy in the treatment of symptomatic youth at high risk for developing bipolar disorder. *Journal of Clinical Psychiatry* 2007;68(5):781–8.
66 Jureidini JN, Doecke CJ, Mansfield PR, Haby MM, Menkes DB, Tonkin AL. Efficacy and safety of antidepressants for children and adolescents. *BMJ* 2004;328(7444):879–83.
67 Berk M, Conus P, Kapczinski F, Andreazza AC, Yücel M, Wood SJ, et al. From neuroprogression to neuroprotection: implications for clinical care. *Medical Journal of Australia* 2010;193(S4):S36–40.
68 Berger G, Dell'Olio M, Amminger P, Cornblatt B, Phillips L, Yung A, et al. Neuroprotection in emerging psychotic disorders. *Early Intervention in Psychiatry* 2007;1(2):114–27.
69 Meldrum BS. Implications for neuroprotective treatments. *Progress in Brain Research* 2002;135:487–95.
70 Berger GE, Wood S, McGorry PD. Incipient neurovulnerability and neuroprotection in early psychosis. *Psychopharmacology Bulletin* 2003;37(2):79–101.
71 Bai O, Wei Z, Lu W, Bowen R, Keegan D, Li XM. Protective effects of atypical antipsychotic drugs on PC12 cells after serum withdrawal. *Journal of Neuroscience Research* 2002;69(2):278–83.
72 Wei Z, Mousseau DD, Richardson JS, Dyck LE, Li XM. Atypical antipsychotics attenuate neurotoxicity of beta-amyloid(25–35) by modulating Bax and Bcl-X(l/s) expression and localization. *Journal of Neuroscience Research* 2003;74(6):942–7.
73 Manji HK, Moore GJ, Chen G. Clinical and preclinical evidence for the neurotrophic effects of mood stabilizers: implications for the pathophysiology and treatment of manic-depressive illness. *Biological Psychiatry* 2000;48(8):740–54.
74 Manji HK, Moore GJ, Chen G. Bipolar disorder: leads from the molecular and cellular mechanisms of action of mood stabilizers. *British Journal of Psychiatry* 2001;41:s107–19.
75 Xu H, Steven Richardson J, Li XM. Dose-related effects of chronic antidepressants on neuroprotective proteins BDNF, Bcl-2 and Cu/Zn-SOD in rat hippocampus. *Neuropsychopharmacology* 2003;28(1):53–62.
76 Seymour CB, Mothersill C, Mooney R, Moriarty M, Tipton KF. Monoamine oxidase inhibitors l-deprenyl and clorgyline protect nonmalignant human cells from ionising radiation and chemotherapy toxicity. *British Journal of Cancer* 2003;89(10):1979–86.
77 Cornblatt BA, Lencz T, Smith CW, Olsen R, Auther AM, Nakayama E, et al. Can antidepressants be used to treat the schizophrenia prodrome? Results of a prospective, naturalistic treatment study of adolescents. *Journal of Clinical Psychiatry* 2007;68(4):546–57.
78 Rosen JL, Miller TJ, D'Andrea JT, McGlashan TH, Woods SW. Comorbid diagnoses in patients meeting criteria for the schizophrenia prodrome. *Schizophrenia Research* 2006;85(1–3):124–31.
79 Lin A, Wood SJ, Nelson B, Beavan A, McGorry P, Yung AR. Outcomes of nontransitioned cases in a sample at ultra-high risk for psychosis. *American Journal of Psychiatry* 2015;172(3):249–58.
80 Fusar-Poli P, Valmaggia L, McGuire P. Can antidepressants prevent psychosis? *Lancet* 2007;370(9601):1746–8.
81 Berk M, Hallam K, Lucas N, Hasty M, McNeil CA, Conus P, et al. Early intervention in bipolar disorders: opportunities and pitfalls. *Medical Journal of Australia* 2007;187(S7):S11–4.

82 Berger GE, Wood SJ, Ross M, Hamer CA, Wellard RM, Pell G, et al. Neuroprotective effects of low-dose lithium in individuals at ultra-high risk for psychosis. A longitudinal MRI/MRS study. *Current Pharmaceutical Design* 2012;18(4):570–5.
83 Peet M, Stokes C. Omega-3 fatty acids in the treatment of psychiatric disorders. *Drugs* 2005;65(8):1051–9.
84 Amminger GP, Schäfer MR, Papageorgiou K, Klier CM, Cotton SM, Harrigan SM, et al. Long-chain omega-3 fatty acids for indicated prevention of psychotic disorders: a randomized, placebo-controlled trial. *Archives of General Psychiatry* 2010;67(2):146–54.
85 Amminger GP, Schäfer MR, Schlögelhofer M, Klier CM, McGorry PD. Longer-term outcome in the prevention of psychotic disorders by the Vienna omega-3 study. *Nature Communications* 2015;6:7934.
86 McGorry PD, Nelson B, Markulev C, Yuen HP, Schäfer MR, Mossaheb N, et al. Effect of ω-3 polyunsaturated fatty acids in young people at ultrahigh risk for psychotic disorders: the NEURAPRO randomized clinical trial. *JAMA Psychiatry* 2017;74(1):19–27.
87 Cadenhead K, Addington J, Cannon T, Cornblatt B, Mathalon D, McGlashan T, et al. Omega-3 fatty acid versus placebo in a clinical high-risk sample from the North American Prodrome Longitudinal Studies (NAPLS) consortium. *Schizophrenia Bulletin* 2017;43(1):S16.
88 Amminger GP, Nelson B, Markulev C, Yuen HP, Schäfer MR, Berger M, et al. The NEURAPRO biomarker analysis: long-chain omega-3 fatty acids improve 6-month and 12-month outcomes in youths at ultra-high risk for psychosis. *Biological Psychiatry* 2020;87(3):243–52.
89 Davies C, Bhattacharyya S. Cannabidiol as a potential treatment for psychosis. *Therapeutic Advances in Psychopharmacology* 2019;9:2045125319881916.
90 Barnes TR, Drake R, Paton C, Cooper SJ, Deakin B, Ferrier IN, et al. Evidence-based guidelines for the pharmacological treatment of schizophrenia: updated recommendations from the British Association for Psychopharmacology. *Journal of Psychopharmacology* 2020;34(1):3–78.
91 Williams AL, Katz D, Ali A, Girard C, Goodman J, Bell I. Do essential fatty acids have a role in the treatment of depression? *Journal of Affective Disorders* 2006;93(1–3):117–23.
92 Osher Y, Belmaker RH. Omega-3 fatty acids in depression: a review of three studies. *CNS Neuroscience & Therapeutics* 2009;15(2):128–33.
93 Nemets H, Nemets B, Apter A, Bracha Z, Belmaker RH. Omega-3 treatment of childhood depression: a controlled, double-blind pilot study. *American Journal of Psychiatry* 2006;163(6):1098–100.
94 Ferraz AC, Kiss A, Araújo RL, Salles HM, Naliwaiko K, Pamplona J, et al. The antidepressant role of dietary long-chain polyunsaturated n-3 fatty acids in two phases in the developing brain. *Prostaglandins, Leukotrienes, and Essential Fatty Acids* 2008;78(3):183–8.
95 Fava M, Borus JS, Alpert JE, Nierenberg AA, Rosenbaum JF, Bottiglieri T. Folate, vitamin B12, and homocysteine in major depressive disorder. *American Journal of Psychiatry* 1997;154(3):426–8.
96 Beydoun MA, Shroff MR, Beydoun HA, Zonderman AB. Serum folate, vitamin B-12, and homocysteine and their association with depressive symptoms among U.S. adults. *Psychosomatic Medicine* 2010;72(9):862–73.
97 Taylor MJ, Carney S, Geddes J, Goodwin G. Folate for depressive disorders. *Cochrane Database of Systematic Reviews* 2003;2:CD003390.
98 Coppen A, Bailey J. Enhancement of the antidepressant action of fluoxetine by folic acid: a randomised, placebo controlled trial. *Journal of Affective Disorders* 2000;60(2):121–30.

99 Godfrey PS, Toone BK, Carney MW, Flynn TG, Bottiglieri T, Laundy M, et al. Enhancement of recovery from psychiatric illness by methylfolate. *Lancet* 1990;336 (8712):392–5.
100 Weng S, Tang J, Wang G, Wang X, Wang H. Comparison of the addition of Siberian ginseng (Acanthopanax senticosus) versus fluoxetine to lithium for the treatment of bipolar disorder in adolescents: a randomized, double-blind trial. *Current Therapeutic Research* 2007;68(4):280–90.
101 Berk M, Dean O, Cotton SM, Gama CS, Kapczinski F, Fernandes BS, et al. The efficacy of N-acetylcysteine as an adjunctive treatment in bipolar depression: an open label trial. *Journal of Affective Disorders* 2011;135(1–3):389–94.

17 Attention-deficit/hyperactivity disorder in youth

David Coghill

Introduction

Attention-deficit/hyperactivity disorder (ADHD) is characterised by a developmentally inappropriate, pervasive (across different situations such as home and school/work) and persistent pattern of significant inattention, hyperactivity and/or impulsivity. Onset is typically in childhood and the symptoms are associated with substantial impairment in social, academic, and/or occupational functioning. The definition of ADHD in DSM-5 is based upon a set of 18 symptoms covering two dimensions, inattention (nine symptoms) and hyperactivity/impulsivity (nine symptoms), and distinguishes three presentations of ADHD: predominantly inattentive presentation (at least six symptoms of inattention, less than six of hyperactivity/impulsivity); predominantly hyperactive/impulsive presentation ($\geq$ 6 hyperactivity/impulsivity, $<$ 6 inattention); combined ($\geq$ 6 hyperactivity/impulsivity and $\geq$ 6 inattention). These symptoms must have persisted for at least six months, must be pervasive across at least two situations (e.g., home, school, work and/or social life) and several of them must have been present before 12 years of age. Whilst formally recognised, this age of onset criterion has been challenged, as it is not uncommon to find youth and adults whose symptoms were less visible in childhood and for whom impairment only became clear later in life.[1]

Although ADHD was traditionally considered a disorder of childhood it is now clear that, in many cases, it persists into youth and adulthood. A recent systematic review of ADHD prevalence during childhood and adolescence based on 102 studies from across all world regions calculated an overall prevalence of ADHD of 5.3%. The prevalence for children was 6.5% and for adolescents 2.7%.[2] ADHD is a global disorder, and differences in reported epidemiological prevalence between countries are mainly accounted for by differences in methodology.[2] Despite concerns that the prevalence of ADHD might be increasing in recent years, this was not supported by a recent meta-analysis that found no evidence for an increased prevalence over the past three decades when standardised diagnostic procedures are followed.[3] There is, however, evidence to suggest that rates of recognition and diagnosis are increasing in most parts of the world. This trend is welcome in most countries where ADHD is currently significantly under diagnosed and treated,[4,5] but is of some concern in the USA where it seems as if rates of diagnosis in most states already exceed epidemiological prevalence rates.[6] In most countries the under-recognition of ADHD is most significant for adults, and treatment rates have been shown to fall sharply during early to mid-adolescence.[7]

Estimates of the prevalence of ADHD in adults suggest a prevalence around 2.5%.[8] The only population study found in the literature assessing ADHD in young adults and using the most recent DSM-5 criteria reported a prevalence of 3.6% (95% CI 2.9–4.1).[9] Although in childhood ADHD is more common in males than females, a more balanced sex ratio is found in samples of youth and adults.

Clinical presentation and course through adolescence

As is the case for most mental health disorders, the clinical presentation of ADHD is highly variable. Some patients have more minor symptoms, while others may have severe impairments. Most authorities agree that the presence of impairment is key to making a clinical diagnosis. In this respect, in clinical practice the precise number of symptoms is probably less important than the presence of clearly *impairing* symptoms. It is also the case that DSM-5 no longer requires the full syndrome be present before age 12 years, only that symptoms were present before this time. Most authorities have welcomed this change as it is not uncommon to meet individuals with clear, current impairment from symptoms that were less impairing earlier in life (usually because of the presence of 'scaffolding' from parents or teachers which is no longer present).

Whilst the core symptoms of ADHD are relatively consistent across development, they do manifest differently at different developmental stages. This is due to a combination of developmental and environmental factors. Perhaps the most frequently discussed change with development is a reduction in observed hyperactivity with increasing age. Whilst this is true, the meaning is often misunderstood. Young people and adults with ADHD certainly appear less overactive, however if asked about 'inner tension' and feelings of restlessness, they almost always indicate that this has increased over time. They therefore still find sitting in one place difficult even though they are sometimes able to hide this. Impulsivity, on the other hand, often continues to be a problem throughout life with continued excessive talking, interrupting others and butting in to their conversations, blurting out ideas and difficulty waiting turn. Similarly, whilst inattention presents differently in children as opposed to youth or adults due to environmental differences (e.g., difference between primary and secondary school and the associated demands, difference between educational and work settings or the demands of unemployment), it continues to be a major obstacle. Symptoms include making careless mistakes; difficulty remaining focused during lectures, conversations or lengthy reading; difficulty listening and following instructions; problems starting and finishing tasks; organisational difficulties; distractibility; forgetfulness in day-to-day tasks and frequently losing things.

The predominantly inattentive presentation is relatively more common in females and, together with the combined presentation, seems to have a higher impact on academic performance. The predominantly hyperactive/impulsive presentation is relatively uncommon outside of early childhood, but when it is present it is associated with more aggressive behaviours. This group also tend to be unpopular and highly rejected by their peers. The combined presentation is associated with all of the issues found in the other presentations, but also with greater overall impairments in global functioning compared with the other two types.

One aspect of ADHD that has been relatively neglected in children but becomes more apparent for youth and adults is subjective experiences of ADHD symptoms. Young people with ADHD often describe excessive mind wandering (or mental restlessness), physical restlessness as noted earlier and mood lability. Whilst not formally included as a core symptom of ADHD (due to its relatively low discriminant validity), high levels of emotional lability and irritability are common, which is often experienced as being just as impairing as the core symptoms.

A large majority (60–85%) of children with ADHD will continue to meet criteria for the disorder during their teenage years, and longitudinal studies have documented that ADHD/HKD (hyperkinetic disorder) persists through childhood into adolescence and adulthood in many cases.[10] The extent to which ADHD persists into adulthood depends heavily on how it is defined. About 65% of children with ADHD experience partial remission in adulthood (with significant clinical impairments), and the full ADHD diagnosis is met in approximately 15% at age 25, when full diagnostic criteria were required.[11] There is, however, considerable variability in those estimates, with recent European data reporting much higher rates of persistence (up to 80%) for children and youth diagnosed with combined type ADHD.[12,13] Either way it is clear that most children with ADHD continue to have problems into adolescence and young adulthood.

Sex differences in the rates of ADHD also change across development.[14,15] Whilst males predominate in childhood, by adulthood rates are much more similar. It is not yet clear whether these changes occur in adolescence or young adulthood. One potential explanation for the predominance of ADHD in males during childhood is the greater hyperactivity/impulsivity in boys compared to girls at this stage of development. However, mean scores for ADHD symptoms in general population samples show that, as a group, boys have higher levels of both inattentive and hyperactive/impulsive symptoms than girls. By late adolescence, while sex differences in inattention appear to remain, the level of hyperactivity/impulsivity in boys seems to decline to the level of the girls such that the expression of core ADHD symptoms is more similar across the sexes in the adult population.[15]

The risk factors that determine the persistence of ADHD diagnosis into adulthood remain unclear. However, some studies suggested that higher persistence is associated with:[16–18]

- A family history of ADHD
- Experience of adversities during childhood (including family adversity)
- Increased severity of ADHD symptoms during childhood
- Presence of comorbidities (e.g., major depressive disorder, high comorbidity, paternal [but not maternal] anxiety mood disorder and parental antisocial personality disorder)

Comorbidity

ADHD is frequently comorbid with other mental health conditions, and in clinical samples rates of comorbidity of around 80% are not uncommon. The pattern of comorbidity changes across development. In childhood the most common comorbidities are oppositional defiant disorder (30–60%) and anxiety (around 25%). These often persist into adolescence where there is also an increase in rates of conduct disorder (10–20%) and depression (10–20%). Rates of substance use also increase from this time and overall are twice as high as in the non-ADHD population, although some of this increase is related to conduct disorder rather than ADHD per se. Tic disorders and Tourette's are also more common in those with ADHD, as are a range of language delays, learning disorders, developmental coordination disorder, sleep problems and other neuropsychological deficits.

Later in youth and into adulthood, rates of bipolar disorder are increased, as are those of borderline personality disorder. These last two comorbidities are particularly important for clinicians in youth mental health services as they are amongst the most common examples of mistaken diagnosis for those with ADHD.[19] Philipsen and colleagues found high rates of ADHD in a group of women seeking treatment for borderline personality disorder (childhood ADHD in 41.5%; adult ADHD 16.1%).[20] Childhood ADHD was associated with higher levels of emotional abuse in childhood and greater severity of adult borderline symptoms. Adult ADHD was associated with greater risk for additional Axis I and II disorders. The presence of any type of personality disorder does not preclude the presence of ADHD and, indeed, in many cases increases the risk. It is therefore important to recognise that in people with a personality disorder, ADHD should be diagnosed in the usual way, with care taken to elicit the symptom criteria, age of onset, pervasiveness and impairment criteria that are used to define ADHD.

Although it was previously precluded to make a diagnosis of ADHD in the presence of autism, this has now been reversed, and DSM now allows a comorbid diagnosis of ADHD and autism spectrum disorder (ASD). Whilst the data is incomplete, it is estimated that around 50% of those with ASD also meet criteria for ADHD. Like ADHD, ASD has traditionally been under-recognised within youth mental health, and it is therefore important that clinicians consider both disorders when making their assessments of patients presenting with symptoms of other disorders. It is not a contest between one disorder, or explanation, and another but a recognition that comorbidity is common and that we should think about it as '*this and that*' rather than '*this or that*'.

Pathogenesis and aetiology

Genetic and environmental causes of ADHD

ADHD is highly heritable, with twin studies suggesting a heritability between 60 and 90%.[21] ADHD is not, however, a genetic disorder in any simple sense. The genetic contribution is likely a combination of common polymorphisms and less common copy number variants.[22] Gene-wide association studies (GWAS) have recently identified 12 independent risk loci that surpass genome-wide significance.[23] These loci are enriched in evolutionarily constrained genomic regions and loss-of-function intolerant genes, and around brain-expressed regulatory marks. The strong concordance with GWAS of continuous population measures of ADHD symptoms supports the notion that the categorically defined clinical diagnosis of ADHD is in fact an extreme expression of continuous heritable traits. Most of these genetic factors appear to be active early in development, and it is not yet clear to what degree genetic variation can influence the development of ADHD during later childhood and adolescence or, indeed, whether genetic factors influence course and remission of ADHD later in life.

Whilst it is generally agreed that environmental factors are very likely to be important in the aetiology of ADHD, their role remains unclear at present. As for genes, it is assumed that their greatest influence will occur prenatally;[24] however, despite demonstration of associations between prenatal risk factors (e.g., prematurity, maternal smoking during pregnancy) and ADHD, there remains insufficient evidence to support a definite causal relationship. Several epidemiological and data linkage studies have made substantial contributions to our understanding of the relationships between genes and environment. In particular, these studies have started to account for some of the genetic and familial confounds that were not considered in the original studies.[25,26] When taken into consideration these new data throw several of the proposed environmental causal data into doubt.[24] Several factors in the post-natal environment have also been proposed to play a role. For instance, diet may play a small but significant role, and there is data from randomised controlled trials that certain food additives increase the risk for ADHD, at least in certain individuals.[27] Social adversity, and more specifically family adversity, appears to be implicated in the course and persistence of the condition rather than in its onset. ADHD is associated with social disadvantage, and rates are higher in those that have been victims of abuse.[28,29] These findings may, however, be due to gene x environment correlations, whereby those with ADHD are more likely to be victimised. There is a clear need for more research into the impact of the environment on the development of ADHD and in particular the complex interactions between genes and environment.

Brain development and ADHD

Neuroimaging

The main avenues for understanding the contribution of differential profiles of brain development on ADHD come from structural and functional neuroimaging and neuropsychological studies. Structural and functional neuroimaging studies have documented developmental abnormalities in brain anatomy and function in individuals with ADHD.[30,31] Meta-analyses of structural studies most consistently show smaller volumes in the ADHD brain, which are most consistent in the basal ganglia.[31] Smaller total intracranial volumes have been described in children with ADHD, while in adults with ADHD, these subcortical volume reductions appear to be less pronounced.[32] Functional imaging studies in children with ADHD have demonstrated hypoactivation in systems involved in executive function (fronto-parietal network) and attention (ventral attentional network). Also, significant hyperactivation was observed in the default, ventral attention and somato-motor networks. In adults, there was also ADHD-related hypoactivation in the fronto-parietal system, while hyperactivation was present in the visual, dorsal attention and default networks.[30] Longitudinal neuroimaging studies from childhood to adulthood are starting to appear. These show that, at a group level, smaller brain volumes and many of the morphometric abnormalities found in children with ADHD tend to persist over time in those with persistent ADHD assessed in childhood, adolescence and early adulthood.[33–35] This includes the cortical thinning that has been described in the medial and dorsolateral prefrontal cortex and the medial and superior prefrontal and precentral regions. Similar findings have been reported for several subcortical regions. Divergent developmental trajectories between persisters and control individuals from childhood to adulthood have been described for the basal ganglia and total cerebellar volume. There are currently few data on the continuity of functional brain alterations in ADHD.

Neurocognition

ADHD is associated with a broad range of cognitive deficits. These include difficulties with working memory, set shifting, inhibition, decision-making and other executive functions, as well as lower-level non-executive memory deficits, delay aversion, reaction time variability and various problems with timing.[36] From a cognitive perspective ADHD is highly heterogeneous, meaning that none of these cognitive domains are necessarily problematic in any one person and indeed only around a third will have a deficit in any particular domain. For this reason, cognitive testing is not helpful in making an ADHD diagnosis. It can, however, help understand someone's particular strengths and weaknesses. When ADHD persists through adolescence into adulthood these deficits seem to remain relatively stable. Whilst there have been theories about relationships between changes in cognition and remission of ADHD, the data on this is somewhat inconsistent.[37] This may reflect a relative dissociation between cognitive performance and ADHD symptoms that has been independently identified by several groups.[38,39] It is therefore not yet clear whether changes in ADHD status across development are related to changes in cognitive processes and skills. There is, however, a developing consensus that impairments in executive function do not distinguish remitters from persisters.[10]

Assessment

Assessment protocols for ADHD have been well described for children, adolescents and adults.[40–42] All emphasise the importance of several key points.

- The diagnosis of ADHD is based on clinical judgement of integrated data gathered from multiple sources.

- ADHD is best assessed by clinical interviews.
- These can be augmented by (but should not be replaced by):
    - questionnaires
    - direct observations
    - neuropsychological measures
- Education of staff at a primary care level and education about ADHD is essential to ensure that those with ADHD are promptly identified and referred.
- A comprehensive assessment for ADHD is complex and often time consuming. Those conducting these assessments need to be well trained.
- The purpose of an 'ADHD assessment' is not only to confirm or exclude the presence of ADHD but also to identify whether there are any other problems or disorders that are causing impairment.
- At the end of the assessment process the clinician should have developed a comprehensive formulation that comprehensively describes the patient's problems.

As ADHD is a complex disorder which is commonly accompanied by comorbid disorders and difficulties it is important to recognise that the assessment of ADHD cannot occur in a vacuum and must be considered as part of a comprehensive assessment process. It must also be recognised that, like all other psychiatric diagnoses, there are no biological tests for ADHD. Rather, it involves the integration of information from different sources and a clinical decision-making process that is able to resolve conflicting observations and information. The diagnosis itself is, however, supported by a strong evidence base, and there are a range of validated questionnaires and interview schedules available to support the assessment process. It is sometimes, but not always, helpful to supplement the information gathered from the child / young person, parents, carers, other family members, teachers and others, with direct observation. A (neuro) psychological assessment can also sometimes be helpful to assess cognitive strengths and difficulties. At the end of the process the clinician will need to determine a principal and differential diagnosis, a judgement about the presence of any comorbid disorders, and develop a formulation that places these diagnoses in context.

For youth the clinical interview can be divided into a general evaluation of the young person, their problems and the context within which they are occurring, and specific questioning about ADHD and its common comorbidities (Box 17.1). Whilst these lists make the distinction between the two tasks seem very clear and orderly, it is important to remember that the patient and their family will often have waited a long time to tell their story 'to someone who understands', and, at the same time, may be quite anxious about the assessment process. It is therefore important that they are allowed space and time to describe the difficulties from their perspective and to vent their frustrations. The assessment can be seen as the start of a relationship between the clinical services and the family, and as those with a diagnosis of ADHD will often require a prolonged period of treatment, it is important to get off on the right foot and start to cultivate a strong therapeutic alliance from the beginning. This will often pay dividends further down the line, where continued concordance and compliance with treatment is likely to be central to success.

Box 17.1 Clinical interview with the patient and their family

General evaluation

- Clarify presenting complaints
- Systematic evaluation of symptoms
- Describe how problems developed
- Developmental history including previous professional reports
- Family history of ADHD
- Pregnancy and birth history (foetal growth, toxaemia, bleeding or severe infections during pregnancy, maternal diabetes or epilepsy, other maternal illness or traumas, poor maternal nutrition, maternal medication, nicotine, alcohol and drug use, gestational age, birth complications, birth weight, neonatal complications)
- Early developmental history (milestones for psychomotor development, language, attachment, sleep and feeding problems, growth and early temperament)
- Medical history (especially tics and epilepsy, psychosis – if adolescent)
- Medication (especially anticonvulsants, antihistamines, sympathetomimetics, steroids)
- Family functioning and family problems
- Social networks and other resources

Specific questioning

- The behaviours that comprise ICD and DSM ADHD diagnoses, and
  - their relationship to current level of development
  - any situational variation
  - ages of onset
  - development over time
  - their presence in other family members
- A rating of impairment across different settings (home, school/college, work)
- Related problems (e.g., behavioural and learning problems, emotional problems, tics, conduct disorder, alcohol problems)
- Self/Parent completed rating scales

Whilst in children the focus of the interview is often the parent, with young people this will start to move towards the young person themselves. The parent will however remain an important source of information. It is they who will be best able to identify when problems started, how pervasive they are/were and the degree of impairment. Even for those not living at home, parent information remains important but can be augmented by that of a partner or friend. If the patient is still at school/college/university is essential to the process, whilst for those at work, information from this context can be extremely helpful. Whilst the collection of personal information from a third party must always be balanced against privacy issues, the importance of a good quality history covering multiple aspects of a person's life cannot be overstated.

Although many clinical assessments will be conducted via a standard clinical history and examination, there are occasions where a more structured assessment is useful. In particular, clinicians who have not had full training in the assessment of ADHD or are just starting to conduct assessments for ADHD may find it useful to use a formal interview schedule to guide this part of the assessment process. There are several reliable interviews available. This is one area where the appropriate tool will differ between adolescents (up to around 18 years / school leaving), for whom child and adolescent interviews such as the semi-structured Kiddie-SADS or the structured Development and Well-being Assessment (DAWBA) – both of which are available to download online – are recommended. These interviews are designed to be conducted with children and adolescents who are still attending school and are less relevant to the older young person at work, university, college or unemployed. For these situations the two most widely used are the Conners' Adult ADHD Diagnostic Interview for DSM-IV (CAADID), which is a licensed instrument, and the Diagnostic Interview for ADHD in Adults (DIVA), which is available online. Both interviews take a similar approach to the systematic evaluation of each of the 18-symptom DSM items for both current symptoms in adulthood and retrospective symptoms from childhood.

Many clinicians worry that ADHD is going to be a difficult disorder to diagnose accurately because of the overlap between the symptoms and impairments of ADHD, those associated with other common mental health disorders, and normal behaviour. However, once clinicians have gained experience of the diagnostic and treatment process they usually realise that the diagnostic problems are no more or less complicated than those found for other mental health conditions.

When distinguishing ADHD symptoms from normal behaviour it is necessary to apply reasonable thresholds on the basis of the level of severity. Severity can be reflected in the degree of personal distress to self and others and levels of functional impairment from the symptoms. Persistence is also an important feature. Unlike episodic disorders from which people can recover, ADHD symptoms are present over extended periods of time (although they will often fluctuate depending on circumstances). For this reason, relatively mild symptoms, experienced on a day-to-day basis, can lead to moderate to severe levels of impairment. It is therefore important to understand the impairments associated with the symptoms rather than just tick off a checklist of symptoms.

The other commonly voiced concern is about distinguishing ADHD from comorbid disorders. These include anxiety, depression, bipolar and borderline personality disorders, as well as substance abuse and antisocial personality disorder. Here it is first essential to ensure that the presentation is not better explained by a single underlying condition. When considering the relationship of ADHD to comorbid conditions, there are three main categories that should be considered:[43]

1 Symptoms of ADHD that mimic other disorders

   a Anxiety: mental restlessness, ceaseless thoughts, restlessness, poor sleep, avoidance of situations (e.g., queues, social situations)
   b Depression: initial insomnia and restless sleep, impulsive eating, low self-esteem, unstable moods, impatience and irritability, concentration problems
   c Borderline personality disorder: chronic symptoms emerge from childhood/adolescence, impulsive behaviour, mood instability, angry outbursts, impaired social relationships
   d Bipolar disorder: mood instability, motor restlessness, mental restlessness and distractible mind, distractibility and difficulty concentration, over-talkativeness

2 Neurodevelopmental disorders that often accompany ADHD, for example, autism, specific learning difficulties (e.g., dyslexia, dyscalculia), general learning difficulties (e.g., low IQ) and developmental coordination disorder (e.g., DCD, dyspraxia)
3 The development of other disorders where ADHD acts as a developmental risk factor

   a Shared genetic and environmental risk factors
   b ADHD generates exposure to risky environments for other disorders (e.g., repeated negative educational experiences leading to low self-esteem and depression)
   c ADHD may enhance the impact of other risk factors, for example, children with ADHD with the COMT genotype are more likely to develop antisocial behavioural problems[44]
   d Multiple risk factors, where the innate characteristics of ADHD combine with environmental exposure to risky environments, for example, substance abuse disorders and ADHD. This association is likely to be multifaceted, including increased exposure to environmental risk factors for addiction, poor self-regulation and impulsivity leading to increased risk-taking behaviours and self-treatment of ADHD symptoms

Treatment and management

At every age the recommended treatment for ADHD should be multimodal.[10] For adolescents and young adults this includes psychoeducation, medication and disorder-orientated psychological treatments including cognitive behavioural therapy and family therapy.

Psychoeducation is the mainstay of all treatment in mental health and should be offered to everyone who has a diagnosis of ADHD. In order to provide high-quality psychoeducation it is essential that all clinicians working in the field make sure that they are up to date with accurate information about causes, course and treatment.

Medication treatments

Stimulant medications including methylphenidate, dexamphetamine and lisdexamfetamine have been known to be efficacious for many years, and more recent studies have demonstrated efficacy for several non-stimulant medications including atomoxetine and guanfacine.[45] Whilst most of these medications have been demonstrated to be effective across the lifespan, guanfacine has not been trialled in adults and is therefore only licensed for children and adolescents. Because of the need to address regulatory requirements, most medications have been trialled in children and adolescents (up to 16–18 years) and then separately in adults. There appear to be some discontinuities in efficacy and tolerability across the age range. As a consequence a recent network meta-analysis and some evidence-based clinical guidelines have made different recommendations for first-line medications in children/adolescents and adults.[45,46] It is, however, generally agreed that the stimulants are usually the first choice medications and that methylphenidate and the amphetamines (including the prodrug lisdexamfetamine) are similar in efficacy. Around 70% of people with ADHD respond well to methylphenidate and 70% to an amphetamine, with between 90–95% responding to one or the other.[47] Atomoxetine and guanfacine are regarded as second-line medications and are generally given when someone has failed to respond to or not tolerated both stimulant classes, although there are some occasions when they may be given as first-line treatments (e.g., where there is active substance abuse, in the presence of tics or where a patient actively refuses treatment with a stimulant). Guanfacine has the added benefit of being able to be safely co-prescribed with a stimulant and is therefore a choice for those patients who respond to a stimulant but still have residual symptoms and for those for whom the dose of stimulant cannot be optimally titrated due to adverse effects. All of the ADHD medications are highly effective with moderate to large effect sizes in children and adolescents and lower but still moderately large effect sizes in adults (Table 17.1).[45] Unfortunately, it was

Table 17.1 Clinician-rated change in ADHD symptoms[45]

Medication	*Children and adolescents*	*Adults*
	SMD (95% CI)	*SMD (95% CI)*
Amphetamines	−1.02 (−1.19 to −0.85)	−0.79 (−0.99 to −0.58)
Atomoxetine	−0.56 (−0.66 to −0.45)	−0.45 (−0.58 to −0.32)
Guanfacine	−0.67 (−0.85 to −0.50)	Not available
Methylphenidate	−0.78 (−0.93 to −0.62)	−0.49 (−0.64 to −0.35)

Note: SMD: Standardised Mean difference; CI: Confidence Interval

not possible in the recent network meta-analysis to give separate outcomes for children and adolescents, primarily because most studies did not report results separately by age group. There appears to be change in efficacy at some point in development (a lower efficacy in adults compared to children and youth), but it is not clear when this occurs. Based on these findings the European ADHD Guidelines Group concluded that the balance of evidence supports methylphenidate as the first-choice treatment for children and adolescents, whilst amphetamines (including lisdexamfetamine) are preferred in adults.[45]

In terms of adverse effects, the most common with stimulants are loss of appetite and sleep problems. Increased pulse and blood pressure appear to be due to direct vasopressor effects of the medications (both stimulant classes and atomoxetine), whereas guanfacine can be associated with lowering of pulse and blood pressure, although rebound hypertension needs to be considered as a possibility when stopping medication.[48] Public concerns that stimulant treatment in childhood and adolescence may increase substance use disorders in adulthood seem unsubstantiated.[49]

Non-pharmacological approaches

Non-pharmacological approaches to the treatment of ADHD have been less well studied in general, and the evidence for effective non-pharmacological treatments for adolescents and adults is particularly scarce.[10] In children and adolescents only supplementation with free fatty acids (omega-3, fish oils) and exclusion of artificial food colours from the diet have been shown to have significant beneficial effects on core ADHD symptoms when rigorous approaches to blinding are enforced, and even then the effects are relatively small.[50] Although behavioural parent training approaches improve positive parenting and reduce oppositionality they do not seem to be efficacious in reducing core ADHD symptoms in children.[50] The first studies of cognitive behavioural therapy in ADHD do, however, suggest that this may be an effective approach for treating adolescents and adults with ADHD.[51,52] There is also emerging evidence that mindfulness-based interventions may be effective in ADHD.[53]

Organising and delivering treatment

Despite the availability of highly efficacious treatments, the reported outcomes for ADHD treated within community clinics is not as good as would be expected or hoped for.[54,55] Evidence from clinical trials and observational studies suggests that the way treatment is organised and delivered may be as important as the treatment itself.[55,56] Coghill and Seth demonstrated that, using a structured, measurement-based care approach, clinical outcomes were improved not only such that they were equivalent to those from clinical trials, but also that these effects could be sustained over many years.[56] Their approach included several key components, including a structured titration for medication treatments that aimed to optimise outcome and minimise adverse effects, a standardised approach to measuring clinical outcomes and adverse effects that was implemented at every visit, structured approaches to assessing response at school and the assessment of 'other problems' (comorbidity and other non-health problems) with the ability to address any issues identified in a separate setting. A full description of this approach has been published along with a sample toolkit and protocols.[56] Of these elements we suspect that the use of a measurement-based care approach is the most effective and would be the first change that could be made to most clinical settings.

Stimulant medications only work on the day that they are taken and then for a maximum of 12–13 hours. It is likely that poor adherence to treatment is one of the main reasons for treatment failure. Evidence suggests that whilst compliance with treatment is an issue for those with ADHD across the lifespan, it is a particular problem in youth. A large study of ADHD medication use in the UK found that by age 20 almost all of those young people taking an ADHD medication had stopped. Other challenges to treating ADHD in youth include increased difficulty assessing treatment effects due to less prominent symptoms, less accurate reporting from parents and teachers, low inter-correlation between parent/teacher and self-report of ADHD symptoms, increased complications in choosing appropriate medication due to comorbidity, increased risk of non-compliance or substance abuse. Various approaches to improving adherence have been suggested. These include patient (youth and parent) education, individualised approaches for tailoring medication (as described by Coghill and Seth),[56] behavioural strategies, and peer support strategies (Box 17.2).

Box 17.2 Approaches to improving compliance in adolescence

Patient (youth and parent) education

- Targeting knowledge and skills
- Discussing aetiology and course of ADHD
- Being open and honest about possible short and long term adverse effects
- Elicit and address misconceptions/misinformation about ADHD and ADHD medications
- Make sure psychoeducation is current, unbiased and accurate

Individualised approaches for tailoring medication

- Find out what outcomes are important for each patient
- Maximal therapeutic benefit and minimal adverse effects
- Target the right times of the day
- Use titration protocols
- Simplify dosing

- Allow for flexibility
- Educate about time to response
- Consider changing preparation/medication

Behavioural strategies

- May require work with parents and/or young person
- Target environmental constraints to adherence, improve the salience of taking medication, address habitual and automatic processes that may influence adherence behaviour, and improve patient self-efficacy in taking medication
- Technology-based approaches
- Alerts and reminders to refill scripts and take meds
- Pill reminder boxes, beepers to remind parents/youth to take medication
- Parent training
- Pill swallowing training
- Behavioural approaches to reduce oppositionality and improve overall compliance

Peer support strategies

- Peers are often effective at engaging similarly situated individuals into services because they are viewed as credible role models who provide hope, empower participants and enhance satisfaction with services
- Further, peer-delivered services decrease isolation, normalise feelings of distress and destigmatise views about mental illness and seeking treatment
- Family advocates – to help parents
- Youth advocates – to help adolescents

Another issue of particular importance is the transition from child and adolescent services to adult services. Whilst much of what has been written about this topic is based on opinion rather than evidence, there are several good critiques available, and several of these make clear recommendations.[57,58] Several of the key points are described in Box 17.3. This is an area where child and youth services that extend the age range up to the mid-twenties potentially have a real advantage, particularly those services that run through childhood, adolescence and into young adulthood. Of course this is dependent on those services developing specialist skills in the management of ADHD that can be employed alongside their other areas of focus (e.g., psychosis, eating disorders, substance use disorders and personality disorders), which unfortunately is not always the case. Whilst these services still need to manage transitions with adult services (and child services for those focussing on young people), they have the advantage of not transitioning at the same time as school finishes and a lot of young people are in the middle of many other life transitions.

Box 17.3 Issues to consider when developing protocols for transition between child/adolescent and adult services for ADHD

- The joint development of clear transition protocols should be developed by commissioners, child and adolescent mental health services (CAMHS)/paediatric services, adult mental health services (AMHS) and primary care.
- These should specify time frames, lines of responsibility, who should be involved, how the young person should be prepared and what should happen if AMHS are not able to accept the referral.
- Protocols should allow for flexibility in the age of transition so as to accommodate developmental needs and stages.
- Ideally, transition should occur at a time of clinical stability. Patients should not have to relapse or have worsening mental health in order to continue to be able to access services.
- Transition protocols should include psychoeducational material that provides high-quality, comprehensive, impartial and appropriately written information for both young people and their parents and carers.
- The needs and wishes of parents/carers should be respected and their ongoing involvement with the young person negotiated.
- Health care jurisdictions should be encouraged to use similar care.

Conclusions

ADHD is most often a lifelong condition. Whilst ADHD may present differently at different developmental and life stages, the core presentation remains rather consistent. Comorbidities increase in complexity during adolescence and into adulthood, but despite often complex presentations ADHD in adolescence and through into adulthood can be reliably diagnosed through careful and structured approaches to assessment. Psychoeducation is the pillar of treatment for ADHD across the lifespan. This requires the clinician to have a comprehensive, up-to-date knowledge of ADHD that allows them to impart clear guidance and support for those who are diagnosed and their families. Medication remains a treatment of choice for most of those with ADHD, with the psychostimulants methylphenidate and lisdexamfetamine considered as first-line treatments by most evidence-based guidelines. Atomoxetine is an effective treatment for adolescents and adults, and guanfacine is licensed for adolescents in many countries. Non-pharmacological treatments are less well studied, but early studies suggest that cognitive behavioural therapy can be helpful for adolescents and adults with ADHD. How care is delivered is as important as what is prescribed, and evidence supports the use of measurement-based care approaches in order for treatment optimisation, rather than simple improvement, to be the goal of treatment. Adherence is a particular issue for adolescents with ADHD, although it is also an issue at other ages and stages of development. Recognition of the risks around times of transition are key to improving adherence and engagement with services for those with ADHD and should be considered early in treatment. Another key to ensuring good engagement with services is to maintain as open a door as possible. As in other aspects of their lives, adolescents often have a rather ambivalent relationship with health care. Facilitating them to move back into care with as little fuss as possible increases opportunities for a good outcome and allows the young person to learn from their experiences, setting up better relationships with providers in the future.

References

1 Coghill D, Asherson P, Faraone SV, Rohde LA. The age of onset of attention-deficit hyperactivity disorder. In de Girolamo G, McGorry PD, Sartorius N (Eds) *Age of onset of mental disorders: etiopathogenetic and treatment implications*. New York: Springer; 2018. p 217–36.

2 Polanczyk G, de Lima MS, Horta BL, Biederman J, Rohde LA. The worldwide prevalence of ADHD: a systematic review and metaregression analysis. *American Journal of Psychiatry* 2007;164(6):942–8.

3 Polanczyk GV, Willcutt EG, Salum GA, Kieling C, Rohde LA. ADHD prevalence estimates across three decades: an updated systematic review and meta-regression analysis. *International Journal of Epidemiology* 2014;43(2):434–42.

4 Raman SR, Man KKC, Bahmanyar S, Berard A, Bilder S, Boukhris T, et al. Trends in attention-deficit hyperactivity disorder medication use: a retrospective observational study using population-based databases. *Lancet Psychiatry* 2018;5(10):824–35.

5 Hinshaw SP, Scheffler RM, Fulton BD, Aase H, Banaschewski T, Cheng W, et al. International variation in treatment procedures for ADHD: social context and recent trends. *Psychiatric Services* 2011;62(5):459–64.

6 Visser SN, Danielson ML, Bitsko RH, Holbrook JR, Kogan MD, Ghandour RM, et al. Trends in the parent-report of health care provider-diagnosed and medicated attention-deficit/hyperactivity disorder: United States, 2003–2011. *Journal of the American Academy of Child and Adolescent Psychiatry* 2014;53(1):34–46.

7 McCarthy S, Asherson P, Coghill D, Hollis C, Murray M, Potts L, et al. Attention-deficit hyperactivity disorder: treatment discontinuation in adolescents and young adults. *British Journal of Psychiatry* 2009;194(3):273–7.

8 Simon V, Czobor P, Bálint S, Mészáros A, Bitter I. Prevalence and correlates of adult attention-deficit hyperactivity disorder: meta-analysis. *British Journal of Psychiatry* 2009;194(3):204–11.

9 Matte B, Anselmi L, Salum GA, Kieling C, Gonçalves H, Menezes A, et al. ADHD in DSM-5: a field trial in a large, representative sample of 18- to 19-year-old adults. *Psychological Medicine* 2015;45(2):361–73.

10 Franke B, Michelini G, Asherson P, Banaschewski T, Bilbow A, Buitelaar JK, et al. Live fast, die young? A review on the developmental trajectories of ADHD across the lifespan. *European Neuropsychopharmacology* 2018;28(10):1059–88.

11 Faraone SV, Biederman J, Mick E. The age-dependent decline of attention deficit hyperactivity disorder: a meta-analysis of follow-up studies. *Psychological Medicine* 2006;36(2):159–65.

12 Cheung CH, Rijdijk F, McLoughlin G, Faraone SV, Asherson P, Kuntsi J. Childhood predictors of adolescent and young adult outcome in ADHD. *Journal of Psychiatric Research* 2015;62:92–100.

13 van Lieshout M, Luman M, Twisk JW, van Ewijk H, Groenman AP, Thissen AJ, et al. A 6-year follow-up of a large European cohort of children with attention-deficit/hyperactivity disorder-combined subtype: outcomes in late adolescence and young adulthood. *European Child & Adolescent Psychiatry* 2016;25(9):1007–17.

14 Kooij SJ, Bejerot S, Blackwell A, Caci H, Casas-Brugué M, Carpentier PJ, et al. European consensus statement on diagnosis and treatment of adult ADHD: the European Network Adult ADHD. *BMC Psychiatry* 2010;10:67.

15 Larsson H, Dilshad R, Lichtenstein P, Barker ED. Developmental trajectories of DSM-IV symptoms of attention-deficit/hyperactivity disorder: genetic effects, family risk and associated psychopathology. *Journal of Child Psychology and Psychiatry* 2011;52(9):954–63.

16 Lara C, Fayyad J, de Graaf R, Kessler RC, Aguilar-Gaxiola S, Angermeyer M, et al. Childhood predictors of adult attention-deficit/hyperactivity disorder: results from the World Health Organization World Mental Health Survey Initiative. *Biological Psychiatry* 2009;65(1):46–54.

17 Biederman J, Petty CR, Clarke A, Lomedico A, Faraone SV. Predictors of persistent ADHD: an 11-year follow-up study. *Journal of Psychiatric Research* 2011;45(2):150–5.

18 Biederman J, Petty CR, O'Connor KB, Hyder LL, Faraone SV. Predictors of persistence in girls with attention deficit hyperactivity disorder: results from an 11-year controlled follow-up study. *Acta Psychiatrica Scandinavica* 2012;125(2):147–56.

19 Asherson P, Young AH, Eich-Höchli D, Moran P, Porsdal V, Deberdt W. Differential diagnosis, comorbidity, and treatment of attention-deficit/hyperactivity disorder in relation to bipolar disorder or borderline personality disorder in adults. *Current Medical Research and Opinion* 2014;30(8):1657–72.

20 Philipsen A, Limberger MF, Lieb K, Feige B, Kleindienst N, Ebner-Priemer U, et al. Attention-deficit hyperactivity disorder as a potentially aggravating factor in borderline personality disorder. *British Journal of Psychiatry* 2008;192(2):118–23.

21 Thapar A, Harrington R, Ross K, McGuffin P. Does the definition of ADHD affect heritability? *Journal of the American Academy of Child and Adolescent Psychiatry* 2000; 39(12):1528–36.

22 Martin J, O'Donovan MC, Thapar A, Langley K, Williams N. The relative contribution of common and rare genetic variants to ADHD. *Translational Psychiatry* 2015;5:e506.

23 Demontis D, Walters RK, Martin J, Mattheisen M, Als TD, Agerbo E, et al. Discovery of the first genome-wide significant risk loci for attention deficit/hyperactivity disorder. *Nature Genetics* 2019;51(1):63–75.

24 Sciberras E, Mulraney M, Silva D, Coghill D. Prenatal risk factors and the etiology of ADHD-review of existing evidence. *Current Psychiatry Reports* 2017;19(1):1.

25 Skoglund C, Chen Q, D'Onofrio BM, Lichtenstein P, Larsson H. Familial confounding of the association between maternal smoking during pregnancy and ADHD in offspring. *Journal of Child Psychology and Psychiatry* 2014;55(1):61–8.

26 Langley K, Heron J, Smith GD, Thapar A. Maternal and paternal smoking during pregnancy and risk of ADHD symptoms in offspring: testing for intrauterine effects. *American Journal of Epidemiology* 2012;176(3):261–8.

27 McCann D, Barrett A, Cooper A, Crumpler D, Dalen L, Grimshaw K, et al. Food additives and hyperactive behaviour in 3-year-old and 8/9-year-old children in the community: a randomised, double-blinded, placebo-controlled trial. *Lancet* 2007;370 (9598):1560–7.

28 Russell G, Ford T, Rosenberg R, Kelly S. The association of attention deficit hyperactivity disorder with socioeconomic disadvantage: alternative explanations and evidence. *Journal of Child Psychology and Psychiatry* 2014;55(5):436–45.

29 McMillen JC, Zima BT, Scott LD Jr, Auslander WF, Munson MR, Ollie MT, et al. Prevalence of psychiatric disorders among older youths in the foster care system. *Journal of the American Academy of Child and Adolescent Psychiatry* 2005;44(1):88–95.
30 Cortese S, Kelly C, Chabernaud C, Proal E, Di Martino A, Milham MP, et al. Toward systems neuroscience of ADHD: a meta-analysis of 55 fMRI studies. *American Journal of Psychiatry* 2012;169(10):1038–55.
31 Frodl T, Skokauskas N. Meta-analysis of structural MRI studies in children and adults with attention deficit hyperactivity disorder indicates treatment effects. *Acta Psychiatrica Scandinavica* 2012;125(2):114–26.
32 Hoogman M, Bralten J, Hibar DP, Mennes M, Zwiers MP, Schweren LSJ, et al. Subcortical brain volume differences in participants with attention deficit hyperactivity disorder in children and adults: a cross-sectional mega-analysis. *Lancet Psychiatry* 2017;4(4):310–9.
33 Castellanos FX, Lee PP, Sharp W, Jeffries NO, Greenstein DK, Clasen LS, et al. Developmental trajectories of brain volume abnormalities in children and adolescents with attention-deficit/hyperactivity disorder. *JAMA* 2002;288(14):1740–8.
34 Shaw P, Lerch J, Greenstein D, Sharp W, Clasen L, Evans A, et al. Longitudinal mapping of cortical thickness and clinical outcome in children and adolescents with attention-deficit/hyperactivity disorder. *Archives of General Psychiatry* 2006;63(5):540–9.
35 Shaw P, Malek M, Watson B, Greenstein D, de Rossi P, Sharp W. Trajectories of cerebral cortical development in childhood and adolescence and adult attention-deficit/hyperactivity disorder. *Biological Psychiatry* 2013;74(8):599–606.
36 Coghill DR, Seth S, Matthews K. A comprehensive assessment of memory, delay aversion, timing, inhibition, decision making and variability in attention deficit hyperactivity disorder: advancing beyond the three-pathway models. *Psychological Medicine* 2014;44(9):1989–2001.
37 O'Neil S, Halperin JM, Coghill D. Neuropsychological functioning and ADHD: a developmental perspective. In Banaschewski T, Coghill D, Zuddas A (Eds) *Oxford textbook of attention deficit hyperactivity disorder*. Oxford: Oxford University Press; 2018. p 118–27.
38 van Lieshout M, Luman M, Twisk JW, Faraone SV, Heslenfeld DJ, Hartman CA, et al. Neurocognitive predictors of ADHD outcome: a 6-year follow-up study. *Journal of Abnormal Child Psychology* 2017;45(2):261–72.
39 Coghill DR, Hayward D, Rhodes SM, Grimmer C, Matthews K. A longitudinal examination of neuropsychological and clinical functioning in boys with attention deficit hyperactivity disorder (ADHD): improvements in executive functioning do not explain clinical improvement. *Psychological Medicine* 2014;44(5):1087–99.
40 Taylor E, Döpfner M, Sergeant J, Asherson P, Banaschewski T, Buitelaar J, et al. European clinical guidelines for hyperkinetic disorder – first upgrade. *European Child & Adolescent Psychiatry* 2004;13(1):17–30.
41 Bolea-Alamañac B, Nutt DJ, Adamou M, Asherson P, Bazire S, Coghill D, et al. Evidence-based guidelines for the pharmacological management of attention deficit hyperactivity disorder: update on recommendations from the British Association for Psychopharmacology. *Journal of Psychopharmacology* 2014;28(3):179–203.
42 NICE. *Attention deficit hyperactivity disorder: diagnosis and management of ADHD in children, young people and adults*. London: National Institute for Health and Clinical Excellence; 2008.
43 Asherson P. ADHD in adults. In Banaschewski T, Zuddas A, Asherson P, Buitelaar J, Coghill D, Danckaerts M, et al. (Eds) *ADHD and hyperkinetic disorder*. Oxford: Oxford University Press; 2015. p 89–111.

44 Caspi A, Langley K, Milne B, Moffitt TE, O'Donovan M, Owen MJ, et al. A replicated molecular genetic basis for subtyping antisocial behavior in children with attention-deficit/hyperactivity disorder. *Archives of General Psychiatry* 2008;65(2):203–10.

45 Cortese S, Adamo N, Del Giovane C, Mohr-Jensen C, Hayes AJ, Carucci S, et al. Comparative efficacy and tolerability of medications for attention-deficit hyperactivity disorder in children, adolescents, and adults: a systematic review and network meta-analysis. *Lancet Psychiatry* 2018;5(9):727–38.

46 NICE. *Attention deficit hyperactivity disorder: diagnosis and management; NICE guideline [NG87]*. London: National Institute for Health and Care Excellence; 2018.

47 Hodgkins P, Shaw M, Coghill D, Hechtman L. Amfetamine and methylphenidate medications for attention-deficit/hyperactivity disorder: complementary treatment options. *European Child & Adolescent Psychiatry* 2012;21(9):477–92.

48 Cortese S, Holtmann M, Banaschewski T, Buitelaar J, Coghill D, Danckaerts M, et al. Practitioner review: current best practice in the management of adverse events during treatment with ADHD medications in children and adolescents. *Journal of Child Psychology and Psychiatry* 2013;54(3):227–46.

49 Dalsgaard S, Mortensen PB, Frydenberg M, Thomsen PH. ADHD, stimulant treatment in childhood and subsequent substance abuse in adulthood – a naturalistic long-term follow-up study. *Addictive Behaviors* 2014;39(1):325–8.

50 Sonuga-Barke EJ, Brandeis D, Cortese S, Daley D, Ferrin M, Holtmann M, et al. Non-pharmacological interventions for ADHD: systematic review and meta-analyses of randomized controlled trials of dietary and psychological treatments. *American Journal of Psychiatry* 2013;170(3):275–89.

51 Antshel KM. Psychosocial interventions in attention-deficit/hyperactivity disorder: update. *Child and Adolescent Psychiatric Clinics of North America* 2015;24(1):79–97.

52 Solanto MV, Marks DJ, Wasserstein J, Mitchell K, Abikoff H, Alvir JM, et al. Efficacy of meta-cognitive therapy for adult ADHD. *American Journal of Psychiatry* 2010; 167(8):958–68.

53 Cairncross M, Miller CJ. The effectiveness of mindfulness-based therapies for ADHD: a meta-analytic review. *Journal of Attention Disorders* 2020;24(5):627–43.

54 Langley K, Fowler T, Ford T, Thapar AK, van den Bree M, Harold G, et al. Adolescent clinical outcomes for young people with attention-deficit hyperactivity disorder. *British Journal of Psychiatry* 2010;196(3):235–40.

55 Swanson JM, Arnold LE, Jensen P, Hinshaw SP, Hechtman LT, Conners CK, et al. Long- term outcomes in the Multimodal Treatment study of Children with ADHD (the MTA): from beginning to end. In Banaschewski T, Coghill D, Zuddas A (Eds) *Oxford textbook of attention deficit hyperactivity disorder*. Oxford: Oxford University Press; 2018. p 315–32.

56 Coghill D, Seth S. Effective management of attention-deficit/hyperactivity disorder (ADHD) through structured re-assessment: the Dundee ADHD Clinical Care Pathway. *Child and Adolescent Psychiatry and Mental Health* 2015;9:52.

57 Young S, Adamou M, Asherson P, Coghill D, Colley B, Gudjonsson G, et al. Recommendations for the transition of patients with ADHD from child to adult healthcare services: a consensus statement from the UK adult ADHD network. *BMC Psychiatry* 2016;16:301.

58 Young S, Murphy CM, Coghill D. Avoiding the 'twilight zone': recommendations for the transition of services from adolescence to adulthood for young people with ADHD. *BMC Psychiatry* 2011;11:174.

18 The mental health of LGBTIQA+ young people

Ashleigh Lin, Penelope Strauss, Dylan Gilbey and Yael Perry

Introduction

LGBTIQA+ is the acronym used to describe people who are lesbian, gay, bisexual, transgender, intersex, queer/questioning, asexual and of other diverse sexual, gender and bodily identities. We use this umbrella term in the broadest possible way to be inclusive of all diverse sexualities, genders and bodily variations. In doing so, we acknowledge that people with LGBTIQA+ identities have in common experiences of discrimination, harassment and marginalisation from society, and the need for safe and inclusive health care. However, we also acknowledge the limitations of LGBTIQA+ language when attempting to speak about the full breadth of people's bodies, genders, relationships, sexualities and lived experiences. Each identity, and within that, every LGBTIQA+ individual, has unique needs, challenges, experiences and strengths.

Many hundreds of terms are used by young people to describe their experience of being LGBTIQA+ in a way that feels right for them, and these terms are constantly changing. Acknowledging the terms chosen by a young person and using them correctly when talking to or about a person is validating and humanising. The term "queer" has historically been used as a slur to describe people of diverse sexuality. However, many young people have reclaimed the term, using it instead to celebrate the diversity of sexual, gender and bodily identities in an inclusive way.

Sexual diversity

Most people are familiar with diverse sexualities such as being lesbian, gay and bisexual (see Box 18.1). Other sexual identities, such as asexual and pansexual, may be less familiar. Asexuality is a sexual orientation characterised by a persistent lack of sexual attraction toward any people of any gender; it is estimated that between 1% and 2% of the population identify as asexual.[1,2] Pansexuality refers to sexual attraction regardless of gender and outside of binary gender definitions. It is also worth noting that not all people with diverse sexualities will necessarily identify with any of these labels, and young people are increasingly eschewing labels for their sexuality entirely. For this reason, among others, estimating the proportion of people in the population with diverse sexualities is difficult and such estimates vary widely; however, there is evidence to suggest that the number of young people expressing diverse sexualities is growing.

Box 18.1 What does sexuality mean?

Sexuality is multifaceted. It is generally thought to consist of at least three dimensions:

- **Attraction:** to whom you're attracted sexually, or have feelings for romantically
- **Behaviour:** with whom you engage in sexual activity or romantic relationships
- **Identity:** the label with which you self-identify, e.g., "lesbian"

These dimensions do not always correlate with one another. For example, a man may identify as bisexual despite having only ever had relationships with women, or a man may identify as straight despite having had passing sexual encounters with other men. Even where people's identification may be incongruent, these identities should always be validated and respected.

Some specific sexual and romantic identities are:

- Gay
- Lesbian
- Bisexual/Bi
- Pansexual/Pan
- Asexual/Ace
- Aromantic

Gender diversity

Trans and gender diverse (TGD) people identify as a gender that does not align with the sex they were assigned at birth (see Box 18.2). Recent estimates suggest that 2.3%–2.7% of high-school aged adolescents identify as TGD,[3,4] and a recent Australian study found that almost half of TGD young people aged 14–25 describe their gender in non-binary terms (neither male nor female gender), such as non-binary, agender and genderqueer.[5]

Box 18.2 What does trans and gender diverse mean?

Trans and gender diverse refers to people whose gender identity does not match the sex assigned to them at birth (that which is on their birth certificate). This contrasts with cisgender people whose gender does match the sex they were assigned at birth. Many trans and gender diverse individuals identify as male or female, while others identify with other genders. Some specific gender identities are:

- Trans Male
- Male
- Trans Female
- Female
- Non-binary
- Genderqueer
- Agender
- Genderfluid

Historically, both gender and sexuality identities that differed from heteronormative and cisnormative roles were classified as disorders in diagnostic manuals. While homosexuality has been removed as a psychiatric diagnosis, diagnoses for gender diversity remain in these manuals. The new ICD-11 lists two "Gender Incongruence" diagnoses as conditions related to sexual health (one for adolescents and adults and another for pre-pubertal children), which replace prior "Gender Identity Disorder" diagnoses from the ICD-10 which was listed as a mental disorder. The DSM-5 uses "Gender Dysphoria" as a diagnosis for all ages including pre-pubertal children, with two miscellaneous categories ("other specified" and "unspecified"). Importantly, not everyone who is TGD will experience gender dysphoria, which refers specifically to the distress experienced by an individual because of the mismatch between the gender identity and the sex characteristics.

Box 18.3 What are pronouns and why should I use them?

Everyone has pronouns, regardless of their gender identity. Using the correct pronouns for someone is important as it validates their identity. The most common pronouns are:

- She/her/hers
- He/him/his
- They/them/theirs

Never assume someone's pronouns based on their appearance, behaviour, name or any other characteristic. It is best practice to ask for someone's pronouns and then use those pronouns. If you make a mistake, apologise, move on, and try not to make the mistake again. Using the incorrect pronouns for someone is a form of *misgendering*.

Bodily diversity

Intersex individuals are people with an intersex variation – a term used to describe individuals who are born with congenital atypical sex traits that may be chromosomal, hormonal and/or anatomical characteristics. It is estimated that 1%–2% of the population has an intersex variation, however this is likely a conservative estimate due to the physical invisibility of many variations and associated lack of awareness by many intersex individuals until later in life.[6] The known proportions of people with intersex variations (or any other LGBTIQA+ people, for that matter) in the population are also likely underestimated due to lack of awareness or experienced stigma and fear of stigma leading to non-disclosure. Intersex characteristics are included under "Disorder of Sex Development" in the ICD-11. Of note, internationally, statements from intersex advocates such as the Malta Declaration and Darlington Statement call for the depathologising of variations in sex characteristics in medical guidelines, protocols and classifications because it is stigmatising and harmful.[7,8]

The aforementioned categories are not mutually exclusive, and any one individual may identify with one or more of these identities. Everyone's sexuality, gender identity and body variation are unique to them, and assumptions about one aspect of a person based on another should be avoided.[9]

Mental health and LGBTIQA+ young people

LGBTIQA+ young people are significantly more vulnerable to mental health difficulties than their peers. Crucially, this is not as a direct result of their LGBTIQA+ identity, but rather the fact that LGBTIQA+ young people are faced with a range of negative experiences including stigma, discrimination, harassment and marginalisation, which place them at higher risk for developing mental health difficulties. There is strong evidence that LGBTIQA+ young people have higher rates of psychological distress, depression and anxiety, and suicidal thoughts than the general population.[6,10–12]

It is well documented that notable disparities exist between the mental health and wellbeing of lesbian, gay or bisexual (LGB) young people and their heterosexual peers. Relative to heterosexual youth, young people who identify as LGB are more likely to express depressive symptomatology, have problems with substance abuse and have a significantly elevated risk of suicidality. Recent international meta-analytic evidence demonstrates that LGB youth are roughly twice more likely than their heterosexual-identifying peers to have at least one suicide attempt. Such disparities have been observed as early as late childhood and are relatively constant into adulthood; however, late adolescence may be a period of particular risk of mental health difficulties for LGB youth. Notably, these disparities are not uniform among LGB youth. Bisexual young people of any gender appear to be at particular risk of mental health difficulties, such as depressive symptomatology and suicidality, over and above that experienced by gay and lesbian young people, and lesbian and bisexual young women may be at particular risk over and above gay and bisexual young men.[13]

TGD young people experience markedly poorer mental health outcomes than the general population and LGB youth. Data from 859 TGD young people aged 14–25 years in the *Trans Pathways* study revealed that this population experiences especially poor mental health. Findings indicated that three in four TGD young people had been diagnosed with depression and/or anxiety, 80% had self-harmed and almost one in two (48.1%) had attempted to end their life by suicide.[5] This suicide attempt rate is approximately 20 times the rate of attempted suicide of a general adolescent population in Australia[14] and is remarkably similar to those reported in young TGD populations in the United Kingdom, where the suicide attempt rate was 45%.[12] As with sexually diverse young people, mental health difficulties and risk of suicidality begin early in this population; for example, in *Trans Pathways* there was no significant difference in the rate of suicide attempts between participants aged under 18 and those who were 18 or older.

There is a critical lack of research with regard to the mental health of intersex young people, due in part to the fact that many individuals only discover their intersex status as an adult, often when the issue of fertility arises. The most common mental health difficulties faced by intersex individuals are depression, anxiety and PTSD. They also face increased risk of self-harm and suicide compared to the general Australian population.[6]

Risk factors for mental health difficulties in LGBTIQA+ young people

Stigma is a significant risk factor for mental health difficulties in LGBTIQA+ young people. Stigma occurs when societal or cultural norms define particular attributes, such as diverse sexuality, gender and/or bodily variations, as abnormal, shameful or otherwise undesirable. This can lead to prejudice and discrimination against people expressing the stigmatised attribute. Another consequence of stigma can be self-stigma, which is the process by which members of stigmatised populations come to internalise and self-identify with the stigma to which they are exposed, that is, agreeing that the way they are is abnormal, shameful or undesirable. By early adolescence, most young people will already be aware of dominant cultural attitudes towards stigmatised attributes such as diverse gender, sexuality or body variations.[15–17] This corresponds to the period in which most people begin to become aware of their developing sexual orientation and in many cases, their gender. As such, early adolescence will typically be when stigma and self-stigma will begin to impact the mental health of LGBTIQA+ young people, although many LGBTIQA+ young people report identifying feelings of difference much earlier in childhood. Importantly, stigma and self-stigma present significant barriers to disclosure and help-seeking and may result in isolation and low self-esteem.[18]

Largely as a result of stigma, LGBTIQA+ young people experience higher rates of bullying and exclusion than their heterosexual and cisgender peers. In addition, many LGBTIQA+ young people feel isolated; this is heightened for young people living in rural and remote regions where stigma may be greater and service access poorer. Many LGBTIQA+ young people are unsupported by peers and family members, making them more likely to leave school and more likely to experience homelessness than youth from the general population.[19,20] Indeed, LGBTIQA+ young people are overrepresented within homeless services, with up to 30% of clients identifying as LGBTIQA+.[19] In addition, LGBTIQA+ young people who experience homelessness are also more likely to be homeless longer. The experience of trauma is also common in LGBTIQA+ young people, ranging from bullying by peers to physical and sexual abuse within and outside of the family. We caution against the assumption that these experiences of abuse are in any way causative of these young peoples' LGBTIQA+ identities. Rather, factors commonly associated with these identities, such as gender nonconformity in childhood or increased sexual risk-taking in adolescence, may increase their likelihood of being targets of maltreatment or abuse.[21]

Intersex individuals may have additional experiences that are likely to impact mental wellbeing. They may experience trauma due to medical interventions (namely surgery) performed often at a young age to "correct" anatomy so that sexual characteristics align with traditional cisnormative ideas of the sexual anatomy of a male or female. Surgical procedures conducted in infancy may be kept secret from the individual, which results in a feeling of the loss of bodily autonomy and associated trauma.[22] Families who are informed of their child's intersex variation may be presented with information by medical staff such that the only solution appears to be surgical intervention, but in order to better support intersex individuals it is crucial that families and the individual are provided with accurate information about the lifelong experiences of people with intersex variations. In general, broader society should be exposed to information about intersex variations to increase understanding and acceptance, and human variation should be recognised as expansive beyond traditional male and female body types.

In addition to mental health difficulties, substance use and problems related to sexual health are prevalent issues faced by LGBTIQA+ young people. LGBTIQA+ young people are more likely to use alcohol, smoke cigarettes and use other drugs than their peers. Research suggests that this could be due to the higher incidence of mental health problems and may serve as a way of dealing with abuse and discrimination, but peer modelling in the LGBTIQA+ community also likely plays a role in the high incidence of substance use in this young population.[23] LGBTIQA+ young people have difficulty accessing relevant sexual health education as it often is focused predominantly on heterosexual relationships and reproduction and does not address gender diversity, same-sex attraction or diversity of bodies sufficiently, or at all. This can lead to misinformation, impacting the sexual health and wellbeing of LGBTIQA+ young people, as well as perpetuating feelings of difference, impacting mental health as well.[24]

Although we cite risk factors here which may help explain additional risk for mental health difficulties in LGBTIQA+ young people overall, we note also that these young people also experience largely the same negative experiences and risk factors for poor mental health as their peers. An LGBTIQA+ person who is seeking help due to experiencing mental health difficulties may therefore be doing so for reasons entirely unrelated to their gender, sexuality or bodily variation or any of the risk factors described earlier.

Experiences with health services

In general, many young people are confronted with barriers to uptake of services, including accessibility, cost, perceived stigma and concerns about the characteristics of the provider. Due to the range of difficulties often experienced by LGBTIQA+ young people discussed previously, such as low parental support and homelessness, some of these barriers to formal help-seeking may be heightened for LGBTIQA+ young people. This problem is further compounded by the presence of additional unique barriers to help-seeking, such as the heteronormative assumptions LGBTIQA+ people face specifically around sexual health needs (for example, providers often assume the gender of the client's sexual partner[s] and are unaware of the sexual health needs of the individual).[25] LGBTIQA+ young people may also fear their confidentiality being compromised by service providers. Expectations of stigma from service providers is also a major barrier to help-seeking in this population. Research has shown that for these reasons, among others, LGBTIQA+ young people commonly do not reach out for help until they are already in crisis.

These problems are especially notable among TGD young people, who face additional obstacles in terms of potential refusal of care, transphobia, discrimination or lack of provider knowledge, experience or sensitivity. One study found that 60% of TGD young people felt isolated from health services and that 42% had reached out to a health service that did not understand, respect or have previous experience with TGD people.[5] From the perspective of TGD youth, this lack of access to competent health care only serves to reinforce their relative unimportance and marginality in society. Optimal health care for TGD young people urgently requires improved service provision to reduce the unacceptable rates of mental health difficulties and suicidality in this population.

There is a lack of research into the experiences of intersex individuals accessing health services; however, intersex individuals also report negative experiences in their interactions with health and education services, employment and other general community settings. Support programs alleviating isolation, hopelessness and anxiety are crucially important.

Improving the mental health of LGBTIQA+ young people

The high rates of poor mental health and suicidality in LGBTIQA+ young people highlight the urgent need for safe and effective prevention and intervention strategies. The risk factors discussed previously suggest some clear targets for intervention, for example, decreasing bullying, targeting potential causes of homelessness such as increasing familial acceptance, and increasing awareness of LGBTIQA+ identities among peers. However, overall, strategies for reducing the mental health disparity between LGBTIQA+ young people and their peers from the general population need to be multifaceted. These approaches should include individual prevention and intervention strategies, family interventions and intervention at societal and structural levels seeking to improve the social environment for LGBTIQA+ young people and reduce the prevalence of the stressors described earlier. Although the focus of this chapter is on working individually with LGBTIQA+ young people who are experiencing mental health difficulties, we must also acknowledge that their increased risk of these difficulties is a product of their stigmatising social environment and that to reduce these disparities in the long term, it is ultimately these social determinants which need to change. Of note, it is now well accepted that "conversion therapies" that attempt to change sexual or gender identities are traumatising and dangerous for the mental wellbeing of LGBTIQA+ people.[26,27]

In terms of individual interventions, one cannot assume that treatments that are evidence based for use in the general population are equally efficacious in LGBTIQA+ populations or appropriate for their specific needs and experiences. Resources that do not mention or portray LGBTIQA+ people are unlikely to lead LGBTIQA+ young people to feel included or acknowledged. At best, this may present a barrier to their engagement with the information or treatment but may even increase feelings of invisibility and exacerbate existing self-stigma and mental health difficulties. For these reasons, many LGBTIQA+ young people have expressed preference for treatment which is specifically LGBTIQA+ centred, although this preference may not be universal. When deciding on or offering intervention for LGBTIQA+ young people, the availability of such targeted resources or treatments should be considered and discussed with the client.[18,24]

Suicide prevention is a particular area that requires additional evidence in LGBTIQA+ youth populations. One study recently showed that LGBT people aged 12–14 represent roughly a quarter of all deaths by suicide in that age group;[28] this significantly outweighs the proportion of LGBTIQA+ people and is likely an underestimate, as many young people may die by suicide before disclosing their LGBTIQA+ identity. We know of no suicide prevention guidelines or interventions developed specifically for LGBTIQA+ young people, even though the level of risk suggests that there is great need for clinical services which serve young people to engage in suicide prevention practices that are appropriate for this group.

There is growing recognition of the utility and value of digital interventions for LGBTIQA+ young people.[29–31] This is due to the strong use of digital technologies among this group, as well as the ability of this mode of treatment to overcome many of the barriers to help-seeking described earlier, such as fear of stigma and accessibility. However, many existing digital interventions are unsuitable for LGBTIQA+ young people because, for example, they assume or imply heterosexuality. To remedy this, there has been increased empirical investigation into the effectiveness of digital interventions targeting sexually diverse youth (see *Rainbow SPARX*, for example),[32] but to date, there remain no evidence-based interventions of this nature aimed specifically at TGD or intersex young people. Whether TGD and intersex young people derive equal or less benefit – or potential harms – from existing programs compared with their peers is unknown. Pending outcomes of empirical investigation, we must establish whether current interventions should be used or adapted, or if novel programs are necessary to achieve meaningful outcomes in LGBTIQA+ populations.

Looking forward, there are several further avenues which could be pursued in terms of improving the mental wellbeing of LGBTIQA+ young people. Given the high rates of trauma (including abuse, discrimination and bullying) in this group, a trauma-informed approach may be worth considering in clinical settings and interventions. Additionally, while many risk factors for mental health are external factors such as abuse and discrimination, internal factors such as self-stigma and self-esteem may also be important factors to consider for interventions with LGBTIQA+ young people. To ensure interventions are informed by the lived experience of those individuals who will use them, the inclusion of LGBTIQA+ young people in the design, development (or adaptation) and implementation of mental health resources will be crucial. Steps to LGBTIQA+ inclusive practice and tips for terminology are included in Box 18.4.

Box 18.4 First steps to inclusive practice

- The *physical environment* of a clinical setting can immediately tell a young person how welcoming the service is. Ways in which you can create an inclusive environment are:
    - Gender neutral bathrooms
    - Inclusive, non-assuming administrative forms
    - Display evidence that it is a safe space (e.g., posters, flags)
- *Consider why you are asking about gender, sexuality or intersex status.* If what you are asking is not directly relevant to the topic at hand, and your client has not brought this up themselves, is there a reason you need to know? These are very personal aspects of a person's identity, and young people may not want to discuss this with you.
- *Do not make assumptions about people's gender and sexuality.* Conversations about gender and sexuality should be approached with openness about the individual's feelings, experiences and identity. We encourage clinicians to tread a balance between awareness and acknowledgment of the unique experiences of LGBTIQA+ young people, without assuming that these experiences are universal to this population, or even why they're seeing you.
- Be aware that *some people may not know that they are intersex*, and many do not learn this about themselves until later in life (e.g., when trying to conceive). Some people who are intersex may have undergone medical procedures as an infant, child or adolescent without their consent, and this experience can be traumatic.

Some tips for inclusive terminology:

- Reflect the language a person has used for themselves (for example, their name that they use may not match their official documents).

- Ask respectfully what name and pronouns a person uses. Consider offering them your pronouns in return, or having your pronouns displayed (e.g., on your email signature or on visible identification).
- Avoid gendering when it's unnecessary – use "they, them, their, theirs" or their name. Other un-gendered language – "parent" "partner" "folks" "sibling" "everyone" "people".
- Don't assume gender identity based on gender expression, sex characteristics or lack of disclosure.
- Avoid generalisations regarding gender, sex & sexuality, and challenge gender roles, myths and stereotypes.

Intersectional identities

The experience of living at the intersection of multiple identities is sometimes not considered by health care providers in their interactions with LGBTIQA+ young people. When assessing or treating a LGBTIQA+ young person, it is vital to consider the intersecting influence of these identities on their mental health, including, but not limited to, age, sexuality, gender, culture, race, ethnicity and religion. Some of these factors may play a role in family acceptance of the young person's identity; this is particularly important because it is well established that parental acceptance is a major protective factor for mental wellbeing in this population. LGBTIQA+ young people with a disability have a different experience to their peers without disabilities and may face "double discrimination" which impacts mental health. Moreover, it is imperative to not assume that the same techniques used with adults will be successful with young people: assessments and interventions should be developmentally appropriate and informed by youth populations. In general, there is a lack of research on how the various intersectional ties impact the social and emotional wellbeing and mental health of LGBTIQA+ young people. Thus, the best understanding of this can be garnered from an in-depth conversation with the young person where these issues are thoroughly explored. Following this, care needs to be provided in a way that is acceptable and safe for the young person. For example, an Indigenous LGBTIQA+ young person has a right to health care that is both culturally appropriate and inclusive of their LGBTIQA+ status.

Box 18.5 Gender-affirmation for TGD young people

The ability to affirm one's gender through social, medical and legal means is beneficial for the mental health of young people.

Social affirmation refers to the changing of appearance (e.g., clothing, hair), name and pronouns to align with gender identity. **Gender-affirming medical intervention** includes hormonal intervention (which can be pubertal suppression or gender-affirming hormones such as oestrogen or testosterone) and/or surgery(ies). **Legal transition** includes changing name and/or gender/sex marker on forms of identification, such as one's birth certificate and passport. Not all TGD people will chose medical intervention; for many, socially affirming their gender is sufficient. Importantly, the ability of a young person to undertake steps towards gender-affirmation is dependent on familial, cultural and legal factors which differ around the world.

Where to from here?

LGBTIQA+ young people represent a significant proportion of the young population and an even more significant proportion of young people experiencing mental health difficulties. Despite this, they have limited access to safe and appropriate health care. In addition to the development and/or validation of interventions for this population, there is clearly a need for practitioners to be aware of the unique issues facing LGBTIQA+ young people. All disciplines involving care of young people (including but not limited to psychology, psychiatry and general medicine) should receive training in their core curricula to equip the future workforce with skills to work with this population.

References

1 Rothblum ED, Krueger EA, Kittle KR, Meyer IH. Asexual and non-asexual respondents from a U.S. population-based study of sexual minorities. *Archives of Sexual Behavior* 2020;49(2):757–67.

2 Bogaert AF. Asexuality: prevalence and associated factors in a national probability sample. *Journal of Sex Research* 2004;41(3):279–87.

3 Fisher CM, Waling A, Kerr L, Bellamy R, Ezer P, Mikolajczak G, et al. *6th national survey of Australian secondary students and sexual health 2018*. Bundoora: Australian Research Centre in Sex, Health & Society, La Trobe University; 2019.

4 Rider GN, McMorris BJ, Gower AL, Coleman E, Eisenberg ME. Health and care utilization of transgender and gender nonconforming youth: a population-based study. *Pediatrics* 2018;141(3):e20171683.

5 Strauss P, Cook A, Winter S, Watson V, Wright Toussaint D, Lin A. *Trans pathways: the mental health experiences and care pathways of trans young people. Summary of results*. Perth: Telethon Kids Institute; 2017.

6 Jones T, Hart B, Carpenter M, Ansara G, Leonard W, Lucke J. *Intersex: stories and statistics from Australia*. Cambridge: Open Book Publishers; 2016.

7 Third International Intersex Forum. *Public statement by the Third International Intersex Forum (Malta Declaration)*. Malta: Third International Intersex Forum; 2013. Retrieved from: http://intersexday.org/en/third-international-intersex-forum/

8 Androgen Insensitivity Syndrome Support Group Australia (AISSGA), Intersex Trust Aotearoa New Zealand (ITANZ), Organisation Intersex International Australia (OIIAU), et al. *Darlington Statement: joint consensus statement from the intersex community retreat in Darlington, March 2017*. Retrieved from: http://darlington.org.au/statement/

9 Grinspan MC, Carpenter M, Ehrt J, Kara S, Narrain A, Patel P, et al. *The Yogyakarta Principles plus 10: additional principles and state obligations on the application of international human rights law in relation to sexual orientation, gender identity, gender expression and sex characteristics to complement the Yogyakarta Principles.* Geneva; 2017. Retrieved from: www.yogyakartaprinciples.org/principles-en/yp10/

10 Andersen JP, Blosnich J. Disparities in adverse childhood experiences among sexual minority and heterosexual adults: results from a multi-state probability-based sample. *PLoS One* 2013;8(1):e54691.

11 Strauss P, Cook A, Winter S, Watson V, Wright Toussaint D, Lin A. Associations between negative life experiences and the mental health of trans and gender diverse young people in Australia: findings from Trans Pathways. *Psychological Medicine* 2020;50(5):808–17.

12 Bradlow J, Bartram F, Guasp A, Jadva V. *School report: the experiences of lesbian, gay, bi and trans young people in Britain's schools in 2017.* London: Stonewall; 2017. Retrieved from: www.stonewall.org.uk/school-report-2017

13 Gilbey D, Mahfouda S, Ohan J, Lin A, Perry Y. Trajectories of mental health difficulties in young people who are attracted to the same gender: a systematic review. *Adolescent Research Review* 2019; in press.

14 Lawrence D, Johnson S, Hafekost J, Boterhoven de Haan K, Sawyer M, Ainley J, et al. *The mental health of children and adolescents: report on the second Australian Child and Adolescent Survey of Mental Health and Wellbeing.* Canberra: Australian Government; 2015.

15 Carney A. Lesbian, gay, and bisexual adolescent suicidality: the impact of social stigma. *Kentucky Nurse* 2014;62(1):4.

16 Gower AL, Valdez CAB, Watson RJ, Eisenberg ME, Mehus CJ, Saewyc EM, et al. First- and second-hand experiences of enacted stigma among LGBTQ youth. *The Journal of School Nursing* 2019; in press.

17 Meyer IH. Minority stress and mental health in gay men. *Journal of Health and Social Behavior* 1995;36(1):38–56.

18 McDermott E, Hughes E, Rawlings V. *Queer futures: understanding lesbian, gay, bisexual and trans (LGBT) adolescents' suicide, self-harm, and help-seeking behaviour.* Lancaster: Lancaster University; 2016.

19 Choi SK, Wilson BDM, Shelton J, Gates G. *Serving our youth 2015: the needs and experiences of lesbian, gay, bisexual, transgender, and questioning youth experiencing homelessness.* Los Angeles: The Williams Institute with True Colors Fund; 2015.

20 Rhoades H, Rusow JA, Bond D, Lanteigne A, Fulginiti A, Goldbach JT. Homelessness, mental health and suicidality among LGBTQ youth accessing crisis services. *Child Psychiatry and Human Development* 2018;49(4):643–51.

21 Xu Y, Zheng Y. Does sexual orientation precede childhood sexual abuse? Childhood gender nonconformity as a risk factor and instrumental variable analysis. *Sexual Abuse* 2017;29(8):786–802.

22 Jones T, Leonard W, Department of Health and Human Services. *Health and wellbeing of people with intersex variations: information and resource paper.* Melbourne: Department of Health and Human Services; 2019.

23 Aromin RA Jr. Substance abuse prevention, assessment, and treatment for lesbian, gay, bisexual, and transgender youth. *Pediatric Clinics of North America* 2016;63(6): 1057–77.

24 McDermott E, Hughes E, Rawlings V. Norms and normalisation: understanding lesbian, gay, bisexual, transgender and queer youth, suicidality and help-seeking. *Culture, Health & Sexuality* 2018;20(2):156–72.

25 Compton DA, Whitehead MB. Educating healthcare providers regarding LGBT patients and health issues: the special case of physician assistants. *American Journal of Sexuality Education* 2015;10(1):101–18.
26 Substance Abuse and Mental Health Services Administration. *Ending conversion therapy: supporting and affirming LGBTQ youth.* Rockville, MD: Substance Abuse and Mental Health Services Administration; 2015.
27 Turban JL, King D, Reisner SL, Keuroghlian AS. Psychological attempts to change a person's gender identity from transgender to cisgender: estimated prevalence across US states, 2015. *American Journal of Public Health* 2019;109(10):1452–4.
28 Ream GL. What's unique about lesbian, gay, bisexual, and transgender (LGBT) youth and young adult suicides? Findings from the National Violent Death Reporting System. *Journal of Adolescent Health* 2019;64(5):602–7.
29 Fleming JB, Hill YN, Burns MN. Usability of a culturally informed mHealth intervention for symptoms of anxiety and depression: feedback from young sexual minority men. *JMIR Human Factors* 2017;4(3):e22.
30 Perry Y, Strauss P, Lin A. Online interventions for the mental health needs of trans and gender diverse young people. *Lancet Psychiatry* 2018;5(2):e6.
31 Strauss P, Morgan H, Wright Toussaint D, Lin A, Winter S, Perry Y. Trans and gender diverse young people's attitudes towards game-based digital mental health interventions: a qualitative investigation. *Internet Interventions* 2019;18:100280.
32 Lucassen MFG, Merry SN, Hatcher S, Frampton CMA. Rainbow SPARX: a novel approach to addressing depression in sexual minority youth. *Cognitive and Behavioral Practice* 2015;22(2):203–16.

19 Eating disorders in young people

Tracey Wade

Introduction

Eating disorders are serious mental illnesses. They result in substantial harm across psychological, physical and social functioning and are associated with elevated mortality compared to other psychiatric disorders, equivalent to substance abuse.[1,2] People with eating disorders have significantly higher rates of suicidality than the general population.[3] Eating disorder symptoms that emerge between 11 and 17 years remain highly stable into early adulthood in the absence of treatment and have significant associations with overweight and worse mental health in adulthood.[4]

Eating disorders have a high prevalence. In 2012, more than 913,000 people had an eating disorder in Australia, with a total socio-economic cost of $69.7 billion.[5] By the age of 20, between 10% and 13% of females will have met criteria for DSM-5 anorexia nervosa (AN), bulimia nervosa (BN), binge eating disorder or other specified feeding and eating disorders and will experience significant impairment compared to young women who have never had an eating disorder.[6–8] The prevalence of eating disorders increases up to age 25, especially those involving bingeing and purging behaviours.[9] In an Australian national cohort study, 23% of women aged 22 to 27 years reported disordered eating that was associated with a significantly reduced quality of life (both mental and physical) over a subsequent 9-year follow-up period.[10]

Individuals with eating disorders have higher health care utilisation than individuals with all other forms of mental illness.[11] BN and AN are the eighth and tenth leading causes of burden of disease and injury respectively in Australian females aged 15 to 24.[12] Cross-sectional epidemiologic and prospective data suggest that binge eating is associated with a higher risk of diabetes, hypertension and dyslipidaemia, all components of the metabolic syndrome, independent of obesity and co-occurring psychiatric disorders.[13–15]

Eating disorders are an overlooked mental illness

Less than one-third of BN cases are detected by health care professionals.[16] This is consistent with other common mental health problems accompanied by comorbid somatic symptoms, which results in reduced likelihood of being diagnosed with a mental health problem.[17] The problem, however, is uniquely exacerbated for eating disorders for at least five reasons, summarised in Table 19.1, including stigma and shame, ambivalence about the disorder and treatment, and lack of encouragement from others to seek help.[18] Patients are more likely to discuss other issues, as indicated by the finding that in general practice, psychological, gastrointestinal or gynaecological complaints are reported at significantly higher levels five years prior to being diagnosed with an eating disorder than people without an eating disorder.[19] Health professionals may fail to ask, or be unfamiliar with the symptoms, and therefore a diagnosis of an eating disorder is not uncommonly delayed.

Eating disorders have also traditionally been neglected in the terms of initiatives that can inform policy and service development in Australia. Eating disorders were excluded from the 2013–2014 replication of the adolescent national survey and have never been included in the adult Australian national mental health surveys. Eating disorders had not made the inclusion list for any previous Australian national mental health plan until the Australian federal minister for health directed that eating disorders be included among populations requiring specific consideration in the Fifth National Mental Health and Suicide Prevention Plan released in 2017.

Table 19.1 Why are so few cases of eating disorders detected by health professionals?

Reasons	*Evidence*
Shame and stigma	"There is still a commonly held view that an eating disorder is a lifestyle choice and that recovery means dropping some negative behaviour." Christine Morgan, Chief Executive Officer, The Butterfly Foundation, 2014
Failure to recognise the severity of disordered eating	"Unfortunately, many people with eating disorders may not think they need treatment." Mayo Clinic, 2018
Ambivalence about the disorder and the treatment	"Soon I'll be thinner than all of you, she swore to herself. And then I'll be the winner. The thinner is the winner." Steven Levenkron, *The Best Little Girl in the World*
Failure of the health professional to ask	"We do know the majority of people with eating disorders have contact with health professionals. They present with apparently unrelated complaints and do not disclose their eating problems. While people may not volunteer information about their eating problem, asking questions and allowing the person to see that their eating habits are important may offer a non-judgemental environment for them to start seeking help."[47]
Unfamiliarity of the health professional with eating disorder symptoms	"Fewer than 60% of the low weight [vignette] presentations received a primary diagnosis of anorexia nervosa [from 154 general practitioners], suggesting a justified reluctance to make a diagnosis based on limited information. However, this conservative approach limits access to specialist treatment, as only 40% of the total sample of low weight cases were immediately referred to mental health services (rising to just 52% after 8 weeks without improvement)."[48]

Development of appropriate policies and systems

Over the last ten years Australian governments at both federal and state levels have been turning their attention to the development of appropriate policies and systems related to eating disorders. The turning point for eating disorders was signified ten years ago by the funding of the National Eating Disorder Collaboration (NEDC) by the federal Department of Health and Ageing. This collaboration has been continuously supported by Labor and Liberal federal governments since that time and, as of April 2019, has just been refunded for another 3-year period. The NEDC is a collaboration of people and organisations with an expertise or interest in eating disorders across Australia. The NEDC aims to improve the health outcomes of people with, or at risk of developing, an eating disorder in Australia, recognising the need to take a long-term approach to promotion, prevention and early intervention for eating disorders. Their vision is threefold: (1) that eating disorders are a priority mainstream health issue in Australia; (2) a healthy, diverse and inclusive Australian society acts to prevent eating disorders; (3) every Australian at risk has access to an effective continuum of eating disorders prevention, care and ongoing recovery support. The NEDC has completed numerous projects over the decade informing the development of appropriate policies and systems related to eating disorders, such as work force development; evidence reviews of prevention, treatment and management of eating disorders; primary health network capacity building and engagement; and implementation of the National Eating Disorders Framework. The most visible output is the NEDC website (www.nedc.com.au), which brings research, expertise and opinion from leaders in the field together in one place, with resources available to those with lived experience of an eating disorder, families, health, educational and sports and fitness professionals.

This work has coincided with increased activity from state governments in the development of policies and systems to enhance the prevention and treatment of eating disorders. In New South Wales and Western Australia, governments have announced significant policy and funding commitments to eating disorders. The Queensland and Victorian governments both fund state-wide coordination and service development centres for eating disorders. In South Australia, the previous state government gave funding for the development of new eating disorders services, and the current state government has committed funding for new paediatric eating disorder services. The current federal government's commitment to deliver a more adequate response for people with eating disorders has resulted in the announcement of new Medicare Benefit Scheme items commencing in November of 2019. This funding will allow patients with severe eating disorders to access a Medicare rebate of up to 40 psychological and 20 dietetic services per year. In addition, the federal government announced funding for the roll-out of residential programs around Australia in the 2019 budget.

The lesson learnt from this increased level of policy and system development is that facilitation of respectful and meaningful partnerships and communication is essential for progress. The establishment of the NEDC has enabled meaningful partnerships between clinicians, those with lived experience, researchers, the health system, and federal and state governments to work on ways of translating our knowledge about eating disorders to real-world settings and of identifying gaps in service provision.

Development of appropriate service models for young people

The patient journey across the developmental spectrum of eating disorders is complex, encapsulating many different trajectories, from brief illness to recurring but different eating disorders with various comorbidities.[20] No one service model can be specified but there are general principles that should guide development of any service models in young people, summarised in Figure 19.1.

Early intervention increases likelihood of recovery

The first important principle is early intervention. The mean time from the development of symptoms to presentation for treatment is more than eight months for children and adolescents with eating disorders[21] and five to six years in young adults.[22] Younger age at detection in primary care predicts recovery in both AN and BN, and early detection is considered of major importance for a favourable outcome in eating disorders.[23] The longer the disruption to nutritional health associated with all eating disorders results in more severe neurobiological sequalae, including greater rigidity in thinking and poorer emotional regulation, both of which can impede interventions. This requires service models that do not require service eligibility for youth to be determined by the presence of an eating disorder that meets diagnostic criteria.

Coordination of services is key plank of any service model

Treatment guidelines recognise that coordination of eating disorder services is key to effective service provision.[24] Transition from child and adolescent services to adult services has long been recognised as causing delays, disruption to care and deterioration.[25] This has led to the call to provide an integrated service across youth to prevent discontinuity of care,[25,26] an issue of particular pertinence to eating disorders where the same evidence-based therapies straddle across childhood to young adulthood, or from adolescence to young adulthood (see Figure 19.1). A successful example of an integrated tertiary eating disorder service provided across all ages for individuals and their families exists in the Dorset National Health Service,[27] removing the need for transitions due to age and leading to changes in care driven by patient need rather than service structure. Seamless transitions and integrated care are also

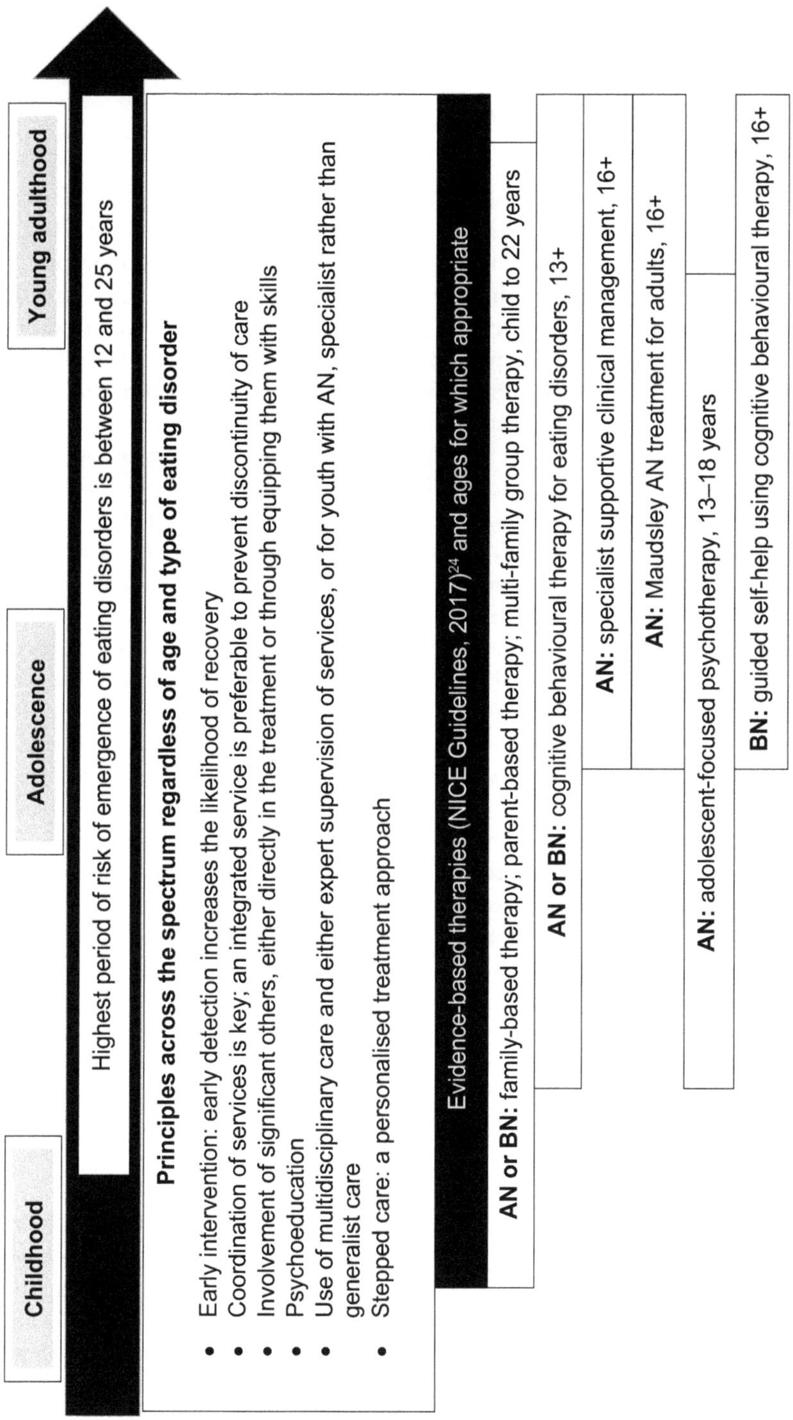

Figure 19.1 Emerging eating disorders in youth: general principles and age appropriate interventions

a key focus of the 2018 model of care for eating disorder services developed in Ireland.[28]

Involvement of significant others in service provision is essential

Utilising the resources of the family and significant others is a key plank in many eating disorder treatments regardless of the age of the person and the type of eating disorder. Family-based, parent-focused and multi-family group therapies for adolescents and young adults with AN rely on families to manage the eating disorder at home to promote recovery.[29,30] Other therapies such as eating disorder–focused cognitive behaviour therapy (CBT-ED) for youth with AN or BN advocate the involvement of significant others to facilitate treatment,[31] where the patient is willing. CBT-ED for adolescents and youth with AN includes routine family involvement in therapy, with nine scheduled shared sessions (covering topics such as the identification of family factors liable to hinder the patient's attempts to change, meal planning, the conduct of mealtimes, and the generation of solutions to foreseeable problems) and additional sessions for family crises or extreme difficulties at mealtimes.[32] The Maudsley Model of Treatment of Adults with AN (MANTRA) also introduces the notion that support from others is important early on in treatment, and patients are encouraged to think who in their social network might be most helpful to them in beating AN and who they therefore might want to invite to join some sessions.[33]

In addition, there is an emphasis on upskilling significant others so that they can feel better equipped to deal with an eating disorder while attending to their own needs. Meta-analytic findings show that group-based carers' skills workshops reduce carer distress, expressed emotion and care-giving burden associated with eating disorder symptoms.[34] Provision of Collaborative Care Skill Training workshops in the Australian context has also been shown to decrease carer distress and burden and carer use of maladaptive coping.[35] Remote interventions can also be helpful: significant others who used workbooks completed in conjunction with 20 minutes of clinician guidance (email or telephone) per week showed significant improvements in anxiety and depression, negative experiences of care-giving, the impact of the eating disorder symptoms and carer-expressed emotion, an effect maintained at 3-month follow-up.[36]

Psychoeducation needs to be an aspect of all interventions

The current National Institute for Health and Care Excellence (NICE) guidelines recognise the importance of communication and information for both those with eating disorders as well as families and significant others involved in supporting the person.[24] This aspect is of importance in work with eating disorders, given the degree of misinformation popularly available about healthy eating and weight, the more technical information about medical impacts of disordered eating and the need to justify the treatment strategies, including an initial focus on restoring nutritional health before psychotherapy can be effective. More recently, a 5-day multi-family group therapy for adults with AN has been developed that incorporates novel approaches to psychoeducation focused on neurobiology and development of skills in significant others to help manage the traits that can contribute to disease chronicity.[37]

Multidisciplinary and expert evidence-based services are associated with better outcomes

Comprehensive eating disorder care requires a multidisciplinary, multi-agency approach involving primary care, mental health and medical services involved in ongoing medical monitoring. Medical admissions to acute hospitals are required for physical stabilisation in severe restricting eating disorders and sometimes BN. Comorbidity with other psychiatric disorders is not an indicator for hospitalisation, as eating disorder treatments, even brief ones, decrease comorbidity.[38] If, however, prior treatment efforts are failing because of interference by comorbidity, then hospitalisation may be indicated. When inpatient treatment is needed it should be brief and focused on medical safety and refeeding. Specialist outpatient eating disorder teams have been associated with faster recovery, higher patient satisfaction, lower costs, lower rates of inpatient admission and better case identification and access compared to care by generalist services.[39–41] Specialist supervision of novice therapists in non-underweight eating disorders can produce similar outcomes to those of experienced therapists.[38]

Stepped care – a personalised treatment approach

Eating disorder treatment should be provided through outpatient, intensive/day and inpatient settings. Day services have good potential as a step-down from inpatient settings, and research indicates that day services for young people, including adolescents, are associated with decreased costs and decreased number of inpatient admissions.[42,43] The treatment setting should be based on patient clinical presentation, with patients stepping up and down in intensity of care as needed, rather than automatically starting patients at the lowest intensity option. Session-by-session evaluation collaboratively shared with the patient is essential, not only for improving outcomes,[44] but also for detecting lack of early change as this predicts poorer outcome across eating disorders and modalities of treatment.[45] Slow response indicates a need for more intense treatment options, for example, more frequent sessions earlier, greater emphasis on the need for early change, use of adjuncts such as imagery rescripting, mindfulness, dialectical skills training, cognitive remediation training, regular dietician or nutritional input, day- or inpatient treatment or multi-family therapy. When slow responders to guided self-help with BN or Binge Eating Disorder were offered more intensive group therapies, they achieved outcomes commensurate with fast responders at end of treatment and at 6- and 12-month follow-up.[46]

Development of appropriate service interventions that would improve mental health outcomes for young people across the world

Traditionally eating disorders have not been serviced well by early intervention approaches, which is particularly pertinent to youth, where most eating disorders emerge between ages 12 and 25. Recent attention on early intervention in eating disorders has resulted in the development of the First Episode and Rapid Early Intervention Service for Eating Disorders (FREED) program,[25] a service model that has been piloted in south London. The program is intended for people aged 15 to 25 years and was modelled on principles of early intervention in psychiatry: designed to prevent onset or alter the course of serious mental illness through delaying or averting unfavourable outcomes, or through avoiding disruption in people's development and associated secondary disabilities. Early intervention critically depends on early detection of a disorder or its precursors (which requires close and collaborative relationships with general practitioners), and the commencement of effective treatment, tailored to the patient's stage of illness. In May 2017 FREED was awarded the British Medical Journal's prize for Mental Health Team of the year. The early indications of outcome include the following: 100% take-up of treatment compared to 73% in the old service model with longer waiting lists; the need to provide inpatient treatment for patients decreased from 14% to 8.9%; at 12 months after assessment, 70% of patients no longer had an eating disorder; for those people with anorexia 60% had returned to a normal BMI at 12-month follow-up, compared to only 16.6% in the old service model.

Aspects of this service model have recently been established in South Australia. In contrast to FREED, which is embedded in a tertiary service, emergED is embedded within primary care and offered at the *headspace* Edinburgh North, Onkaparinga and Port Adelaide Centres. The services are built on the same five components that distinguish FREED, described in Table 19.2. The emergED model is currently being evaluated. This is an important service initiative that has the capacity to substantially improve outcomes in eating disorders for youth, given few *headspace* Centres currently offer services for eating disorders and the lack of early intervention services in Australia. This is an important area of growth for eating disorder treatment over the next decade.

Conclusion

Eating disorders are common and serious mental disorders. They are associated with high levels of psychological and physical morbidity, including reduced quality of life and high rates of suicidality. They typically begin in adolescence. Early detection and intervention are key to improving outcomes in people with eating disorders. However, eating disorders are often not identified early as young people may not think they have a problem, may feel shame or stigma in asking for help and health professionals may not recognise or may fail to ask about the symptoms, especially when the young person presents with a different problem.

Table 19.2 The five components of the early intervention service model for eating disorders

Component	*Description*
1	Early detection in primary care settings; raising awareness and practitioner skills in general practice, schools and youth service organisations; and provision of a clear, easy referral pathway with an associated website. Encouragement of early referrals rather than watchful waiting.
2	Active outreach and rapid engagement with young people and their families. Self-referral, initial contact by flexible, relaxed means such as text, phone, email, met with a normalising and reassuring engagement style. No waiting lists, an assessment appointment is offered within three weeks.
3	Patient- and family-centred biopsychosocial assessment focused on strengths and resources. There will be a motivational and optimistic outlook, and the emphasis will be on early full recovery. The clinician liaises with the State-wide Eating Disorder Services as needed to develop a developmentally tailored care plan with appropriate treatment options.
4	Psychoeducation and nutritional management focused on the malleability of illness-related biological and brain changes during the early stage of illness and the importance of early nutritional action to remedy these.
5	"Brokering" for the provision of low- and high-intensity psychological interventions for the individual or family-based interventions, offered within 6 weeks of assessment. In some cases, these interventions will be offered by the clinician, but in many cases, they will be offered by other clinicians at *headspace* or by clinicians in other services. Interventions will be matched to the patient's stage of illness and conform to the NICE guidelines.[24]

Close collaboration between primary care, mental health and medical services are needed for optimal care of people with eating disorders. Continuity of care between adolescent and adult services is vital to avoid patients disengaging with treatment. Including families and other support people in management and a multidisciplinary, multi-agency approach is essential if we are to improve outcomes for these highly disabling illnesses.

References

1 Arcelus J, Mitchell AJ, Wales J, Nielsen S. Mortality rates in patients with anorexia nervosa and other eating disorders. a meta-analysis of 36 studies. *Archives of General Psychiatry* 2011;68(7):724–31.

2 Harris E, Barraclough B. Excess mortality of mental disorder. *British Journal of Psychiatry* 1998;173:11–53.

3 Pisetsky EM, Thornton LM, Lichtenstein P, Pedersen NL, Bulik CM. Suicide attempts in women with eating disorders. *Journal of Abnormal Psychology* 2013;122(4):1042–56.

4 Herpertz-Dahlmann B, Dempfle A, Konrad K, Klasen F, Ravens-Sieberer U, BELLA study group. Eating disorder symptoms do not just disappear: the implications of adolescent eating-disordered behaviour for body weight and mental health in young adulthood. *European Child & Adolescent Psychiatry* 2015;24(6):675–84.

5 Paxton S, Hay P, Touyz SW, Forbes D, Madden S, Girosi F, et al. *Paying the price: the economic and social impact of eating disorders in Australia.* Australia: Butterfly Foundation; 2012.

6 Stice E, Marti CN, Rohde P. Prevalence, incidence, impairment, and course of the proposed DSM-5 eating disorder diagnoses in an 8-year prospective community study of young women. *Journal of Abnormal Psychology* 2013;122(2):445–57.
7 Fairweather-Schmidt AK, Wade TD. DSM-5 eating disorders and other specified eating and feeding disorders: is there a meaningful differentiation? *International Journal of Eating Disorders* 2014;47(5):524–33.
8 Allen KL, Bryne SM, Oddy WH, Crosby RD. DSM-IV-TR and DSM-5 eating disorders in adolescents: prevalence, stability, and psychosocial correlates in a population-based sample of male and female adolescents. *Journal of Abnormal Psychology* 2013;122(3): 720–32.
9 Hudson JI, Hiripi E, Pope HG, Kessler RC. The prevalence and correlates of eating disorders in the National Comorbidity Survey Replication. *Biological Psychiatry* 2007;61(3):348–58.
10 Wade TD, Wilksch SM, Lee C. A longitudinal investigation of the impact of disordered eating on young women's quality of life. *Health Psychology* 2012;31(3):352–9.
11 Striegel-Moore RH, DeBar L, Wilson GT, Dickerson J, Rosselli F, Perrin N, et al. Health services use in eating disorders. *Psychological Medicine* 2008;38(10):1465–74.
12 Australian Institute of Health and Wellbeing (AIHW). *Young Australians: their health and wellbeing 2007*. Canberra: AIHW; 2007.
13 Olguin P, Fuentes M, Gabler G, Guerdjikova AI, Keck PE, McElroy SL. Medical comorbidity of binge eating disorder. *Eating and Weight Disorders* 2017;22(1):13–26.
14 Thornton LM, Watson HJ, Jangmo A, Welch E, Wiklund C, von Hausswolff-Juhlin Y, et al. Binge-eating disorder in the Swedish national registers: somatic comorbidity. *International Journal of Eating Disorders* 2017;50(1):58–65.
15 Hudson JI, Lalonde JK, Coit CE, Tsuang MT, McElroy SL, Crow SJ, et al. Longitudinal study of the diagnosis of components of the metabolic syndrome in individuals with binge-eating disorder. *American Journal of Clinical Nutrition* 2010;91(6):1568–73.
16 Keski-Rahkonen A, Hoek HW, Linna MS, Raevuori A, Sihvola E, Bulik CM, et al. Incidence and outcomes of bulimia nervosa: a nationwide population-based study. *Psychological Medicine* 2009;39(5):823–31.
17 Wilhelm KA, Finch AW, Davenport TA, Hickie IB. What can alert the general practitioner to people whose common mental health problems are unrecognised? *Medical Journal of Australia* 2008;188(S12):S114–8.
18 Ali K, Farrer L, Fassnacht DB, Gulliver A, Bauer S, Griffiths KM. Perceived barriers and facilitators towards help-seeking for eating disorders: a systematic review. *International Journal of Eating Disorders* 2017;50(1):9–21.
19 Ogg EC, Millar HR, Pusztai EE, Thom AS. General practice consultation patterns preceding diagnosis of eating disorders. *International Journal of Eating Disorders* 1997;22(1):89–93.
20 Milos G, Spindler A, Schnyder U, Fairburn CG. Instability of eating disorder diagnoses: prospective study. *British Journal of Psychiatry* 2005;187:573–8.
21 Nicholls DE, Lynn R, Viner RM. Childhood eating disorders: British national surveillance study. *British Journal of Psychiatry* 2011;198(4):295–301.
22 Rosenvinge JH, Kuhlefelt Klusmeier A. Treatment for eating disorders from a patient satisfaction perspective: a Norwegian replication of a British study. *European Eating Disorders Review* 2000;8(4):293–300.
23 van Son GE, van Hoeken D, van Furth EF, Donker GA, Hoek HW. Course and outcome of eating disorders in a primary care-based cohort. *International Journal of Eating Disorders* 2010;43(2):130–8.

24 National Institute for Health and Care Excellence (NICE). *Eating disorders: recognition and treatment.* London: NICE; 2017.
25 Schmidt U, Brown A, McClelland J, Glennon D, Mountford VA. Will a comprehensive, person-centered, team-based early intervention approach to first episode illness improve outcomes in eating disorders? *International Journal of Eating Disorders* 2016;49(4):374–7.
26 Raballo A, Poletti M, McGorry P. Architecture of change: rethinking child and adolescent mental health. *Lancet Psychiatry* 2017;4(9):656–8.
27 THRIVEin Dorset. *Children and young people's mental health and wellbeing Dorset: local transformation plan.* Retrieved from: www.dorsetccg.nhs.uk/wp-content/uploads/2018/04/draft-dorset-cyp-ltp.pdf
28 National Working Group and Clinical Advisory Group of College of Psychiatrists of Ireland. *Eating disorder services. HSE model of care for Ireland.* Dublin: National Clinical Programme for Eating Disorders; 2018.
29 Le Grange D, Hughes EK, Court A, Yeo M, Crosby RD, Sawyer SM. Randomized clinical trial of parent-focused treatment and family-based treatment for adolescent anorexia nervosa. *Journal of the American Academy of Child and Adolescent Psychiatry* 2016;55(8):683–92.
30 Eisler I, Simic M, Hodsoil J, Asen E, Berelowitz M, Connan F, et al. A pragmatic randomised multi-centre trial of multifamily and single family therapy for adolescent anorexia nervosa. *BMC Psychiatry* 2016;16(1):422.
31 Fairburn CG. *Cognitive behaviour therapy and eating disorders.* New York: Guilford Press; 2008.
32 Dalle Grave R, Calugi S, Doll HA, Fairburn CG. Enhanced cognitive behaviour therapy for adolescents with anorexia nervosa: an alternative to family therapy? *Behaviour Research and Therapy* 2013;51(1):R9–12.
33 Schmidt U, Wade TD, Treasure J. The Maudsley Model of Anorexia Nervosa Treatment for Adults (MANTRA): development, key features and preliminary evidence. *Journal of Cognitive Psychotherapy* 2014;28(1):48–71.
34 Hibbs R, Rhind C, Leppanen J, Treasure J. Interventions for caregivers of someone with an eating disorder: a meta-analysis. *International Journal of Eating Disorders* 2015;48(4):349–61.
35 Pépin G, King R. Collaborative care skill training workshop: how Australian carers support a loved one with an eating disorder. *Advances in Eating Disorders* 2016;4(1):47–58.
36 Grover M, Williams C, Eisler I, Fairbairn P, McCloskey C, Smith G, et al. An off-line pilot evaluation of a web-based systemic cognitive-behavioral intervention for carers of people with anorexia nervosa. *International Journal of Eating Disorders* 2011;44(8):708–15.
37 Wierenga CE, Hill L, Knatz Peck S, McCray J, Greathouse L, Peterson D, et al. The acceptability, feasibility, and possible benefits of a neurobiologically-informed 5-day multifamily treatment for adults with anorexia nervosa. *International Journal of Eating Disorders* 2018;51(8):863–9.
38 Pellizzer ML, Waller G, Wade TD. A pragmatic effectiveness study of 10-session cognitive behavioural therapy (CBT-T) for eating disorders: targeting barriers to treatment provision. *European Eating Disorders Review* 2019;27(5):557–70.
39 Gowers SG, Clark AF, Roberts C, Byford S, Barrett B, Griffiths A, et al. A randomised controlled multicentre trial of treatments for adolescent anorexia nervosa including assessment of cost-effectiveness and patient acceptability – the TOuCAN trial. *Health Technology Assessment* 2010;14(15):1–98.
40 Hay PJ, Claudino AM, Touyz S, Abd Elbaky G. Individual psychological therapy in the outpatient treatment of adults with anorexia nervosa. *Cochrane Database of Systematic Reviews* 2015;7:CD003909.

41 House J, Schmidt U, Craig M, Landau S, Simic M, Nicholls D, et al. Comparison of specialist and nonspecialist care pathways for adolescents with anorexia nervosa and related eating disorders. *International Journal of Eating Disorders* 2012;45(8):949–56.
42 Herpertz-Dahlmann B, Schwarte R, Krei M, Egberts K, Warnke A, Wewetzer C, et al. Day-patient treatment after short inpatient care versus continued inpatient treatment in adolescents with anorexia nervosa (ANDI): a multicentre, randomised, open-label, non-inferiority trial. *Lancet* 2014;383(9924):1222–9.
43 Ornstein RM, Lane-Loney SE, Hollenbeak CS. Clinical outcomes of a novel, family-centered partial hospitalization program for young patients with eating disorders. *Eating and Weight Disorders* 2012;17(3):e170–7.
44 Lambert MJ, Whipple JL, Vermeersch DA, Smart DW, Hawkins EJ, Nielsen SL, et al. Enhancing psychotherapy outcomes via providing feedback on client progress: a replication. *Clinical Psychology and Psychotherapy* 2002;9(2):91–103.
45 Vall E, Wade TD. Predictors of treatment outcome in individuals with eating disorders: a systematic review and meta-analysis. *International Journal of Eating Disorders* 2015;48(7):946–71.
46 Chen EY, Cacioppo J, Fettich K, Gallop R, McCloskey MS, Olino T, et al. An adaptive randomized trial of dialectical behavior therapy and cognitive behavior therapy for binge-eating. *Psychological Medicine* 2017;47(4):703–17.
47 National Eating Disorders Collaboration. *Eating disorders: a professional resource for general practitioners.* 2nd ed. New South Wales: National Eating Disorders Collaboration; 2015.
48 Currin L, Waller G, Treasure J, Nodder J, Stone C, Yeomans M, et al. The use of guidelines for dissemination of "best practice" in primary care of patients with eating disorders. *International Journal of Eating Disorders* 2007;40(5):476–9.

Part IV

Future directions

20 Future directions in youth mental health

Alison R. Yung, Cristina Mei and Patrick D. McGorry

Introduction

Young people are at risk of, and are often heavily impacted by, the onset of a mental illness. The vast majority of mental disorders emerge during the developmentally sensitive transition period between childhood and adulthood.[1] It is now recognised that this period extends well into the third decade of life.[2,3] This lengthened period of transition, termed emerging adulthood, reflects a range of complex interplays between biological, maturational and societal factors.[2,4–7] Changes in brain structure and functional connectivity, pubertal hormones, developmental challenges of achieving independence from the family of origin, peer and romantic relationships and educational and vocational issues all converge in this period to make it uniquely vulnerable to the onset of mental illness.[8]

Mental disorders that begin in childhood or adolescence tend to be more severe than those with onsets in later adulthood. They are also frequently undetected early in the illness. Secondary problems are then likely to occur on this background of prolonged, unidentified primary mental disorder, for example, depression following anxiety.[9] It is not surprising, therefore, that mental illness in young people is often associated with ongoing disability, including impaired social functioning, poor educational achievement, unstable employment, substance abuse and victimisation.[10,11] These may all lead to a cycle of dysfunction and disadvantage that can be difficult to reverse. The often poor outcomes that are associated with early onset of mental disorders also highlight the need for early intervention to minimise disability, prevent onset of secondary problems and promote recovery.

The youth mental health approach recognises the importance of understanding and appropriately responding to the full range of mental health and social needs of young people aged 12 to 25 years.[12] Since it began in Australia, youth mental health service reform has expanded to many countries, improving access to care and the outcomes of young people with mental disorders.[13–17] However, this transformation remains an area of ongoing development and refinement. There is still an urgent need for discoveries that transform the outcomes of young people and reduce the avertable burden of mental disorders on young people, families and society more broadly.

This chapter will explore areas in youth mental health that have achieved broad consensus and the uncertainties, challenges and opportunities that the field faces, and it will propose some key priority areas for future research. Box 20.1 describes areas of broad consensus.

Box 20.1 Areas in which there is broad consensus

- Becoming an adult is a lengthened process. The age of 18 no longer represents the commencement of adulthood, with mature adulthood now achieved around the mid to late 20s.[2,3] This is reflected in the World Health Organization's definition of young people (10–24 years).
- Mental disorders are common among young people. Most disorders develop between childhood and young adulthood, prior to 24 years of age.[1]
- Mental illness in young people is often associated with ongoing disability, including impaired functioning, social isolation, reduced educational and vocational attainment, substance abuse, and victimisation.[10,11]
- The traditional configuration of mental health services based on a paediatric-adult split (i.e., child and adolescent mental health services versus adult mental health services) is a design flaw.[18] It fails to reflect the pattern of mental illness onset and impact as well as the developmental and cultural needs of young people.
- Treatment in the earliest stages of mental illness can improve outcomes, particularly for psychotic disorders but also for depression, borderline personality disorder and other diagnoses.[17,19–25]
- The course and functional impacts of even the most serious forms of mental illness can be positively altered through early intervention.[22,26]
- Integrated mental health services for young people can improve service access, symptomatic and functional recovery, and patient satisfaction.[16,17]
- There are economic benefits in investing in youth mental health. It can deliver a substantial return on investment while achieving positive health and social benefits.[27]

Challenges and knowledge gaps

Mechanisms of mental disorders

Despite numerous research attempts, there is limited understanding of the causes of mental disorders and the factors that predict treatment response. A limitation of the evidence base is that research efforts have not sufficiently focused on the early stages of mental illness.

Transdiagnostic clinical staging

Clinical staging is a new diagnostic method in psychiatry that links diagnosis with treatment and acknowledges the continuum of mental disorders (from asymptomatic to chronic illness) that is not captured by current diagnostic systems.[28,29] Clinical staging has become increasingly popular among researchers; however, a consensus approach has not been achieved, leading to inconsistency in how staging has been applied.

Prevention, mental health promotion and epidemiology

The extensive evidence accumulated over the past three decades has challenged the historic, and now obsolete, view that mental disorders could not be prevented. A current gap is identifying modifiable risk and protective factors that can be effectively targeted by preventive interventions.

Treatment and novel interventions

Available therapies predominately target acute symptoms of mental disorders rather than long-term relapse prevention and functioning. This is reflected by their limited short and long-term outcomes. One-third to half of young people with a mental disorder do not respond to first-line treatments and approximately 50% experience multiple episodes.[10,30,31] To improve these outcomes, the development of effective novel interventions is needed.

New technologies

Preliminary evidence supports the effectiveness of digital mental health interventions.[32–34] However, its translation into current models of care remains a challenge due to low patient and clinician uptake, the design of interventions, and ineffective implementation strategies.[35,36] The right balance between digital and existing service delivery platforms requires investigation.

Socio-cultural factors

Socio-cultural factors can influence mental illness onset as well as an individual's access to treatment. These factors are complex, and greater research is needed to determine how they can be addressed within specific communities, such as Indigenous populations, minority ethnic groups and the homeless.

Service delivery and innovation

Integrated youth mental health services, such as *headspace*, improve access to care and yield favourable recovery outcomes; however, there is not yet a single integrated service delivery model that is regarded as the gold standard.[17]

Improving access to care

Despite increased provision of youth-specific models of care, seeking help for a mental disorder can be a challenging and complex process for young people. Mechanisms and strategies that improve young people's awareness of mental health issues and how, when and where to seek help are needed. Research on stigma reduction intersects with these issues and is also needed.

Translation and implementation

A significant body of knowledge and evidence has been built in youth mental health on the components of care and youth-friendly service models, as well as effective interventions and treatments, particularly for psychosis and vocational programs.[19,22,26,37–39] However, major gaps exist in access, knowledge translation and implementation science. This has impacted the routine delivery of evidence-based strategies for early diagnosis and treatment.[40–42] Strategies and resources need to be developed and made available to the whole sector (both research and service delivery) to effectively translate relevant findings into practice in a timely and consistent manner.

Challenges in conducting youth mental health research

Lack of funding

To effectively implement national and global change, adequate investment in youth mental health research and care is critical. Research into the prevention, diagnosis and treatment of mental illness, particularly for children and young people, is significantly underfunded,[43] obstructing progress in mental health care.[44]

Reinforcing youth mental health as a discrete sector

The progress achieved in creating a youth mental health paradigm needs to be built upon to ensure that it is distinct from child and adolescent mental health, which has not achieved the same level of research output. Better integration is needed between the research sector and various health service delivery levels (e.g., primary, tertiary care, mental health, physical health and substance use services). This will benefit young people and minimise the likelihood that they fall between the gaps and will enhance research capacity and translation.

Insufficient workforce

The critical mass of researchers needed to support further progress in youth mental health and early intervention is currently lacking. Strategies to attract and retain researchers and to support clinicians to engage in research are required.

Engaging vulnerable populations

Mental health research into vulnerable populations, such as First Nations people, culturally and linguistically diverse and homeless young people, is challenging due to difficulties in engaging with these populations. To improve recruitment and retention of participants, strategies are needed that target specific barriers and facilitators.

Lack of common tools to assess mental health symptoms

There is a need to develop a standardised assessment toolkit that can be used nationally and internationally. This would enable the generation of large datasets that could be used to answer critical research questions. What should be measured and how is an area requiring consensus and should involve young people and carers.

Opportunities

The International Association for Youth Mental Health (IAYMH) was established in 2012. It aims to bring together professionals, researchers, young people and carers. The mission of IAYMH is to change the way the global community thinks about young people and their mental health. IAYMH hosts an international conference every two years which is planned and delivered in partnership with young people. The International Youth Mental Health Research Network (IYMHRN) is a subprogram within IAYMH that aims to bring together researchers and research institutions with an interest in youth mental health from across the world. The aims of this network are shown in Box 20.2.

Box 20.2 Aims of the International Youth Mental Health Research Network

1. Establish a set of international research priorities in youth mental health in collaboration with young people and carers.
2. Enable the generation of new knowledge through innovation and the exchange of research outcomes.
3. Establish an evidence-based case for increased funding and investment in youth mental health research and service delivery.
4. Identify, nurture and professionally develop a team of high-quality researchers and research leaders.
5. Consult with young people and families in framing and progressing IYMHRN's aims, principles and priorities.

The network currently consists of approximately 130 international youth mental health researchers. The global coverage and expertise of the IYMHRN places it in a strong position to generate significant gains in youth mental health research through collaborations that capitalise on the wealth of data collected to date, whilst also fostering opportunities for new and innovative discoveries.[45]

This network has made substantial progress that provides major opportunities for youth mental health research, including:

- The **identification of critical research gaps** (noted previously)
- The **development of a set of global research priorities** for youth mental health (see next part)
- Establishment of a **Lancet Psychiatry Commission on Youth Mental Health**[46]
- Development of an **international consensus statement on clinical staging for young people**[47]

Future research directions

Following its second major meeting in 2018, IYMHRN developed a set of global research priorities for youth mental health. This was published in the journal *Early Intervention in Psychiatry*.[45] The recommended priorities are directed towards areas that are likely to generate the greatest impact on youth mental health nationally and internationally (see Table 20.1).

Table 20.1 Research priorities for youth mental health[45]

Research area	*Research priorities*
Prevention, mental health promotion & epidemiology	• Identify malleable risk and protective factors for preventive interventions. • Develop an accepted common language and terminology for positive mental health and mental illness. • Focus on high-risk groups, notably LGBTIQ, refugees, Indigenous populations, culturally and linguistically diverse populations, and young people in out-of-home and statutory care. • Conduct international comparative population and cohort studies. • Develop an internationally standardised toolkit of assessment and outcome measures for youth mental health, including a core instrument or set of instruments that is used transnationally to evaluate and compare service outcomes and to identify effective or ineffective service features.
Neuroscience & development	• Conduct biomarker studies in broader transdiagnostic samples of patients from the earliest stages of mental ill-health, using multiple methods and more potent statistical tools. • Enable the better prediction of outcome in young people with mental ill-health by developing relevant developmental trajectory curves (including brain and epigenetic age, and cognitive development) that can use neurobiological data combined with clinical and functional data to map the impact of treatments. • Proactively link to general population neurological and development research and build on these findings with a focus on mental health.

Research area	*Research priorities*
Transdiagnostic clinical staging	• Develop an international consensus statement for clinical staging in youth mental health that will enhance clinical practice, support youth mental health service planning, and can provide a framework for research.
Treatment & novel interventions	• Accelerate the development of new and novel interventions and the translation of knowledge through sector networking, knowledge sharing and supporting study designs. • Re-engage with the pharmaceutical industry to support the creation of new biological therapies. • Build on virtual technologies by investing in research and development for psychosocial therapies that incorporate virtual or augmented reality.
The role of new technologies in youth mental health	• Build new service delivery models that incorporate technology and ensure these models can (1) promptly and effectively adapt to technological advances and (2) be supported by rapid and iterative development and evaluation approaches, using methodologies such as co-design with young people to ensure their involvement in the process of continuous improvement.
Socio-cultural factors & youth mental health in low- & middle-income countries (LMICs)	• Capitalise on the already existing broader global health and mental health sector (that is already significantly funded by organisations such as Grand Challenges Canada and the National Institutes of Health) by becoming more involved in and partnering with initiatives and organisations already working in these areas. • Investigate the opportunities to conduct a World Health Survey focused on young people that includes a wider range of LMICs given the large population of young people within these nations.
Services, delivery & innovation	• Develop robust trial methodologies that are applicable across a range of mental health systems (i.e., established or minimally established) and would allow the youth mental health sector to make more definitive statements about the key aspects of the ideal youth mental health service delivery model. • Transnationally test a consensus model of care that can be implemented in a range of high-income countries (HICs) and LMIC settings and that accounts for all countries' financial and infrastructure constraints. This includes models utilising lay health workers within LMICs, which may also be applied to certain settings within HICs (i.e., remote and low-resource areas, indigenous communities).
Translation & implementation	• Model consumer and stakeholder preferences for knowledge translation, transfer and exchange approaches to determine what works for whom. • Build the capacity of youth mental health researchers to conduct translational research and develop a technical assistance centre to support researchers internationally in developing and delivering implementation science. • Invest in training and education to build the capacity of the broader youth mental health workforce (including fellowships, global exchanges) for knowledge translation and implementation. • Develop online courses, including massive open online courses, to facilitate knowledge transfer and translation at a global level.

Source: Reproduced from Mei et al. with permission.[45]

Conclusion

The youth mental health field has emerged and matured over the last two decades. To capitalise on this growth, it is crucial that the sector develops a strategy that addresses critical research gaps and explores effective methods to implement findings that deliver improved outcomes for young people. Youth mental health research requires adequate coordination, planning and funding. Increased investment in youth mental health care is a 'best buy' as it will generate a major return on investment. Early intervention and sustained, evidence-based care is the building block needed for major service redesign and reform. This reform focus can only be progressed and sustained if it is powered by evidence, which in turn can only result from sophisticated and high-quality mental health research. This includes research that aims to maximise the translation of research findings into improvements in health and social services and increases in the quality of life of young people.

References

1 Kessler RC, Berglund P, Demler O, Jin R, Merikangas KR, Walters EE. Lifetime prevalence and age-of-onset distributions of DSM-IV disorders in the National Comorbidity Survey Replication. *Archives of General Psychiatry* 2005;62(6):593–602.
2 Arnett JJ, Žukauskienė R, Sugimura K. The new life stage of emerging adulthood at ages 18–29 years: implications for mental health. *Lancet Psychiatry* 2014;1(7):569–76.
3 Sawyer SM, Azzopardi PS, Wickremarathne D, Patton GC. The age of adolescence. *Lancet Child and Adolescent Health* 2018;2(3):223–8.
4 Lebel C, Beaulieu C. Longitudinal development of human brain wiring continues from childhood into adulthood. *Journal of Neuroscience* 2011;31(30):10937–47.
5 Twenge JM, Park H. The decline in adult activities among U.S. adolescents, 1976–2016. *Child Development* 2019;90(2):638–54.
6 Australian Institute of Health and Welfare. *Australia's welfare 2017*. Canberra: AIHW; 2017.
7 Parent AS, Teilmann G, Juul A, Skakkebaek NE, Toppari J, Bourguignon JP. The timing of normal puberty and the age limits of sexual precocity: variations around the world, secular trends, and changes after migration. *Endocrine Reviews* 2003;24(5):668–93.
8 Paus T, Keshavan M, Giedd JN. Why do many psychiatric disorders emerge during adolescence? *Nature Reviews: Neuroscience* 2008;9(12):947–57.
9 Beesdo K, Bittner A, Pine DS, Stein MB, Höfler M, Lieb R, et al. Incidence of social anxiety disorder and the consistent risk for secondary depression in the first three decades of life. *Archives of General Psychiatry* 2007;64(8):903–12.
10 Gibb SJ, Fergusson DM, Horwood LJ. Burden of psychiatric disorder in young adulthood and life outcomes at age 30. *British Journal of Psychiatry* 2010;197(2):122–7.
11 Dean K, Laursen TM, Pedersen CB, Webb RT, Mortensen PB, Agerbo E. Risk of being subjected to crime, including violent crime, after onset of mental illness: a Danish national registry study using police data. *JAMA Psychiatry* 2018;75(7):689–96.
12 McGorry PD, Goldstone SD, Parker AG, Rickwood DJ, Hickie IB. Cultures for mental health care of young people: an Australian blueprint for reform. *Lancet Psychiatry* 2014;1(7):559–68.
13 Malla A, Iyer S, McGorry P, Cannon M, Coughlan H, Singh S, et al. From early intervention in psychosis to youth mental health reform: a review of the evolution and

transformation of mental health services for young people. *Social Psychiatry and Psychiatric Epidemiology* 2016;51(3):319–26.
14 McGorry P, Bates T, Birchwood M. Designing youth mental health services for the 21st century: examples from Australia, Ireland and the UK. *British Journal of Psychiatry* 2013;54:s30–5.
15 Fusar-Poli P. Integrated mental health services for the developmental period (0 to 25 years): a critical review of the evidence. *Frontiers in Psychiatry* 2019;10:355.
16 Hilferty F, Cassells R, Muir K, Duncan A, Christensen D, Mitrou F, et al. *Is headspace making a difference to young people's lives? Final Report of the independent evaluation of the headspace program.* Sydney: Social Policy Research Centre, UNSW; 2015.
17 Hetrick SE, Bailey AP, Smith KE, Malla A, Mathias S, Singh SP, et al. Integrated (one-stop shop) youth health care: best available evidence and future directions. *Medical Journal of Australia* 2017;207(10):S5–18.
18 McGorry PD. The specialist youth mental health model: strengthening the weakest link in the public mental health system. *Medical Journal of Australia* 2007;187(S7):S53–6.
19 van der Gaag M, Smit F, Bechdolf A, French P, Linszen DH, Yung AR, et al. Preventing a first episode of psychosis: meta-analysis of randomized controlled prevention trials of 12 month and longer-term follow-ups. *Schizophrenia Research* 2013;149(1–3): 56–62.
20 Bertelsen M, Jeppesen P, Petersen L, Thorup A, Øhlenschlaeger J, le Quach P, et al. Five-year follow-up of a randomized multicenter trial of intensive early intervention vs standard treatment for patients with a first episode of psychotic illness: the OPUS trial. *Archives of General Psychiatry* 2008;65(7):762–71.
21 Hegelstad WT, Larsen TK, Auestad B, Evensen J, Haahr U, Joa I, et al. Long-term follow-up of the TIPS early detection in psychosis study: effects on 10-year outcome. *American Journal of Psychiatry* 2012;169(4):374–80.
22 Correll CU, Galling B, Pawar A, Krivko A, Bonetto C, Ruggeri M, et al. Comparison of early intervention services vs treatment as usual for early-phase psychosis: a systematic review, meta-analysis, and meta-regression. *JAMA Psychiatry* 2018;75(6):555–65.
23 Chanen AM, McCutcheon L. Prevention and early intervention for borderline personality disorder: current status and recent evidence. *British Journal of Psychiatry* 2013;54:s24–9.
24 Clarke GN, Hawkins W, Murphy M, Sheeber LB, Lewinsohn PM, Seeley JR. Targeted prevention of unipolar depressive disorder in an at-risk sample of high school adolescents: a randomized trial of a group cognitive intervention. *Journal of the American Academy of Child and Adolescent Psychiatry* 1995;34(3):312–21.
25 Stockings E, Hall WD, Lynskey M, Morley KI, Reavley N, Strang J, et al. Prevention, early intervention, harm reduction, and treatment of substance use in young people. *Lancet Psychiatry* 2016;3(3):280–96.
26 Killackey E, Allott K, Jackson HJ, Scutella R, Tseng YP, Borland J, et al. Individual placement and support for vocational recovery in first-episode psychosis: randomised controlled trial. *British Journal of Psychiatry* 2019;214(2):76–82.
27 Mental Health Australia, KPMG. *Investing to save: the economic benefits for Australia of investment in mental health reform.* Australia: Mental Health Australia; 2018.
28 McGorry PD, Hickie IB, Yung AR, Pantelis C, Jackson HJ. Clinical staging of psychiatric disorders: a heuristic framework for choosing earlier, safer and more effective interventions. *Australian and New Zealand Journal of Psychiatry* 2006;40(8):616–22.
29 McGorry PD, Hickie IB. *Clinical staging in psychiatry: making diagnosis work for research and treatment.* Cambridge: Cambridge University Press; 2019.

30 Ginsburg GS, Becker EM, Keeton CP, Sakolsky D, Piacentini J, Albano AM, et al. Naturalistic follow-up of youths treated for pediatric anxiety disorders. *JAMA Psychiatry* 2014;71(3):310–8.
31 Maalouf FT, Atwi M, Brent DA. Treatment-resistant depression in adolescents: review and updates on clinical management. *Depression and Anxiety* 2011;28(11):946–54.
32 Calear AL, Christensen H, Mackinnon A, Griffiths KM, O'Kearney R. The Youth-Mood Project: a cluster randomized controlled trial of an online cognitive behavioral program with adolescents. *Journal of Consulting and Clinical Psychology* 2009;77(6):1021–32.
33 Alvarez-Jimenez M, Bendall S, Lederman R, Wadley G, Chinnery G, Vargas S, et al. On the HORYZON: moderated online social therapy for long-term recovery in first episode psychosis. *Schizophrenia Research* 2013;143(1):143–9.
34 Firth J, Torous J, Nicholas J, Carney R, Pratap A, Rosenbaum S, et al. The efficacy of smartphone-based mental health interventions for depressive symptoms: a meta-analysis of randomized controlled trials. *World Psychiatry* 2017;16(3):287–98.
35 Mohr DC, Riper H, Schueller SM. A solution-focused research approach to achieve an implementable revolution in digital mental health. *JAMA Psychiatry* 2018;75(2):113–4.
36 Torous J, Nicholas J, Larsen ME, Firth J, Christensen H. Clinical review of user engagement with mental health smartphone apps: evidence, theory and improvements. *Evidence-Based Mental Health* 2018;21(3):116–9.
37 Rickwood D, Paraskakis M, Quin D, Hobbs N, Ryall V, Trethowan J, et al. Australia's innovation in youth mental health care: the headspace centre model. *Early Intervention in Psychiatry* 2019;13(1):159–66.
38 Modini M, Tan L, Brinchmann B, Wang MJ, Killackey E, Glozier N, et al. Supported employment for people with severe mental illness: systematic review and meta-analysis of the international evidence. *British Journal of Psychiatry* 2016;209(1):14–22.
39 Fusar-Poli P, McGorry PD, Kane JM. Improving outcomes of first-episode psychosis: an overview. *World Psychiatry* 2017;16(3):251–65.
40 Nielssen O, McGorry P, Castle D, Galletly C. The RANZCP guidelines for schizophrenia: why is our practice so far short of our recommendations, and what can we do about it? *Australian and New Zealand Journal of Psychiatry* 2017;51(7):670–4.
41 McGorry P. Youth mental health and mental wealth: reaping the rewards. *Australasian Psychiatry* 2017;25(2):101–3.
42 McGorry PD, Ratheesh A, O'Donoghue B. Early intervention – an implementation challenge for 21st century mental health care. *JAMA Psychiatry* 2018;75(6):545–6.
43 MQ: Transforming Mental Health. *UK mental health research funding 2014–2017*. London: MQ: Transforming Mental Health; 2019.
44 Batterham PJ, McGrath J, McGorry PD, Kay-Lambkin FJ, Hickie IB, Christensen H. NHMRC funding of mental health research. *Medical Journal of Australia* 2016; 205(8):350–1.
45 Mei C, Fitzsimons J, Allen N, Alvarez-Jimenez M, Amminger GP, Browne V, et al. Global research priorities for youth mental health. *Early Intervention in Psychiatry* 2020;14(1):3–13.
46 McGorry P. Building the momentum and blueprint for reform in youth mental health. *Lancet Psychiatry* 2019;6(6):459–61.
47 Shah JL, Scott J, McGorry PD, Cross SPM, Keshavan MS, Nelson B, et al. Transdiagnostic clinical staging in youth mental health: a first international consensus statement. *World Psychiatry* 2020;19(2):233–42.

Index

Note: Numbers in **bold** indicate a table. *Italics* indicate a figure.

For Product Safety Concerns and Information please contact our EU
representative GPSR@taylorandfrancis.com
Taylor & Francis Verlag GmbH, Kaufingerstraße 24, 80331 München, Germany

www.ingramcontent.com/pod-product-compliance
Ingram Content Group UK Ltd.
Pitfield, Milton Keynes, MK11 3LW, UK
UKHW020145200926
475702UK00005B/927

* 9 7 8 0 3 6 7 2 5 0 6 1 4 *